Type 2 Diabetes: Role of Diet and Nutrition

Type 2 Diabetes: Role of Diet and Nutrition

Editor: Vanessa Artiga

AMERICAN
MEDICAL PUBLISHERS
www.americanmedicalpublishers.com

AMERICAN
MEDICAL PUBLISHERS
www.americanmedicalpublishers.com

Cataloging-in-Publication Data

Type 2 diabetes : role of diet and nutrition / edited by Vanessa Artiga.
p. cm.
Includes bibliographical references and index.
ISBN 978-1-63927-818-3
1. Type 2 diabetes. 2. Type 2 diabetes--Diet therapy. 3. Type 2 diabetes--Nutritional aspects.
4. Diabetics--Nutrition. 5. Diet in disease. I. Artiga, Vanessa.
RC662.18 .T97 2023
616.462--dc23

American Medical Publishers,
41 Flatbush Avenue,
1st Floor, New York,
NY 11217, USA

ISBN 978-1-63927-818-3 (Hardback)

Contents

Preface

In my initial years as a student, I used to run to the library at every possible instance to grab a book and learn something new. Books were my primary source of knowledge and I would not have come such a long way without all that I learnt from them. Thus, when I was approached to edit this book; I became understandably nostalgic. It was an absolute honor to be considered worthy of guiding the current generation as well as those to come. I put all my knowledge and hard work into making this book most beneficial for its readers.

Diabetes refers to a group of metabolic disorders that are characterized by having high blood sugar level over a long time. Type 2 diabetes (T2D) is a type of diabetes which is characterized by relative lack of insulin, high blood sugar and insulin resistance. The usual symptoms of T2D are frequent urination, unexplained weight loss and increased thirst. There can be other symptoms such as fatigue, increased hunger and sores which do not heal easily. Symptoms usually occur gradually. Long-term complications of high blood sugar may lead to several diseases such as strokes, diabetic retinopathy, heart disease, kidney failure and poor blood flow. There are various preventive measures for T2D, which include consuming a healthy diet, maintaining a normal weight and exercising regularly. Treatment of T2D includes dietary changes and exercise. This book aims to understand the clinical perspectives of type 2 diabetes. It strives to provide a fair idea about role of diet and nutrition in T2D and to help develop a better understanding for its clinical management. Those with an interest in this disease would find this book helpful.

I wish to thank my publisher for supporting me at every step. I would also like to thank all the authors who have contributed their researches in this book. I hope this book will be a valuable contribution to the progress of the field.

Editor

1

Long Term Dietary Restriction of Advanced Glycation End-Products (AGEs) in Older Adults with Type 2 Diabetes Is Feasible and Efficacious-Results from a Pilot RCT

Roni Lotan [1,2,*], Ithamar Ganmore [2,3,4,5], Shahar Shelly [2,6], Moran Zacharia [2], Jaime Uribarri [7], Paul Beisswenger [8], Weijing Cai [7], Aron M. Troen [1] and Michal Schnaider Beeri [2,7]

1 The Nutrition and Brain Health Laboratory, The Institute of Biochemistry, Food and Nutrition Science, The Robert H. Smith Faculty of Agriculture Food and the Environment, The Hebrew University of Jerusalem, 7610001 Rehovot, Israel; aron.troen@mail.huji.ac.il

2 The Joseph Sagol Neuroscience Center, Sheba Medical Center, 5265601 Tel Hashomer, Israel; thamar.Ganmore@sheba.health.gov.il (I.G.); Shelly.Shahar@mayo.edu (S.S.); moran281093@gmail.com (M.Z.); michal.beeri@mssm.edu (M.S.B.)

3 Memory Clinic, Sheba Medical Center, 5265601 Tel Hashomer, Israel

4 Sheba Medical Center, Neurology Department, 5265601 Tel Hashomer, Israel

5 Sackler Faculty of Medicine, Tel Aviv University, 6997801 Tel Aviv, Israel

6 Department of Neurology, Mayo Clinic, Rochester, MN 55905, USA

7 Icahn School of Medicine at Mount Sinai, New York, NY 10029, USA; jaime.uribarri@mountsinai.org (J.U.); weijing.cai@mssm.edu (W.C.)

8 PreventAGE Healthcare, Lebanon, NH 03766, USA; pjb@preventagehealthcare.com

* Correspondence: Roni.lotan@mail.huji.ac.il

Abstract: Introduction: High serum concentrations of advanced glycation end-products (AGEs) in older adults and diabetics are associated with an increased risk of cognitive impairment. The aim of this pilot study was to assess the feasibility of long-term adherence to a dietary intervention designed to decrease intake and exposure to circulating AGEs among older adults with type 2 diabetes. Methods: Herein, 75 participants were randomized to either a standard of care (SOC) control arm or to an intervention arm receiving instruction on reducing dietary AGEs intake. The primary outcome was a change in serum AGEs at the end of the intervention. Secondary and exploratory outcomes included adherence to diet and its association with circulating AGEs. Cognitive function and brain imaging were also assessed but were out of the scope of this article (ClinicalTrials.gov Identifier: NCT02739971). Results: The intervention resulted in a significant change over time in several serum AGEs compared to the SOC guidelines. Very high adherence (above 80%) to the AGE-lowering diet was associated with a greater reduction in serum AGEs levels. There were no significant differences between the two arms in any other metabolic markers. Conclusions: A long-term dietary intervention to reduce circulating AGEs is feasible in older adults with type 2 diabetes, especially in those who are highly adherent to the AGE-lowering diet.

Keywords: type 2 diabetes; advanced glycation end-products; diet; randomized controlled trial; adherence

1. Introduction

Advanced glycation end-products (AGEs) are a class of chemical compound that are created by the non-enzymatic reaction between reducing sugars and free amino groups. This reaction occurs endogenously in the body during the course of normal cellular metabolism [1,2]. AGEs tend to be more abundant in the tissue of older humans rather than younger humans [3], as well as under conditions where the precursors for the reaction, such as circulating glucose, are in excess [1,2]. Thus, older adults with type 2 diabetes (T2D) tend to have higher levels of systemic AGEs.

In addition to the endogenous creation of AGEs, exogenous sources such as pre-formed AGEs from food contribute significantly to the body's pool of AGEs. AGEs exist in most foods, but they are particularly abundant in animal-derived foods. Exposure to high temperatures (i.e., grilling, broiling, roasting, searing, and frying) and long cooking times can greatly increase the amount of AGEs in food [4,5].

AGEs affect cellular functions by binding to the receptor for advanced glycationend-products (RAGE), resulting in the activation of inflammatory and oxidative stress cascades [2,6]. High AGE levels are associated with a wide range of chronic diseases, such as T2D [7], atherosclerosis [8], ocular diseases [9], cancer [10], and kidney disease [11]. Increasing evidence also suggests the involvement of AGEs in neurodegenerative disorders [12], especially Alzheimer's disease (AD).

T2D has been consistently shown to increase the risk ofAD [13]; diabetic individuals have relatively high levels of AGEs, in part due to high circulating glucose levels. In turn, AGEs have been shown to cross-link beta amyloid [14], the hallmark pathology of AD. Thus, increased chronic exposure to AGEs may provide a mechanistic explanation for the higherrisk of AD experienced by diabetic adults compared to non-diabetic older adults. If so, then achieving a lasting reduction of circulating AGEs by reducing dietary intake should reduce the associated risk or severity of disease. Current dietary guidelines for people with diabetes are designed to improve glycemic control but are not specifically designed to decrease AGEs. Short-term clinical trials have shown that middle-aged patients with T2D [15] and chronic kidney disease [16] can significantly reduce their circulating AGEs concentrations and improve biomarkers of disease severity (e.g., less insulin resistance in diabetes) by changing their cooking methods that reduce their dietary AGE intake [17]. Such encouraging findings underscore the importance of rigorously evaluating whether reducing dietary AGE intake can reduce cognitive risk. However, before this can be definitively tested in a randomized controlled clinical trial, it must be shown that such dietary changes will be acceptable and effective in older adults with diabetes, who have a high dementia risk, but may find it difficult to adapt to the necessary dietary changes, and who may show a different biological response to intervention.Therefore, we designed this pilot study to assess whether a six month intervention to decrease dietary AGEs would improve serum AGE levels relative to the dietary standard of care for older adults with T2D based on the American Diabetes Association (ADA) dietary recommendations [18].

2. Materials and Methods

The study was designed according to the CONSORT criteria extension to pilot trials [19] and was approved by the Helsinki Committee of the Sheba Medical Center, Israel (2206-15-SMC). All participants gave signed informed consent. The study was registered at www.clinicaltrials.gov (NCT02739971).

2.1. Screening

Minimum inclusion criteria to participate in the study included being age > 65, a diagnosis ofT2Dand subjective memory complaints. T2D was defined by the use of medications for T2D, health records indicating a diagnosis of T2D, or tworecent routine blood tests indicating fasting glucose above 126 mg/dl. Candidates with any existing neurological condition that can affect cognition were excluded (e.g., dementia, Parkinson's disease, schizophrenia, traumatic head injury, etc.). All participants were required to have a family member as an informant. The study was advertised using mass mailing to recruit volunteers from among people who had previously agreed to receive health-related emails and by advertising through websites and social media forums for clinical trials, dementia, and diabetes. Interested candidates were contacted by telephone to ascertain age and T2D status and were invited to a face-to-face screening visit where cognition and nutritional status were assessed. Participants were eligible if they met the following criteria at the screening visit: a clinical dementia rating scale (CDR) <1 (i.e., normal cognition or questionable dementia, but no frank dementia) [20], Montreal Cognitive Assessment (MoCA) >18 (no dementia) [21], and geriatric depression scale (GDS) <6 (no clinical depression) [22]. In addition, a short dietary questionnaire was administered to assess AGEs intake using a translated version of a validated 7-day questionnaire with comparable food items that are frequently consumed in Israel and are rich in AGEs (e.g., meat, fish, poultry, cheese, egg yolk, fats, fast foods, and convenience breakfast and snack foods) [16]. Each item wasassigned an AGE equivalent based on a database of ~560 food AGE values [5]. Habitual AGE intake wasestimated from the frequency at which these items were reportedly consumed during the past week, after taking into account the portion sizes and the cooking methods (i.e., boiling, roasting, broiling/grilling, frying, or canned). The results wereexpressed as AGEs Eq/day, where 1 AGE equivalent = 1000 kilounits). To increase the likelihood of achieving a significant reduction of dietary AGEs intake, we followed a protocol used in similar trials whereby only participants with estimated AGEs intakes greater than 13 kU/day were invited to participate in the study [3].

2.2. *Intervention*

Upon enrollment, participants were assigned by a computerized random sequence generator to follow one of two diets for 6 months. The standard of care (SOC) arm was instructed to follow dietary guidelines for achieving good glycemic control [18]. The AGE-lowering arm received additional instruction on reducing dietary AGE intake. At the baseline visit, participants from both arms were provided dietary guidance by a registered dietitian. The main focus of the guidelines for good glycemic control for both arms was the intake of carbohydrates, including information on serving sizes, counting, and quality. Recommendations were given for carbohydrate intake from vegetables, fruits, whole grains, legumes, and low-fat dairy products while reducing the consumption of refined sugars. In addition, participants were advised to choose food items rich in mono and poly unsaturated fatty acids compared to saturated and trans fatty acid, as well as to consume lean meat, low sodium, and low processed food items. Other guidelines for good glycemic control were individualized based on the participants' metabolic and nutritional needs, habits, preferences, willingness, and ability to make behavioral changes.

Participants were asked to follow the instructions of the study for 6 months and to avoid any new diet or life-style program during this period. Those assigned the AGE-lowering arm were provided the same guidance on glycemic control, but in addition were taught how to reduce their dietary AGEs intake by modifying the cooking methods and reducing cooking time and temperature without changing the nutrient composition of their food). They were advised to boil, poach, stew, or steam and to avoid frying, baking, or grilling anyanimal-derived products [5]. All participants also received the guidelines in writing. Informants were asked to join the nutritional counseling in case of a shared house with the participant. If the informant could not attend, the dietitian called and instructed him or her by phone. All participants in both arms were called once a week to ascertain and encourage adherence to their diet. Participants from the SOC arm were asked general questions about their nutrition during the week (e.g., "did you manage to follow the guidelines for your diabetes?"). Participants from the AGE-lowering arm were also asked specifically about their attempts to maintain low AGE intake, asking whether and how many times they cooked using methods that produce higher AGEs since the last call. If a participant reported consuming food items rich in AGEs, the dietitian repeated the instructions to lower AGEs by cooking modification of animal products to both the participant and the informant. Each follow-up call included personalized questions related to prior calls regarding personal challenges (such as preventing hypoglycemia or eating on holidays and special events) and progress (such as self-monitoring of fasting glucose). A summary of each telephone call was registered by the study dietitian including the date of the call and the main issues that arose. Failure to reach the participant was also registered.

2.3. *Operational Measurement of Adherence with the Diet*

To minimize potential bias, the study dietitian categorized participants' self-reported adherence upon completion of the study but before serum AGEs results were available and before analyzing any outcomes. Each phone call scored 0 for a negative answer and 1 for a positive answer to the following questions:

1. Did the participant report fully maintaining the guidelines for good glycemic control since the previous call (yes/no for all participants)? As carbohydrates intake is a key strategy in achieving glycemic control [18], the answer for maintaining guidelines for good glycemic control was focused on the intake of food items from this group.
2. Did the participant report using any cooking methods that they wereadvised to avoid for animal derived food items since the previous call? (yes/no for AGE-lowering arm only).

Scores (0/1) obtained from each telephone call were summed for two adherence scales: A T2D adherence scale for all participants and a low AGEs adherence scale for the AGE-lowering arm only. The total score for each scale was divided by the average number of calls and was presented in percentage of "positive answers" reflecting adherence to the guidelines. A 1–5 Likert scale with the following categorization was built: A score of 1 represented participants who maintained the dietary instructions above 80% of phones call ("very high adherence"), a score of 2 represented those who complied with the diet between 60–80% of the calls (good adherence), and a score of 3 referred to adherence of between 40–60% ("partial adherence"). For adherence lower than 40%, participants were asked if they wished to continue participating in the study. A score of 4 represented those compliant below 40% of the calls but with a desire to continue participating in the study("lack of adherence but desire to continue"), and finally, a score of 5 referred to those who had below 40% adherence and who wished to withdraw from the study ("lack of adherence and desire to withdraw"). If the total number of phone calls with the participant was below the 5th quintiles (=less than 14 phone call), another point was added to the final score of the adherence scale, as not answering phone reflect low adherence.

2.4. *Assessments, Outcomes, and Measures*

Identical assessments were repeated at baseline and post-intervention (after 6 months). A fasting blood sample was drawn to analyze markers related to diabetes (glucose, HbA1c, insulin), lipid profile (triglycerides [TG], high-density lipoprotein [HDL], low-density lipoprotein [LDL], total cholesterol), kidney function (Urea, Creatinine), the inflammatory marker C reactive protein (CRP), and a complete blood count. The Homeostatic Model Assessment of Insulin Resistance (HOMA-IR) was calculated according to the following equation: insulin (mu/l) Xglucose (mg/dl)/405 [23]. HOMA-IR was not calculated for participants using insulin (N = 18). Creatinine clearance was calculated using the Cockcroft–Gault equation: ((140−age) Xweight)/72XCreatinine (mg/dl) X 0.85 for females [24]. Blood was centrifuged and serum was separated and stored at −80 °C for subsequent AGEs analysis.

2.5. *Serum AGEs Analysis*

AGEs were measured in a blinded fashion by liquid chromatography–mass spectrometry (LC-MS) using an Agilent model 6490 Triple Quadrupole MS with a 1290 Rapid Resolution LC system and stable heavy isotope substituted internal standards, as described elsewhere [25] (PreventAGE Healthcare Technology, Lebanon, NH, USA). Briefly, duplicate serum samples were centrifuged through a 10-K cutoff Amicon filter. The filtrate contains free AGEs and peptides of various sizes, as well as the analytical method measures the free products. AGEs were separated using a Waters X-select HSS T3 column (2.5 mm, 2.1 3 150 mm) with a mobile phase gradient of methanol and water with 0.20% heptafluorobutyric acid. Five dicarbonyl-derived AGEs were assessed: Ne-carboxymethyl lysine (CML), Ne-carboxyethyl lysine (CEL), glyoxalhydroimidazolone (G-H1), methylglyoxalhydroimidazolone (MG-H1), and 3-deoxyglucosone hydroimidazolone (3DG-H1) [25].

2.6. Nutritional Assessment

General habitual dietary quality and nutritional intake was assessed with a validated Hebrew food frequency questionnaire (FFQ), which was specifically designed to assess nutrition in older adultsand is commonly used in this population [26]. The questionnaire includes 126 items and was administrated by the study dietitian. Dietary AGEs intake was assessed with the short AGEs questionnaire described above.

2.7. Other Measurements

Anthropometrics: Weight, height, and waist circumference (measured in centimeters at the level of the umbilicus) were assessed by the study dietitian. Participants wore their shoes and clothing to avoid discomfort but were asked to leave only basic clothing during measurements. Demographic information: year of birth, years of education, profession, and family status. Lifestyle: physical activity was assessed using the Minnesota Leisure Time Physical Activity Questionnaire [27] and smoking habits were recorded.

2.8. Blinding

Although diet allocation could not be concealed from the participants and study dietitian, care was taken to blind all other research staff to the arm assignments, including the neuropsychologist, the MRI technician, the lab technician where the blood tests were analyzed, and the research assistant who entered the data.

2.9. Statistical Analysis

The primary analysis of the effect of the intervention used intent-to-treat (ITT) methods and secondary analyses used per-protocol (PP) methods. The ITT analysis included all randomized participants who finished 6 months of follow-up. For the PP analysis, participants were considered to be fully compliant if they were at least 80% adherent to their assigned diet as assessed by weekly phone interviews (categorized as "very high adherence" on the adherence scale).

Baseline demographic and clinical characteristics are presented descriptively as proportions or as means with standard deviations. Comparison between arms was analyzed by χ^2 test for categorical outcomes, *t*-test for continuous outcomes distributed normally, and by Mann–Whitney tests for non-normal distributions.

Changes in serum AGEconcentrations from baseline to 6 months were analyzed with paired *t* test or Wilcoxon tests for within-arm changes and by 2 sided *t*-test or Mann–Whitney for the between-arms analysis. Alpha of 0.05 was used for significance levels. SPSS version 23 (IBM Corp., Armonk, NY, USA) was used forall analyses.

3. Results

3.1. Baseline Characteristics and Retention

In total, 75 eligible participants were randomized to enter the study. Baseline characteristics of arms randomized to the AGE-lowering and SOC diet are shown in Table 1. There were no statistically significant differences between the arms at baseline for any variable, indicating that randomization was successful. The mean age was 71.6 ± 4.07 and 74.7% were males. Participants' baseline macronutrient consumption did not differ by arm. Further, 24% used insulin and the average HbA1C% of 6.67 ± 0.67 in the entire sample is indicative of a diabetic population with good control of their blood glucose.

Table 1. Baseline characteristic ($n = 75$).

Variable	AGEsLowering Arm ($n = 35$)	SOC Arm ($n = 40$)	p
Age (years)	71.91 ± 4.20	71.42 ± 3.99	0.57
Gender n (%)	8 (22.9)	11 (27.5)	
Female			0.64
Male	27(77.1)	29 (72.5)	
Education (years)	13.89 ± 2.88	14.93 ± 2.62	0.10
Family history of dementia			
n (%)	23 (65.7)	24(60)	0.61
No family history			
Smoking n (%)	19 (54.3)	15 (37.5)	
Never	14 (40)	23 (57.5)	0.31
In the past	2 (5.7)	2 (5)	
Current			
Medication for T2D n (%)			
All but insulin	29 (82.9)	29(72.5)	0.32
Insulin included	6 (17.1)	9(22.5)	
Diet only	0	2(5)	
MoCA	23.14 ± 2.18	23.25 ± 2.23	0.80
GDS	2.37 ± 1.71	2.53 ± 1.66	0.69
ADL	99.43 ± 2.35	99.75 ± 1.10	0.84
Physical activity (METS/day)	148.75 ± 130.92	118.63 ± 115.61	0.22
Waist circumference (cm)	106.74 ± 10.77	106.05 ± 10.81	0.78
BMI (kg/m^2)	30.02 ± 4.28	29.55 ± 3.58	0.75
CRP (mg/l)	4.79 ± 5.28	3.48 ± 4.22	0.10
Insulin (mU/l) ($n = 57$)[1]	15.24 ± 10.97	15.11 ± 9.41	0.64
HbA1C %	6.63 ± 0.72	6.71 ± 0.67	0.59
HOMA-IR ($n = 57$)[1]	5.04 ± 4.12	4.53 ± 2.35	0.81
Creatinine clearance(ml/min)	84.75 ± 26.27	85.86 ± 22.35	0.84
Estimated AGEs intake (kU/day)	23.25 ± 6.48	22.14 ± 6.50	0.46
Protein (g)	94.89 ± 27.71	96.15 ± 27.44	0.73
Fat (g)	83.21 ± 25.08	82.70 ± 30.78	0.62
Carbohydrates(g)	232.94 ± 66.67	241.75 ± 60.45	0.53
Energy (kcal)	2012.26 ± 488.83	2059.03 ± 553.68	0.86
Serum CML (nmole/L)	127.91 ± 51.06	115.15 ± 39.43	0.26
Serum 3DG (nmole/L)	376.51 ± 202.44	377.92 ± 232.56	0.84
Serum CEL (nmole/L)	104.61 ± 42.04	93.15 ± 38.07	0.18
Serum G-H1 (nmole/L)	12.08 ± 5.21	10.46 ± 2.70	0.12
Serum MG-H1 (nmole/L)	271.41 ± 164.68	216.71 ± 158.51	0.05

All values expressed as Mean ± SD. Abbreviations and explanation: AGEs: Advanced glycation end products; SOC: Standard of care; T2D: Type 2 diabetes; MoCA: Montreal cognitive assessment; GDS: Geriatric depression scale; ADL: Activity of daily living; BMI: Body max index; CRP: C reactive protein; HbA1C: glycated hemoglobin; HOMA-IR: Homeostatic model assessment of insulin resistance; CML: Ne-carboxymethyl lysine; 3DG-H1: 3-deoxyglucosone hydroimidazolone; CEL: Ne-carboxyethyl lysine; G-H1: glyoxalhydroimidazolone; MG-H1: methylglyoxalhydroimidazolone. [1] insulin mean and HOMA-IR include only participants who do not take insulin.

During the 6 month follow-up period, only five participants withdrew, 3 from the SOC arm and 2 assigned to the AGE-lowering diet so that 70 (93%) had complete data for analysis at the 6 months follow-up visit. The average number of completed phone calls was 16.5 calls per patient, with no significant difference in call rates between the two arms ($p = 0.12$) indicating that the extent of patient-dietitian interactions did not differ by arm.

3.2. *Effect of Intervention on Nutritional Intake*

Energy intake (Kcal) declined in both arms by 15.5% on average with no difference between the 2 diet arms ($p = 0.34$). The relative proportion of macronutrients at baseline was similar between the 2 diet arms and remained the same at follow-up, as it was at baseline for each diet, indicating that the decline in energy reflected a decrease in the amount of food consumed rather than a shift in food preferences (Table 2). Estimated AGEs intake reduced significantly in both arms; however, when comparing the between-arm differences in the magnitude of the effect of each diet, the AGE-lowering arm achieved more than twice the reduction in AGEs intake than the controls (−11.8 kU/day vs. −4.6 kU/day, $p < 0.01$; Table 2). Dietary AGEs density was calculated by dividing estimated AGEs intake by the total energy intake. In contrast to the SOC diet, whose dietary AGEs density did not change significantly over the 6 months of the study, the AGE-lowering arm had a significant decline and this difference between the arms was significant (−0.004 kU/kcal vs. −0.0006 kU/kcal p value = 0.001; Table 2).

Table 2. Nutritional intake at baseline and follow-up.

	AGE-Lowering Arm (n = 33)				SOC Arm (n = 37)				
	Baseline	Follow-Up	Delta	p [1]	Baseline	Follow-Up	Delta	p [1]	p [2]
Energy (kcal)	2020.74 ± 493.16	1648 ± 381.32	−372.74 ± 410.73	<0.001	2069.66 ± 574.35	1804.09 ± 503.20	−265.57 ± 511.03	<0.001	0.34
Protein (g)	95.13 ± 28.53	76.63 ± 19.84	−18.50 ± 21.80	<0.001	96.56 ± 27.99	86.95 ± 28.51	−9.60 ± 26.35	0.03	0.13
Fat (g)	83.94 ± 25.26	68.1 ± 18.05	−15.84 ± 25.20	<0.001	84.01 ± 31.38	71.46 ± 23.97	−12.54 ± 24.23	<0.001	0.57
Carbohydrates (g)	232.62 ± 67.73	193.02 ± 57.39	39.60 ± 51.38	<0.001	240.50 ± 61.57	211.57 ± 58.40	−28.92 ± 65.66	0.01	0.45
% Carbohydrates	45.9 ± 7.1	46.7 ± 7.3	0.8 ± 5.5	0.41	47.5 ± 6.1	47.4 ± 6.4	0.4 ± 4.8	0.62	0.74
% Protein	18.8 ± 3	18.6 ± 2.6	−0.2 ± 3.1	0.68	18.7 ± 2.8	19.2 ± 3.3	0.5 ± 3.1	0.29	0.30
% Fat	37.2 ± 5.7	37.5 ± 5.8	−0.2 ± 5.4	0.8	36 ± 5.1	35.3 ± 4.4	0.7 ± 4.6	0.33	0.66
Estimate dAGEs intake (kU/day)	23.51 ± 6.57	11.72 ± 4.98	−11.78 ± 7.09	<0.001	22.65 ± 6.49	18.06 ± 5.91	−4.58 ± 7.56	<0.001	<0.001
AGEs density [3] (kU/Kcal)	0.012 ± 0.003	0.0074 ± 0.003	−0.0047 ± 0.005	<0.001	0.011 ± 0.002	0.010 ± 0.003	−0.0006 ± 0.004	0.385	0.001

All values expressed as mean or % ± SD. Abbreviations and explanation: AGEs: Advanced glycation end products; SOC; Standard of care. p [1] change between baseline and 6 months visit within group; p [2] difference in mean change between AGE-lowering vs. SOC groups. [3] AGEs density was calculated as estimated dietary AGE intake divided by energy intake.

3.3. *Effect of Intervention on Circulating AGEs*

The effect of the intervention on the five serum AGEs (CML, CEL, G-H1, MG-H1, 3DG-H1) is shown in Table 3. The ITT analysis shows that in control participants, all of the measured AGEs tended to increase from the baseline to the follow-up, with statistically significant increases for G-H1 ($p < 0.001$) and MG-H1 ($p = 0.015$). In contrast, in the AGE-lowering arm, circulating AGE concentrations tended to be relatively stable with slight declines that were not statistically significant. Between-arm comparisons of the diet-induced change in AGE serum levels was statistically significant for CEL (The AGE-lowering arm declined by 10% compared to a 4% increase in the SOC arm; $p = 0.044$) and MG-H1 (8% decline in the AGE-lowering arm and 27% increase in the SOC arm; $p = 0.034$).

3.4. *Effect of Intervention on Metabolic Status*

Participants assigned to both the SOC diet and the AGE-lowering diet improved in several metabolic parameters (Table 4). In the SOC arm, insulin and HOMA-IR decreased significantly without significant differences in any other metabolic markers. In the AGE-lowering arm, body mass index (BMI) significantly decreased without significant changes toany other metabolic markers.

3.5. *Per-Protocol Analysis of Adherence to the AGE-Lowering Diet on Study Outcomes*

We further analyzed if the reduction of AGE biomarkers in the AGE-lowering arm wasassociated with their level of adherence. In total, 19participants (57%) were classified as "very highly adherent", 10 (30.9%) had "good adherence", 4 (12.1%) had "partial adherence", and none of the participants were classified as having "low adherence". Since the "partial adherence" category had a small number of participants, we analyzed it together with the "good adherence" category. On average, all serum AGEs declined in the very highly adherent group, while they increased in those classified as having only good or partial adherence. The differences in the very high vs. good and partially adherent groups were statistically significant for CML (−10.7% vs. +8.7% respectively; $p = 0.035$), 3DGH (−10.9% vs. +31.7% respectively; $p = 0.021$), and MG-H1 (−30.2% vs. +23.6% respectively; $p = 0.022$) (Table 5).

Similarly, when metabolic markers were analyzed by adherence, only the very highly adherent group experienced a significant decrease in BMI of 0.77 kg/m^2 ($p = 0.012$). Estimated AGE, energy, protein, carbohydrate, and fat intake all declined significantly in both groups. However, the decrease in estimated AGE intake was significantly greater in the very highly adherent group compared to the good and partially adherent group (−14.64 kU/day in the very high adherence vs. −7.91 kU/day in the good and partially adherent group $p = 0.005$).Other metabolic biomarkers tended to show a greater improvement in the very highly adherent vs. the less adherent groups but this was not statistically significant: HOMA-IR (-1.38 ± 3.07 vs. -0.53 ± 1.99; $p = 0.41$, respectively) and creatinine clearance ($+1.10 \pm 14.47$ vs. -4.11 ± 11.50; $p = 0.27$ respectively). No other metabolic or nutritional differences were observed.

Table 3. Effect of intervention on serum AGEs concentration (ITT analysis).

	AGE-Lowering Arm (n = 33)				SOC Arm (n = 37)				
Measured AGEs (nmole/L)	Baseline	Follow-Up	Change (%)	p^1	Baseline	Follow-Up	Change (%)	p^1	p^2
CML	128.2 ± 52.5	124.8 ±45.4	−2.5 ± 31.5	0.6	112.5 ± 35.6	122.5 ± 52.2	+8.8 ± 39.6	0.1	0.5
3DGH	372.0 ± 207.3	397.2 ± 223.6	+6.7 ± 52.8	0.7	352.6 ± 169.9	372.9 ± 174.2	+5.7 ± 57.4	0.4	0.9
CEL	105.2 ± 43.1	94.6 ± 42.5	−9.9 ± 43.7	0.09	88.3 ± 29.8	91.9 ± 38.0	+3.9 ± 33.3	0.1	0.04
G-H1	12.0 ± 5.3	12.0 ± 5.7	+1.6 ± 4.1	0.9	10.2 ± 2.5	13.3 ± 7.7	+30.3 ± 68.6	<0.01	0.1
MG-H1	270.5 ± 169.5	248.8 ± 172.0	−8.0 ± 67.1	0.3	193.1 ± 92.7	265.7 ± 170.0	+37.3 ± 92.9	0.01	0.03

All values expressed as mean change ± SD. Abbreviations and explanation: AGEs: Advanced glycation end products; SOC; Standard of care; ITT: Intention to treat analysis; CML: Ne-carboxymethyl lysine; 3DGH: 3-deoxyglucosone hydroimidazolone; CEL: Ne-carboxyethyl lysine; G-H1: glyoxalhydroimidazolone; MG-H1: methylglyoxalhydroimidazolone. p^1 change between baseline and 6 months visit within arm; p^2 difference in mean change between AGE-lowering vs. SOC arms.

Table 4. Mean change in metabolic markers after 6 months (ITT).

	AGE-Lowering Arm (n = 33)				SOC Arm (n = 37)				
	Baseline	Follow-Up	Delta	p^1	Baseline	Follow-Up	Delta	p^1	p^2
Insulin (mU/L)	14.74 ± 10.86	12.44 ± 8.96	(n = 25) * 2.28 ± 6.87	0.10	14.05 ± 5.90	11.61 ± 5.09	(n = 27) * −2.09 ± 4.43	0.04	0.90
HbA1C%	6.61 ± 0.68	6.58 ± 0.81	−0.03 ± 0.46	0.20	6.72 ± 0.66	6.71 ± 0.61	−0.01 ± 0.51	0.78	0.84
Glucose (mg/dL)	131.12 ± 23.31	125.06 ± 21.49	−6.06 ± 23.75	0.15	126.97 ± 33.90	121.54 ± 22.75	−5.43 ± 27.53	0.23	0.91
HOMA-IR	4.90 ± 4.14	3.97 ± 3.32	(n = 25) * −0.94 ± 2.55	0.08	4.42 ± 1.9	3.44 ± 1.47	(n = 27) * −0.872 ± 1.74	0.02	0.87
Creatinine Clearance (mL/min)	85.52 ± 26.93	84.08 ± 25.06	−1.18 ± 13.31	0.61	88.23 ± 18.52	85.55 ± 18.78	−2.17 ± 7.76	0.10	0.70
BMI (kg/m^{2})	30.05 ± 4.30	29.54 ± 4.25	−0.50 ± 1.11	0.02	29.36 ± 3.63	28.93 ± 3.77	−0.42 ± 1.38	0.05	0.94
Waist (cm)	107.03 ± 10.62	106.13 ± 9.08	−0.89 ± 5.31	0.17	105.70 ± 10.97	105.16 ± 11.27	−0.83 ± 5.42	0.22	0.74
Physical activity (METs/day)	150.53 ± 131.83	143.13 ± 107.75	−7.39 ± 94.96	0.62	118.43 ± 117.72	153.31 ± 139.57	34.88 ± 132.62	0.12	0.12

All values expressed as mean ± SD. Abbreviations and explanation: ITT: Intention to treat analysis; AGEs: Advanced glycation end products; SOC; Standard of care; HbA1C: glycated hemoglobin HOMA-IR: Homeostatic model assessment of insulin resistance; BMI: Body max index. * Insulin and HOMA-IR include only participants who do not use insulin. p^1 change between baseline and 6 months visit within arm; p^2 difference in mean change between AGE-lowering vs. SOC arms.

Table 5. Mean change in AGEs levels between baseline and 6 months follow-up by level of adherence to the dietary instructions (AGEs-lowering arm).

	Very High Adherence (n = 19)				Good/Partial Adherence (n = 14)				
Measured AGEs (nmole/L)	Baseline	Follow-Up	Change (%)	p [1]	Baseline	Follow-Up	Change (%)	p [1]	p [2]
CML	131.68 ± 57.47	117.09 ± 42.03	−11.0 ± 25.0	0.15	123.58 ± 46.62	135.40 ± 49.28	+9.5 ± 37	0.35	0.035
CEL	109.45 ± 49.98	88.07 ± 42.90	−19.5 ± 43.8	0.04	99.43 ± 32.67	103.57 ± 41.99	+4.1 ± 40.4	0.7	0.11
3DGH	378.40 ± 235.55	337 ± 196.78	−10.9 ± 34.9	0.19	363.35 ± 169.79	478.90 ± 238.85	+31.8 ± 64.9	0.09	0.021
GH1	12.26 ± 6.55	11.28 ± 3.97	−7.9 ± 30.5	0.42	11.72 ± 3.33	13.11 ± 7.55	+11.7 ± 54.1	0.43	0.27
MG-H1	276.30 ± 198.21	192.82 ± 118.60	−30.2 ± 53.0	0.02	262.66 ± 127.54	324.78 ± 206.34	23.65 ± 75.4	0.27	0.022

All values expressed as mean change ± SD. Abbreviations and explanation: AGEs: Advanced glycation end products; CML: Ne-carboxymethyl lysine; 3DGH: 3-deoxyglucosone hydroimidazolone; CEL: Ne-carboxyethyl lysine; G-H1: glyoxalhydroimidazolone; MG-H1: methylglyoxalhydroimidazolone. p [1] change between baseline and 6 months visit within arm; p [2] difference in mean change between AGE-lowering vs. SOC arms.

4. Discussion

Our results show that dietary reduction of AGE intake in older diabetics can have the additional benefit of decreasing circulating AGE levels, beyond that which can be achieved by following the standard of care diet for good glycemic control. As expected, reductions in serum AGEs were more prominent in individuals who were highly adherent to the diet. We designed our intervention based on several earlier randomized controlled trials of dietary AGE reduction, which had demonstrated that limiting dietary AGE intake by modification of cooking methods could reduce circulating AGEs, specifically CML and MG, in healthy individuals [17], as well as in patients with metabolic syndrome [28], diabetes [15], and renal failure [16]. Moreover, those studies yielded a 23–35% reduction of CML and MG, and we observed a more modest reduction of 8–10% of serum CEL and MG-H1. Several considerations might account for the relatively modest reduction in AGEs concentrations that we achieved. First, we considered a priori that older adults with T2D may respond differently to dietary AGE-lowering than younger diabetics. The average age in the earlier clinical trials was 60–62 [15,29,30], whereas our participants were on average a decade older. AGE concentrations increase with age and diabetes, and renal clearance of AGE decreases with age [3]. Because the concentration of circulating AGEs reflects the balance of intake, endogenous production, enzymatic removal, and clearance, the relative contribution of dietary intake to overall circulating AGEs may be relatively less important than other factors in this population.

Of interest, participants in the SOC arm showed a tendency for all serum AGEs to increase over time reaching statistical significance for G-H1 (+30%) and MG-H1 (+33%).Other trials with participants with the metabolic syndrome and diabetes have also documented that participants who didnot follow the AGE-lowering diet hada tendency to increase serum AGE levels [15,28]. Our results suggest that a higher reduction of AGE intake may be needed in order to have a biological response in circulating AGEs in this population. It is also important to note that we assessed serum AGE concentrations using mass spectrometry in contrast to most other AGE clinical trials that used ELISA. The two methods are different and results may not be comparable.

In contrast to other trials, dietary AGE-lowering did not improve HOMA-IR in our population. This might simply reflect the relatively modest reduction of circulating AGEs in our study and the older age of our population. Of note, our average baseline HbA1c at 6.6% wasrelatively low for older adults with T2D, thus indicating good glycemic possibly that could explainthe lack of effect of the low AGE diet on metabolic markers. Moreover, 24% of our patients did not have assessment of HOMA because they were medicated with insulin and the number of participants might have not been large enough to demonstrate an effect of AGE change. This together with the high education level, low drop-out rate, and high adherence to diet may indicate selection bias towards a relatively well educated, diet-conscious, motivated, and resilient study population.

Future clinical trials should include participants with more severe T2D as they may be amenable to a greater reduction in metabolic markers so the possible "floor effect" of good glycemic control found in our sample may be avoided. In addition, as reported in previous trials in participants with T2D [15,29], the levels of HbA1c were not improved following the intervention of AGEs reduction nor by the SOC diet. While this could be the result of the relatively stable population as discussed above, it indicates that the improvement in the circulating AGEs in the intervention arm is attributed primarily to the reduction of the dietary AGEs and not the glycation process. Lastly, we can notrule out the possibility of aninterviewer biasthatmay have led the participants to reporta lower AGE intake than what actually was eaten. In order to assess the scope of this bias, we aimed to analyze the validity of the participant's reportsby assessing if the effect on circulating AGEs wasaffected by adherence. The greater improvement in circulating AGEs among those who reported greater adherence to the low AGE diet suggests that this bias was at least somewhat limited. The study dietitian spoke to participants approximately weekly with a structured questionnaire that reviewed the prior week's eating habits in relation to the diet, providing suggestions to improve the diet for the following weeks. That allowed for a semi quantitative measurement of adherence to the diet. In the AGE-lowering arm, there were significant and robust declines in serum AGEs levels in the very high adherence subgroup (over 80%), which comprised 57% of the AGE-lowering arm, suggesting that a high proportion of individuals wereable and willing to commit to a low AGE diet closely supervised by a nutritionist. These results emphasize that maintaining adherence may be a crucial component of a future RCT study design. In contrast, in the subgroup with good/partial adherence, there was in fact an increase in serum AGE levels during the intervention, pointing out that such a diet should be carefully followed in order to reach a beneficial effect. The adherence scale that we constructed for this study may be useful for "predicting" the extent of circulating AGE reduction and might be tested for other nutritional biomarkers as well. In future trials, and in clinical practice, working with a quantitative scale during an intervention phase can help find participants that need closer support and monitoring by a dietitian to increase adherence associated with improved clinical biomarkers and outcomes.

Our study has several limitations including that by the nature of the design (explicit dietary interventions) neither the investigators nor the patients were blind to the intervention. The dropout rate in this clinical trial was relatively low (6.7%) and the two arms did not differ neither in number nor cause of dropout. Yet, it is possible that the relatively high adherence to the low-AGE diet was related to its novelty. The novelty of a dietary approach may increase adherence, at least in the short-term. We attempted to minimize this by providing tailored (rather than general) recommendations for T2D [18] for the participants in the SOC arm, which may have provided a sense of novelty in this arm as well. In addition, the sample size of our study might not have been large enough to demonstrate an effect of AGEs reduction on metabolic markers in older adults with T2D.

The study has several strengths. The number and length of phone calls with the two arms was essentially identical limiting the placebo effect. In addition, the study used MS for the measurements of AGEs, which is more precise than ELISA used in the most RCT in the field. Lastly, our low dropout rates emphasize the feasibility of such programs in older adults with T2D.

5. Conclusions

The current study provides new evidence that dietary AGE restriction is feasible in older adults with T2D and that there are modest decreases in specific serum AGE levels resulting from a low AGE diet unrelated to changes in other metabolic markers. These decreases occur primarily in individuals who are highly adherent to the diet. Larger and longer-term studies are required to ascertain the health benefits of low AGEs diet in older adults with T2D. The ability of participants from a clinical trial setting to maintain such dietary guidelines for long term should also be tested.

Author Contributions: Conceptualization: M.S.B. and A.M.T.; methodology: R.L., M.S.B., A.M.T., J.U., and W.C.; formal analysis: R.L., M.S.B., A.M.T.; investigation: R.L., I.G., S.S., M.S.B., and A.M.T.; data curation, M.Z.; writing—original draft preparation, R.L.; writing—review and editing, M.S.B., A.M.T., J.U., W.C., and P.B.; supervision: M.S.B., A.M.T., and R.L.; funding acquisition: M.S.B. All authors have read and agreed to the published version of the manuscript.

References

1. Poulsen, M.W.; Hedegaard, R.V.; Andersen, J.M.; de Courten, B.; Bugel, S.; Nielsen, J.; Skibsted, L.H.; Dragsted, L.O. Advanced glycation endproducts in food and their effects on health. *Food Chem. Toxicol.* **2013**, *60*, 10–37. [CrossRef] [PubMed]
2. Kellow, N.J.; Coughlan, M.T. Effect of diet-derived advanced glycation end products on inflammation. *Nutr. Rev.* **2015**, *73*, 737–759. [CrossRef] [PubMed]
3. Vlassara, H.; Cai, W.; Goodman, S.; Pyzik, R.; Yong, A.; Chen, X.; Zhu, L.; Neade, T.; Beeri, M.; Silverman, J.M.; et al. Protection against loss of innate defenses in adulthood by low advanced glycation end products (AGE) intake: Role of the antiinflammatory AGE receptor-1. *J. Clin. Endocrinol. Metab.* **2009**, *94*, 4483–4491. [CrossRef] [PubMed]
4. Goldberg, T.; Cai, W.; Peppa, M.; Dardaine, V.; Baliga, B.S.; Uribarri, J.; Vlassara, H. Advanced glycoxidation end products in commonly consumed foods. *J. Am. Diet. Assoc.* **2004**, *104*, 1287–1291. [CrossRef]
5. Uribarri, J.; Woodruff, S.; Goodman, S.; Cai, W.; Chen, X.; Pyzik, R.; Yong, A.; Striker, G.E.; Vlassara, H. Advanced glycation end products in foods and a practical guide to their reduction in the diet. *J. Am. Diet. Assoc.* **2010**, *110*, 911–916.e912. [CrossRef]
6. Bierhaus, A.; Humpert, P.M.; Morcos, M.; Wendt, T.; Chavakis, T.; Arnold, B.; Stern, D.M.; Nawroth, P.P. Understanding RAGE, the receptor for advanced glycation end products. *J. Mol. Med.* **2005**, *83*, 876–886. [CrossRef]
7. Ahmed, N. Advanced glycation endproducts–role in pathology of diabetic complications. *Diabetes Res. Clin. Pract.* **2005**, *67*, 3–21. [CrossRef]
8. Hartog, J.W.; Voors, A.A.; Bakker, S.J.; Smit, A.J.; van Veldhuisen, D.J. Advanced glycation end-products (AGEs) and heart failure: Pathophysiology and clinical implications. *Eur. J. Heart Fail.* **2007**, *9*, 1146–1155. [CrossRef]
9. Stitt, A.W. Advanced glycation: An important pathological event in diabetic and age related ocular disease. *Br. J. Ophthalmol.* **2001**, *85*, 746–753. [CrossRef]
10. van Heijst, J.W.; Niessen, H.W.; Hoekman, K.; Schalkwijk, C.G. Advanced glycation end products in human cancer tissues: Detection of Nepsilon-(carboxymethyl)lysine and argpyrimidine. *Ann. N. Y. Acad. Sci.* **2005**, *1043*, 725–733. [CrossRef]
11. Uribarri, J.; Peppa, M.; Cai, W.; Goldberg, T.; Lu, M.; Baliga, S.; Vassalotti, J.A.; Vlassara, H. Dietary glycotoxins correlate with circulating advanced glycation end product levels in renal failure patients. *Am. J. Kidney Dis.* **2003**, *42*, 532–538. [CrossRef]
12. Salahuddin, P.; Rabbani, G.; Khan, R.H. The role of advanced glycation end products in various types of neurodegenerative disease: A therapeutic approach. *Cell. Mol. Biol. Lett.* **2014**, *19*, 407–437. [CrossRef] [PubMed]
13. Cukierman, T.; Gerstein, H.C.; Williamson, J.D. Cognitive decline and dementia in diabetes–systematic overview of prospective observational studies. *Diabetologia* **2005**, *48*, 2460–2469. [CrossRef] [PubMed]
14. Vitek, M.P.; Bhattacharya, K.; Glendening, J.M.; Stopa, E.; Vlassara, H.; Bucala, R.; Manogue, K.; Cerami, A. Advanced glycation end products contribute to amyloidosis in Alzheimer disease. *Proc. Natl. Acad. Sci. USA* **1994**, *91*, 4766–4770. [CrossRef]
15. Uribarri, J.; Cai, W.; Ramdas, M.; Goodman, S.; Pyzik, R.; Chen, X.; Zhu, L.; Striker, G.E.; Vlassara, H. Restriction of advanced glycation end products improves insulin resistance in human type 2 diabetes: Potential role of AGER1 and SIRT1. *Diabetes Care* **2011**, *34*, 1610–1616. [CrossRef] [PubMed]
16. Uribarri, J.; Peppa, M.; Cai, W.; Goldberg, T.; Lu, M.; He, C.; Vlassara, H. Restriction of dietary glycotoxins reduces excessive advanced glycation end products in renal failure patients. *J. Am. Soc. Nephrol.* **2003**, *14*, 728–731. [CrossRef]
17. Uribarri, J.; Cai, W.; Pyzik, R.; Goodman, S.; Chen, X.; Zhu, L.; Ramdas, M.; Striker, G.E.; Vlassara, H. Suppression of native defense mechanisms, SIRT1 and PPARgamma, by dietary glycoxidants precedes disease in adult humans; relevance to lifestyle-engendered chronic diseases. *Amino Acids* **2014**, *46*, 301–309. [CrossRef]

18. Evert, A.B.; Boucher, J.L.; Cypress, M.; Dunbar, S.A.; Franz, M.J.; Mayer-Davis, E.J.; Neumiller, J.J.; Nwankwo, R.; Verdi, C.L.; Urbanski, P.; et al. Nutrition therapy recommendations for the management of adults with diabetes. *Diabetes Care* **2014**, *37*, S120–S143. [CrossRef]
19. Eldridge, S.M.; Chan, C.L.; Campbell, M.J.; Bond, C.M.; Hopewell, S.; Thabane, L.; Lancaster, G.A.; Group, P.C. CONSORT 2010 statement: Extension to randomised pilot and feasibility trials. *BMJ* **2016**, *355*, i5239. [CrossRef]
20. Morris, J.C.; Ernesto, C.; Schafer, K.; Coats, M.; Leon, S.; Sano, M.; Thal, L.J.; Woodbury, P. Clinical dementia rating training and reliability in multicenter studies: The Alzheimer's Disease Cooperative Study experience. *Neurology* **1997**, *48*, 1508–1510. [CrossRef]
21. Lifshitz, M.; Dwolatzky, T.; Press, Y. Validation of the Hebrew version of the MoCA test as a screening instrument for the early detection of mild cognitive impairment in elderly individuals. *J. Geriatr. Psychiatry Neurol.* **2012**, *25*, 155–161. [CrossRef] [PubMed]
22. Bass, D.S.; Attix, D.K.; Phillips-Bute, B.; Monk, T.G. An efficient screening tool for preoperative depression: The Geriatric Depression Scale-Short Form. *Anesth Analg* **2008**, *106*, 805–809, table of contents. [CrossRef] [PubMed]
23. Matthews, D.R.; Hosker, J.P.; Rudenski, A.S.; Naylor, B.A.; Treacher, D.F.; Turner, R.C. Homeostasis model assessment: Insulin resistance and beta-cell function from fasting plasma glucose and insulin concentrations in man. *Diabetologia* **1985**, *28*, 412–419. [CrossRef] [PubMed]
24. Cockcroft, D.W.; Gault, M.H. Prediction of creatinine clearance from serum creatinine. *Nephron* **1976**, *16*, 31–41. [CrossRef]
25. Saulnier, P.J.; Wheelock, K.M.; Howell, S.; Weil, E.J.; Tanamas, S.K.; Knowler, W.C.; Lemley, K.V.; Mauer, M.; Yee, B.; Nelson, R.G.; et al. Advanced Glycation End Products Predict Loss of Renal Function and Correlate With Lesions of Diabetic Kidney Disease in American Indians With Type 2 Diabetes. *Diabetes* **2016**, *65*, 3744–3753. [CrossRef]
26. Shahar, D.; Fraser, D.; Shai, I.; Vardi, H. Development of a food frequency questionnaire (FFQ) for an elderly population based on a population survey. *J. Nutr* **2003**, *133*, 3625–3629. [CrossRef]
27. Richardson, M.T.; Leon, A.S.; Jacobs, D.R., Jr.; Ainsworth, B.E.; Serfass, R. Comprehensive evaluation of the Minnesota Leisure Time Physical Activity Questionnaire. *J. Clin. Epidemiol* **1994**, *47*, 271–281. [CrossRef]
28. Vlassara, H.; Cai, W.; Tripp, E.; Pyzik, R.; Yee, K.; Goldberg, L.; Tansman, L.; Chen, X.; Mani, V.; Fayad, Z.A.; et al. Oral AGE restriction ameliorates insulin resistance in obese individuals with the metabolic syndrome: A randomised controlled trial. *Diabetologia* **2016**, *59*, 2181–2192. [CrossRef]
29. Cai, W.; He, J.C.; Zhu, L.; Peppa, M.; Lu, C.; Uribarri, J.; Vlassara, H. High levels of dietary advanced glycation end products transform low-density lipoprotein into a potent redox-sensitive mitogen-activated protein kinase stimulant in diabetic patients. *Circulation* **2004**, *110*, 285–291. [CrossRef]
30. Vlassara, H.; Cai, W.; Crandall, J.; Goldberg, T.; Oberstein, R.; Dardaine, V.; Peppa, M.; Rayfield, E.J. Inflammatory mediators are induced by dietary glycotoxins, a major risk factor for diabetic angiopathy. *Proc. Natl. Acad. Sci. USA* **2002**, *99*, 15596–15601. [CrossRef]

2

Identification of Inflammatory and Disease-Associated Plasma Proteins that Associate with Intake of Added Sugar and Sugar-Sweetened Beverages and Their Role in Type 2 Diabetes Risk

Stina Ramne *, Isabel Drake, Ulrika Ericson, Jan Nilsson, Marju Orho-Melander, Gunnar Engström and Emily Sonestedt

Department of Clinical Sciences Malmö, Lund University, 214 28 Malmö, Sweden; isabel.drake@med.lu.se (I.D.); ulrika.ericson@med.lu.se (U.E.); jan.nilsson@med.lu.se (J.N.); marju.orho-melander@med.lu.se (M.O.-M.); gunnar.engstrom@med.lu.se (G.E.); emily.sonestedt@med.lu.se (E.S.)

* Correspondence: stina.ramne@med.lu.se

Abstract: It has been suggested that high intake of added sugar and sugar-sweetened beverages (SSBs) increase the level of circulating inflammatory proteins and that chronic inflammation plays a role in type 2 diabetes (T2D) development. We aim to examine how added sugar and SSB intake associate with 136 measured plasma proteins and C-reactive protein (CRP) in the Malmö Diet and Cancer–Cardiovascular Cohort (n = 4382), and examine if the identified added sugar- and SSB-associated proteins associate with T2D incidence. A two-step iterative resampling approach was used to internally replicate proteins that associated with added sugar and SSB intake. Nine proteins were identified to associate with added sugar intake, of which only two associated with T2D incidence ($p < 0.00045$). Seven proteins were identified to associate with SSB intake, of which six associated strongly with T2D incidence ($p < 6.9 \times 10^{-8}$). No significant associations were observed between added sugar and SSB intake and CRP concentrations. In summary, our elucidation of the relationship between plasma proteome and added sugar and SSB intake, in relation to future T2D risk, demonstrated that SSB intake, rather than the total intake of added sugar, was related to a T2D-pathological proteomic signature. However, external replication is needed to verify the findings.

Keywords: added sugar; sugar-sweetened beverages; inflammation; inflammatory proteins; proteomics; type 2 diabetes

1. Introduction

Different dietary components or food items could serve either as pro-inflammatory or anti-inflammatory, and the link between diet and chronic low-grade inflammation could be either direct or mediated through other factors, such as the gut microbiota [1]. The main direct pro-inflammatory effects of diet are induced by positive energy balance and accumulating adiposity [2]. Further, epigenetic changes or excess formulation of reactive oxygen species are examples of mechanisms in which the nutrients and foods we consume may promote inflammation [2].

High intake of added sugars and sugar-sweetened beverages (SSBs) has been hypothesized to promote chronic inflammation. Increased levels of inflammatory markers after high sugar interventions have been observed in a few randomized trials [3,4], while not in other trials [5–7]. The stress of a high postprandial plasma glucose is suggested as an additional potential reason [1]. Glycemic index and load have by some been observed to associate with inflammatory markers, but the overall evidence is inconclusive [8]. However, this is highly dependent on which inflammatory biomarkers are assessed [1]. Therefore, it is of great importance to investigate a wide range of inflammatory and disease-associated plasma proteins. Among the typical inflammatory markers, C-reactive protein (CRP) is best studied in relation to intake of added sugar and SSBs, and there is a lack of studies investigating other disease-associated plasma proteins.

SSB intake has in meta-analyses been shown to associate with increased type 2 diabetes (T2D) risk [9–11], while epidemiological investigations of sugar intake and T2D risk often show no association [12–22]. As far as we are aware, only three out of 14 studies have shown a significant positive association with T2D incidence [16,23,24]. These associations were, however, only found when intake of fructose or glucose were studied specifically, never when intake of sucrose, total sugar or added sugar were studied. Some studies have even shown significant inverse associations [23,25].

The role of chronic inflammation for T2D development is well acknowledged [26,27], and several meta-analyses have observed increased incidence in T2D with higher levels of circulating inflammatory markers [28,29].

All in all, a role of chronic inflammation as a link between added sugar and SSB intake and T2D risk is hypothesized, but associations between added sugar and SSB intake and both inflammatory proteins and T2D are inconsistent in the epidemiological research and limited to a few inflammatory proteins. Therefore, the aim of this explorative study was to examine how added sugar or SSB intake associate with inflammatory and disease-associated plasma proteins and CRP, and if the identified added sugar- and SSB-associated proteins prospectively associate with incidence of T2D.

2. Materials and Methods

2.1. Study Sample

The Malmö Diet and Cancer–Cardiovascular Cohort (MDC-CC) is a deeply phenotyped sub-cohort within the population-based prospective Malmö Diet and Cancer (MDC) cohort, conducted in the city of Malmö in southern Sweden between 1991 and 1996. Participants were recruited by advertisements in public areas and by a personal invitation letter sent to all men born between 1923 and 1945 and all women born between 1923 and 1950 inhabiting the Malmö city area. From the recruited participants in MDC, 6103 were randomly recruited to the MDC-CC during 1991–1994 and fasting blood samples were obtained from the 5540 participants. In total, 4865 blood samples were sent for analysis of plasma proteins, out of which 4742 analyzed samples passed quality control. From these, 301 individuals with a diagnosed diabetes or cardiovascular disease at baseline were excluded from the current study sample, as well as those with missing data on dietary intake ($n = 26$) or model covariates ($n = 33$), resulting in a total sample of 4382 participants. All participants signed written informed consent prior to entering the study, which was approved by the Lund University Ethical Committee (LU 51/90) in accordance with the Declaration of Helsinki.

2.2. Dietary Intake Assessment

To assess dietary intake, a combination of a seven-day food record of all cooked meals, cold beverages (including SSBs) and dietary supplements; a 168 item food frequency questionnaire covering all food items belonging to non-cooked meals spanning over the previous year; and a dietary interview elucidating food choices, cooking methods and portion sizes (with the help of a booklet of photographs of various portions sizes) were applied. The portion size estimation in the food frequency questionnaire was also aided by the booklet of photographs of various portion sizes. The energy and nutrient content of the collected food intake data were obtained from the MDC food database, which was based upon the Swedish national food database from the Swedish National Food Agency. Added sugar intake was estimated from the sum of sucrose and monosaccharides, subtracted for the sum of sucrose and monosaccharides naturally occurring in fruit, vegetables and fruit juices. This has been described in detail in a previous publication [30]. Added sugar intake was investigated as the percentage of non-alcohol energy intake (E%), both as a continuous variable and categorized into six previously studied categories [30]. The E% intake coming from SSBs was estimated on the assumption that all SSBs have a mean sugar content of 10 g per 100 g, based on that the sugar content in soft drinks varies between 10–13 g/100 g and cordial/squash contains approximately 8 g/100 g sugar. The contribution to the added sugar intake (E%) from SSB intake was also calculated. For statistical analyses, the SSB intake (E%) variable was either log transformed (with a constant of 0.1 added), due to its skewed distribution and large proportions of zero consumers, or divided into five categories of 0E%, >0–2E%, >2–3E%, >3–5E% and >5E%.

2.3. Plasma Protein Assessment

Fasting blood samples from baseline examinations were stored at −80 °C until analysis of plasma protein concentrations in 2015. A total of 149 plasma proteins were measured by the SciLifeLab (Uppsala, Sweden) with the Olink Proseek Multiplex proximity extension assays Cardiovascular 1 and Oncology 1 (Olink Proteomics, Uppsala, Sweden). For each protein, the proximity extension technology uses pairs of antibodies marked with oligonucleotides that bind pair-wise with the protein to be measured. When the oligonucleotides reach proximity, paired DNA strings are formed, which are quantified with qPCR. Values are presented as normalized protein expression units (real-time qPCR cycle values on the log2 scale). For statistical analysis, we excluded those proteins that were available in less than 75% of the individuals in the present study sample ($n = 13$), giving 136 plasma proteins analyzed at study samples ranging between 3351 and 4382 individuals. A full list of all 136 plasma proteins is available in Table S1.

Measurements of CRP were performed by the Tina-quant® CRP latex high sensitivity assay (Roche Diagnostics, Basel, Switzerland) on an ADVIA 1650 Chemistry System (Bayer Healthcare, Tarrytown, NY, USA). The values are the means of measurements read in 6 s intervals over 1 min after 5 min of incubation. Within our study sample ($n = 4382$), measured CRP was available in 4291 individuals.

2.4. Covariate Assessment

In a self-administered questionnaire, medical history, medication use, socioeconomic factors such as education (assessed on a five-level scale) and lifestyle factors were assessed. The lifestyle factors included leisure time physical activity (LTPA) (five categories of metabolic equivalent hours per week based on the time spent engaging in 17 different activities and their metabolic equivalent intensity factor), alcohol habits (quintiles of consumers with one category of non-consumers) and smoking status (current smokers, former smokers and never smokers). A trained nurse measured body weight and height. Body mass index (BMI) was calculated as weight (kg)/height (m)^2. Fasting plasma glucose was measured using standard procedures.

Low and high energy reporters were determined using Goldberg and Black's cutoffs for the discrepancy between reported energy intake and estimated energy requirements [31]. Additionally, past diet changers were identified at baseline with the questionnaire question "Have you substantially changed your eating habits because of illness or some other reasons?".

2.5. Outcome Assessment

Participants were followed from baseline examinations until incidence of T2D, date of either death or emigration or until 31 December 2016, whichever came first. Diabetes diagnosis was ascertained by the Swedish National Diabetes Register, the regional Diabetes 2000 register of the Scania region, the Malmö HbA1c (glycated hemoglobin) register, the Swedish in- and outpatient registers, the Swedish cause of death register and the Swedish drug prescription register, or in the re-examinations of the MDC-CC in 2007–2012 and the Malmö Preventive Project in 2002–2006 as previously described [32]. Dates of physician-made diagnosis were obtained from the Swedish National Diabetes Register and the Diabetes 2000 register. The Malmö HbA1c register identified individuals with two or more HbA1c measurements ≥ 6.0%. The in- and outpatient registers and the cause of death register identified those with the ICD10 codes E10–E14 and O244–O249, and the drug prescription register identified those who have obtained anti-diabetic medication. In our study sample, a total of 767 individuals were considered as incident diabetes cases, out of which 17 were confirmed to not be of type 2 and 310 were confirmed to be of type 2. For the remaining 440 diabetes cases, type was not specified. However, due to the high age of the population, these diabetes cases were assumed to be of type 2, resulting in a total of 750 cases of T2D.

2.6. Statistical Analyses

Statistical analyses were performed in Stata/SE (version 15, StataCorp LLC, College Station, TX, USA). Baseline characteristics were examined across six categories of added sugar intake and across five categories of SSB intake. Categorical variables were expressed as percentages and continuous variables were expressed as mean (SD) or median (IQR).

Associations between added sugar and SSB intake (E%, continuous variables, SSB log transformed) and plasma proteins were studied with multivariable linear regression, adjusted for age, sex, season, screening date, total energy intake, education level, smoking status, alcohol habits and LTPA. For internally replicating our discovery of proteins associating with added sugar and SSB intake, we adopted a two-step iterative resampling (TSIR) approach based on reasoning by Kang et al. [33]. The authors concluded that for gene discovery in genome-wide association studies, a 70:30 split into discovery and replication cohort and a replication in 20 out of 100 iterations provide satisfying balance between risk of type 1 and type 2 errors. In our study, the study sample was divided into 100 random discovery cohorts (2/3 of the study sample) and the remaining (1/3) was used as replication cohorts. The first step was performed in the discovery cohorts, where we identified the proteins that associated with added sugar and SSB intake (E%) at three different significance levels: $\alpha_1 < 0.05$, $\alpha_1 < 0.01$ and α_1 corresponding to p-values adjusted for false discovery rate (FDR) of 0.05 using the Benjamini–Hochberg method. In step two, the identified proteins' associations with added sugar and SSBs were then examined in the replication cohorts, where an α_2 of 0.05 was always applied as cutoff. A protein was considered internally replicated if it was associated in the same direction in both the discovery and replication cohort in at least 20 out of 100 of the randomly generated discovery and replication cohorts. For plotting purposes, we standardized the added sugar and the logSSB variables to make ß-coefficients comparable.

Longitudinal associations between internally replicated plasma proteins with T2D incidence were examined using Cox proportional hazards regression with standardized proteins and using follow-up time as the time metric. The model was adjusted for age, sex, education level, smoking status, alcohol habits and LTPA, as well as in additional models with further adjustment for baseline BMI, fasting glucose and CRP. A Bonferroni corrected p-value of 0.003 (0.05/16) was applied as the significance level in this analysis of 16 proteins. We also studied potential interactions between the 136 plasma proteins (standardized) and added sugar and logSSB intake on T2D risk, in which the following diet-related covariates were further included in the regression models: total energy intake, season and start date. In these interaction analyses, Bonferroni corrected p-values of $0.05/136 = 0.00037$ were applied. Correlations between all TSIR-identified plasma proteins were studied with pair-wise correlations, and pathways between the identified proteins were explored using the STRING database 11.0 [34].

The association between categories of added sugar and SSB intake and CRP (linear regression) and T2D incidence (Cox proportional hazards regression) were adjusted for age, sex, season, screening date, total energy intake, education level, smoking status, alcohol habits and LTPA. The CRP variable was log transformed due to the skewed nature of it. The predicted marginal means of CRP levels across intake categories were exponentiated back for presentation. We further analyzed the interaction effect of CRP on added sugar and SSB intake (in categories) on their association with T2D incidence. Plotting of interaction effects were performed using marginal predictions at five levels of CRP; −2SD, −1SD, mean, +1SD and +2SD and with mean-centered continuous covariates. Sensitivity analyses excluding low and high energy reporters and past diet changers were performed on the associations between added sugar and SSB intake and T2D and CRP.

3. Results

3.1. Baseline Characteristics

The study population of 4382 participants had a mean age of 57 years (range 45–68) and mean BMI of 25.5 kg/m^2. Added sugar intake contributed on average to 10% of the energy intake, out of which 10% on average came from intake of SSBs. However, 46% of the study population had not reported any intake of SSBs in the seven-day food record, making the median contribution of SSBs to the added sugar intake <1%. As presented in Table 1, with increasing added sugar intake, the proportion of individuals with a university degree and high alcohol consumers appeared to be decreasing. The proportions of current smokers and those eventually getting a T2D diagnosis, as well as fasting glucose and CRP levels, were the highest in both the highest and lowest intake groups of added sugar. BMI appeared to be decreasing with increasing added sugar intake, while reported total energy intake and intake of SSBs were increasing. Table 2 shows how the proportion of women, individuals with a university degree and high alcohol consumers appears to decrease with increasing SSB intake. BMI, fasting glucose, CRP and T2D incidence appear to increase with increasing SSB intake, as well as total energy intake, added sugar intake and contribution of SSBs to added sugar intake.

Table 1. Baseline characteristics of study participants across six categories of added sugar intake.

Added Sugar	≤5E%	>5–7.5E%	>7.5–10E%	>10–15E%	>15–20E%	>20E%
n = 4382	392	842	1129	1544	382	93
Sex, % women	60.5	62.7	61.0	62.1	61.0	54.8
University degree, %	15.1	14.6	13.4	10.2	5.8	6.5
Current smoker, %	32.7	26.1	24.9	24.6	28.3	41.9
Q5 alcohol, %	24.0	20.2	16.9	12.8	12.0	12.9
Incidence T2D, %	20.4	16.3	16.5	16.9	17.3	21.5
Age, years	56.0 (5.8)	56.5 (5.8)	57.7 (6.0)	57.7 (6.0)	58.1 (5.8)	57.7 (5.9)
BMI, kg/m^2	26.2 (4.4)	25.7 (3.9)	25.4 (3.6)	25.4 (3.8)	25.0 (3.8)	25.2 (4.2)
Fasting glucose, mmol/L	5.66 (0.69)	5.65 (0.81)	5.58 (0.65)	5.60 (0.74)	5.60 (0.77)	5.65 (0.72)
CRP [1,2], nmol/L	1.5 (0.7–2.9)	1.3 (0.7–2.8)	1.2 (0.6–2.6)	1.2 (0.6–2.5)	1.4 (0.6–2.9)	1.65 (0.7–3.2)
Energy intake, kcal	2095 (718)	2225 (643)	2298 (636)	2381 (660)	2507 (708)	2572 (784)
SSB intake [1], E%	0 (0–0)	0 (0–0.5)	0 (0–1.1)	0.65 (0–2.3)	2.2 (0.4–4.9)	5.5 (1.4–11.1)
SSB:added sugar [1], E%	0 (0–0)	0 (0–8.3)	0 (0–12.3)	5.5 (0–18.4)	12.9 (2.4–29.8)	24.0 (6.2–45.0)

Data are expressed as percentages (categorical variables) or mean (SD) (continuous variables) unless stated otherwise. [1] Expressed as median (IQR). [2] n = 4291. BMI, body mass index; CRP, C-reactive protein; E%, percent of energy intake; IQR, interquartile range; SSB, sugar-sweetened beverage; T2D, type 2 diabetes; Q5, quintile 5 of consumers.

Table 2. Baseline characteristics of study participants across five categories of SSB intake.

SSBs	0E%	>0–2E%	>2–3E%	>3–5E%	>5E%
n = 4382	2039	1471	310	307	255
Sex, % women	62.7	61.5	64.2	57.0	54.5
University degree, %	13.5	11.7	8.4	8.5	7.5
Current smoker, %	27.1	24.3	30.0	25.7	28.2
Q5 alcohol, %	16.8	17.0	16.5	14.0	9.4
Incidence T2D, %	16.2	17.9	17.1	17.3	20.0
Age, years	57.6 (5.9)	57.0 (6.1)	56.9 (6.0)	57.2 (5.9)	57.4 (5.9)
BMI, kg/m^2	25.4 (3.8)	25.3 (3.7)	25.6 (3.9)	25.8 (3.8)	26.2 (4.3)
Fasting glucose, mmol/L	5.60 (0.68)	5.59 (0.72)	5.63 (0.74)	5.64 (0.87)	5.75 (0.93)
CRP [1,2], nmol/L	1.3 (0.7–2.7)	1.2 (0.6–2.5)	1.35 (0.7–2.9)	1.4 (0.7–2.6)	1.5 (0.7–3.0)
Energy intake, kcal	2211 (649)	2422 (677)	2341 (636)	2456 (696)	2391 (711)
Added sugar intake, E%	8.6 (3.6)	9.99 (3.49)	11.5 (3.5)	13.0 (3.5)	16.4 (4.4)
SSB:added sugar [1], E%	0 (0–0)	8.22 (4.3–13.1)	22.2 (17.7–27.8)	29.6 (24.5–36.2)	47.3 (37.8–58.4)

Data are expressed as percentages (categorical variables) or mean (SD) (continuous variables) unless stated otherwise. [1] Expressed as median (IQR). [2] n = 4291. BMI, body mass index; CRP, C-reactive protein; E%, percent of energy intake; IQR, interquartile range; SSB, sugar-sweetened beverage; T2D, type 2 diabetes; Q5, quintile 5 of consumers.

3.2. *Plasma Proteins Associated with Added Sugar Intake*

As presented in Table 3 and Figure 1a, at $\alpha_1 < 0.05$, nine proteins were internally replicated to associate with added sugar intake: epididymial secretory protein E4 (HE4), folate receptor alpha (FRalpha), tumor necrosis factor receptor superfamily member 4 (TNFRSF4), inducible T cell costimulator ligand (ICOGSL), CD40 ligand (CD40L), cadherin 3 (CDH3), C-X-C motif chemokine 13 (CXCL13), melanoma-derived growth regulatory protein (MIA) and resistin (RETN). Of these, HE4, FRalpha and TNFRSF4 remained internally replicated at $\alpha_1 < 0.01$, and HE4 was the only protein internally replicated at $\alpha_1 <$ FDR0.05. Out of these nine plasma proteins, all except one (CD40L) were positively associated with added sugar intake.

Table 3. The number of times proteins associated with added sugar intake and SSB intake, respectively, out of 100 iterations of random discovery and replication cohorts at various α_1 levels using a TSIR approach. A protein must be replicated at least 20 times to pass internal replication.

Added Sugar, E%	Replicated at $\alpha_1 < 0.05$	Replicated at $\alpha_1 < 0.01$	Replicated at $\alpha_1 <$ FDR0.05
Epididymial secretory protein E4 (HE4)	69	56	20
Folate receptor alpha (FRalpha)	60	37	5
Tumor necrosis factor receptor superfamily member 4 (TNFRSF4)	51	27	3
Cadherin 3 (CDH3)	46	17	1
Inducible T Cell Costimulator Ligand (ICOSLG)	46	14	1
C-X-C motif chemokine 13 (CXCL13)	41	14	0
Melanoma-derived growth regulatory protein (MIA)	40	11	0
CD40 ligand (CD40L)	37	4	0
Resistin (RETN)	23	0	0
Immunoglobulin-like transcript 3 (ILT3)	19	0	0
Interleukin 12 (IL12)	17	0	0
Prostasin (PRSS8)	16	0	0
Matrix metalloproteinase-10 (MMP10)	12	1	0
C-X-C motif chemokine 1 (CXCL1)	3	0	0
Transforming growth factor alpha (TGFalpha)	2	0	0
Interleukin-1 receptor antagonist (IL1ra)	2	0	0
Adrenomedullin (AM)	1	0	0
Renin (REN)	1	0	0
Agouti-related protein (AGRP)	1	0	0
Cathepsin L1 (CTSL1)	1	0	0
Furin (FUR)	1	0	0
SSB, E%			
Interleukin-1 receptor antagonist (IL1ra)	60	46	5
Hepatocyte growth factor (HGF)	44	25	0
Interleukin 12 (IL12)	46	12	0
Prostasin (PRSS8)	31	1	0
Tissue-type plasminogen activator (tPA)	21	5	0
Furin (FUR)	24	0	0
Chitinase-3-like protein 1 (CHI3L1)	22	0	0
Cathepsin D (CTSD)	8	0	0
Tartrate-resistant acid phosphatase type 5 (TRAP)	1	0	0
Parkinson disease protein 7 (PARK7)	1	0	0
Proteinase-activated receptor 1 (PAR1)	1	0	0
Prolactin (PRL)	1	0	0
Lectin-like oxidized LDL receptor 1 (LOX1)	1	0	0
Myoglobin (MB)	1	0	0
C-X-C motif chemokine 1 (CXCL1)	1	0	0

Linear regressions were adjusted for age, sex, season, screening date, total energy intake, education, smoking, alcohol and LTPA. With the TSIR approach, the cutoff was always set to $\alpha_2 < 0.05$ in the replication cohorts. SSB intake is log transformed. FDR, false discovery rate; LTPA, leisure time physical activity; SSB, sugar-sweetened beverage; TSIR, two-step iterative resampling.

3.3. Plasma Proteins Associated with SSB Intake

As presented in Table 3 and Figure 1b, at $\alpha_1 < 0.05$, seven proteins were internally replicated to associate with SSB intake: interleukin-1 receptor antagonist (IL1ra), hepatocyte growth factor (HGF), interleukin 12 (IL12), tissue-type plasminogen activator (tPA), prostasin (PRSS8), furin (FUR) and chitinase-3-like protein 1 (CHI3L1). IL1ra and HGF remained internally replicated at $\alpha_1 < 0.01$ and none of the proteins were internally replicated at $\alpha_1 <$ FDR0.05. No protein was internally replicated to associate with both added sugar and SSB intake.

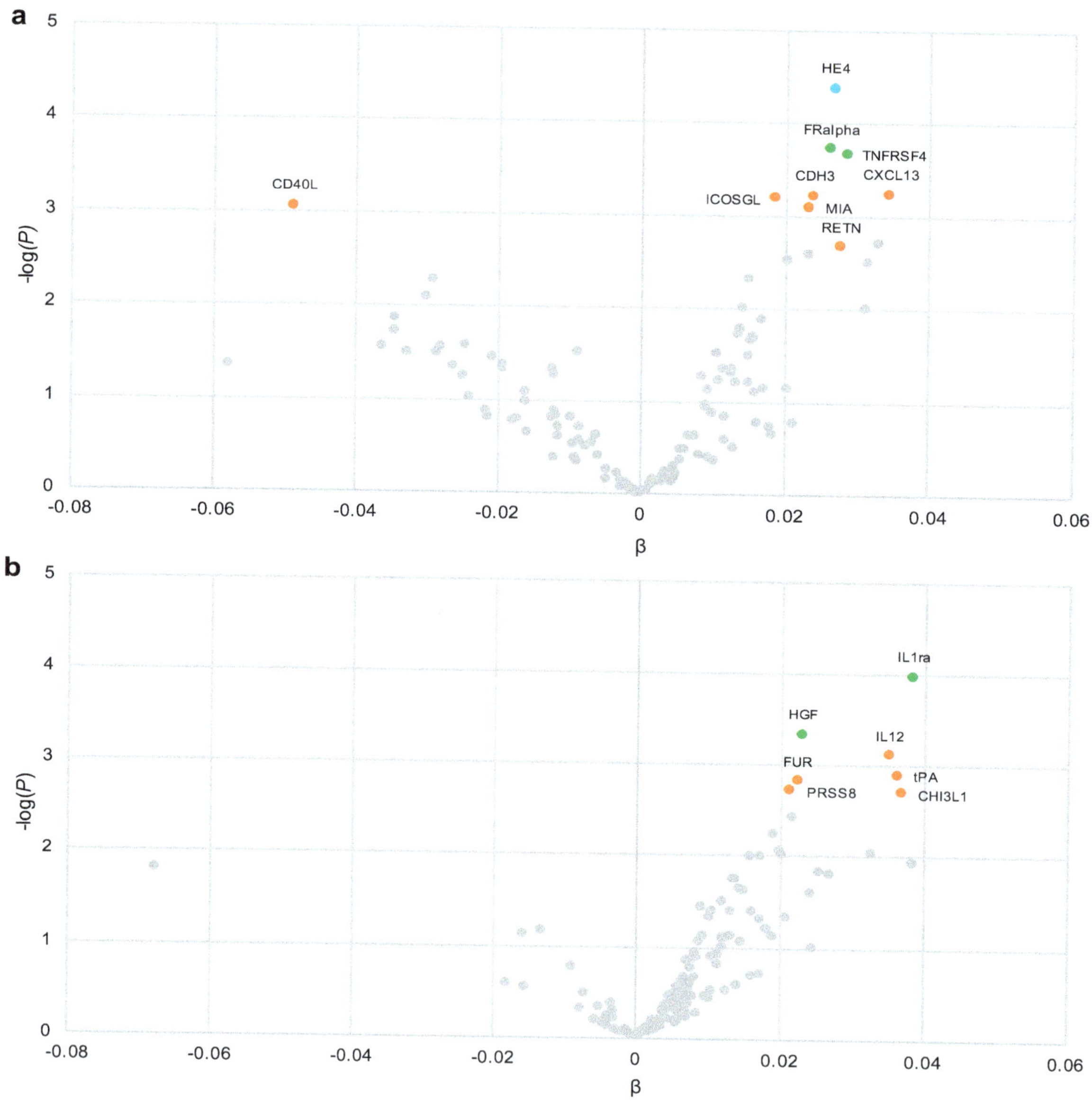

Figure 1. Volcano plot of associations between (**a**) added sugar intake (standardized) and (**b**) SSB intake (log transformed and standardized) and 136 plasma proteins in full sample analysis (n = 3351–4382). Linear regressions were adjusted for age, sex, season, screening date, total energy intake, education, smoking, alcohol and LTPA. Blue, TSIR replicated at $\alpha_1 <$ FDR0.05; green, TSIR replicated at $\alpha_1 < 0.01$; orange, TSIR replicated at $\alpha_1 < 0.05$; grey, not TSIR replicated. FDR, false discovery rate; LTPA, leisure time physical activity; SSB, sugar-sweetened beverage; TSIR, two-step iterative resampling.

All 16 internally replicated proteins correlated significantly and positively with each other, with correlation coefficients ranging from 0.05 to 0.72, $p < 0.001$. A correlation matrix heatmap of all internally replicated proteins can be found in Figure S1. Figure S2 displays the potential pathways between the 16 identified proteins using the STRING database. A known interaction exists between

RETN and CHI3L1, and co-expression occurs between HE4 and PRSS8, IL1ra and RETN, as well as between CD40L, TNFRSF4, CXCL13 and ICOSLG.

3.4. Associtions of Plasma Proteins with T2D Incidence

All seven proteins that were internally replicated to associate with SSB intake except for IL12 were strongly associated with increased T2D incidence (p-values of 6.9×10^{-8} to 2.8×10^{-46}) (Table 4). Among the nine proteins associated with added sugar intake, CD40L and CXCL13 associated significantly with increased T2D incidence (p-values of 0.00045 and 0.00023). Notably, the highest significance for the added sugar-associated proteins (based on the p-value) was observed for CD40L, which was identified to associate inversely with added sugar intake. The associations were in general attenuated after adding baseline BMI and fasting glucose as covariates in the regression models (Table 4), but additional covariate adjustment for CRP only had minor impact (data not shown).

Table 4. Associations with T2D incidence for proteins internally replicated to associate with added sugar intake and SSB intake.

Added Sugar	n	Lifestyle Adjustments		Lifestyle Adjustments + BMI		Lifestyle Adjustments + BMI + Fasting Glucose	
		HR (95% CI)	p	HR (95% CI)	p	HR (95% CI)	p
HE4	4253	1.01 (0.93–1.10)	0.77	1.06 (0.97–1.16)	0.16	1.02 (0.93–1.11)	0.69
FRalpha	4253	0.94 (0.88–1.02)	0.15	1.00 (0.93–1.08)	0.98	0.92 (0.85–0.99)	0.029
TNFRSF4	4175	1.01 (0.93–1.09)	0.84	0.97 (0.90–1.05)	0.52	0.87 (0.81–0.95)	0.0012 *
CDH3	4241	0.96 (0.89–1.03)	0.23	0.98 (0.91–1.05)	0.52	0.94 (0.87–1.01)	0.11
ICOSLG	4253	1.04 (0.96–1.12)	0.35	1.06 (0.98–1.14)	0.15	0.95 (0.88–1.03)	0.25
CXCL13	4175	1.14 (1.06–1.22)	0.00045 *	1.12 (1.04–1.21)	0.0033	1.07 (0.98–1.16)	0.12
MIA	4252	0.96 (0.89–1.04)	0.34	1.01 (0.94–1.09)	0.79	0.99 (0.91–1.07)	0.74
CD40L	4382	1.15 (1.07–1.24)	0.00023 *	1.13 (1.05–1.22)	0.0012 *	1.08 (1.00–1.16)	0.047
RETN	4382	1.11 (1.03–1.19)	0.0057	1.08 (1.01–1.17)	0.031	1.12 (1.04–1.21)	0.0021 *
SSBs							
IL1ra	3761	1.51 (1.42–1.61)	4.6×10^{-37} *	1.35 (1.26–1.45)	2.1×10^{-16} *	1.27 (1.18–1.37)	6.6×10^{-10} *
HGF	4382	1.65 (1.53–1.77)	2.6×10^{-38} *	1.48 (1.37–1.60)	1.0×10^{-22} *	1.37 (1.27–1.48)	5.2×10^{-15} *
IL12	4252	1.05 (0.97–1.13)	0.24	0.98 (0.90–1.06)	0.55	0.87 (0.81–0.95)	0.0014 *
PRSS8	4252	1.43 (1.31–1.55)	7.7×10^{-17} *	1.34 (1.23–1.46)	8.2×10^{-12} *	1.14 (1.05–1.24)	0.0030 *
tPA	4382	1.44 (1.34–1.55)	8.1×10^{-22} *	1.33 (1.23–1.43)	5.6×10^{-13} *	1.18 (1.09–1.28)	4.6×10^{-5} *
FUR	4253	1.78 (1.64–1.92)	2.8×10^{-46} *	1.54 (1.42–1.68)	4.9×10^{-24} *	1.30 (1.20–1.42)	2.2×10^{-9} *
CHI3L1	4370	1.22 (1.13–1.31)	6.9×10^{-8} *	1.17 (1.09–1.26)	2.1×10^{-5} *	1.17 (1.09–1.26)	1.5×10^{-5} *

Plasma proteins are standardized. Cox proportional hazards regressions were adjusted for age, sex, education, smoking, alcohol and LTPA (and BMI and fasting glucose in the additional models). * Significant after Bonferroni correction, $p = 0.05/16 = 0.003$. BMI, body mass index; HR, hazard ratio; LTPA, leisure time physical activity; SSB, sugar-sweetened beverage; T2D, type 2 diabetes.

In an additional exploratory analysis aimed at finding potential interaction effects between added sugar and SSB intake, respectively, and the 136 plasma proteins on T2D risk, no significant interaction were observed after Bonferroni correction for multiple testing (Table S2).

3.5. Associations of Added Sugar and SSB Intake with CRP and T2D Incidence

As presented in Figure 2, no significant linear associations were observed between either added sugar intake or SSB intake and T2D risk (p-trend of 0.51 and 0.28, respectively) or CRP concentrations (p-trend of 0.41 and 0.09, respectively). Regarding added sugar intake, the lowest CRP concentrations and HRs for T2D incidence were observed in the middle intake categories, while for SSB intake, the associations appeared more linearly positive. In sensitivity analyses, excluding low and high energy reporters and past diet changers from these aforementioned analyses, the lowest T2D risk and CRP level were still observed in the middle categories of added sugar intake, suggesting U-shaped associations between added sugar intake and T2D and CRP (Table S3). Furthermore, a significant positive interaction between added sugar and CRP was observed on the association with T2D incidence ($p = 0.01$), where added sugar intake was positively associated with T2D at high CRP levels, but not associated at low CRP levels. A similar tendency was observed for SSB intake, but this interaction was not significant ($p = 0.11$).

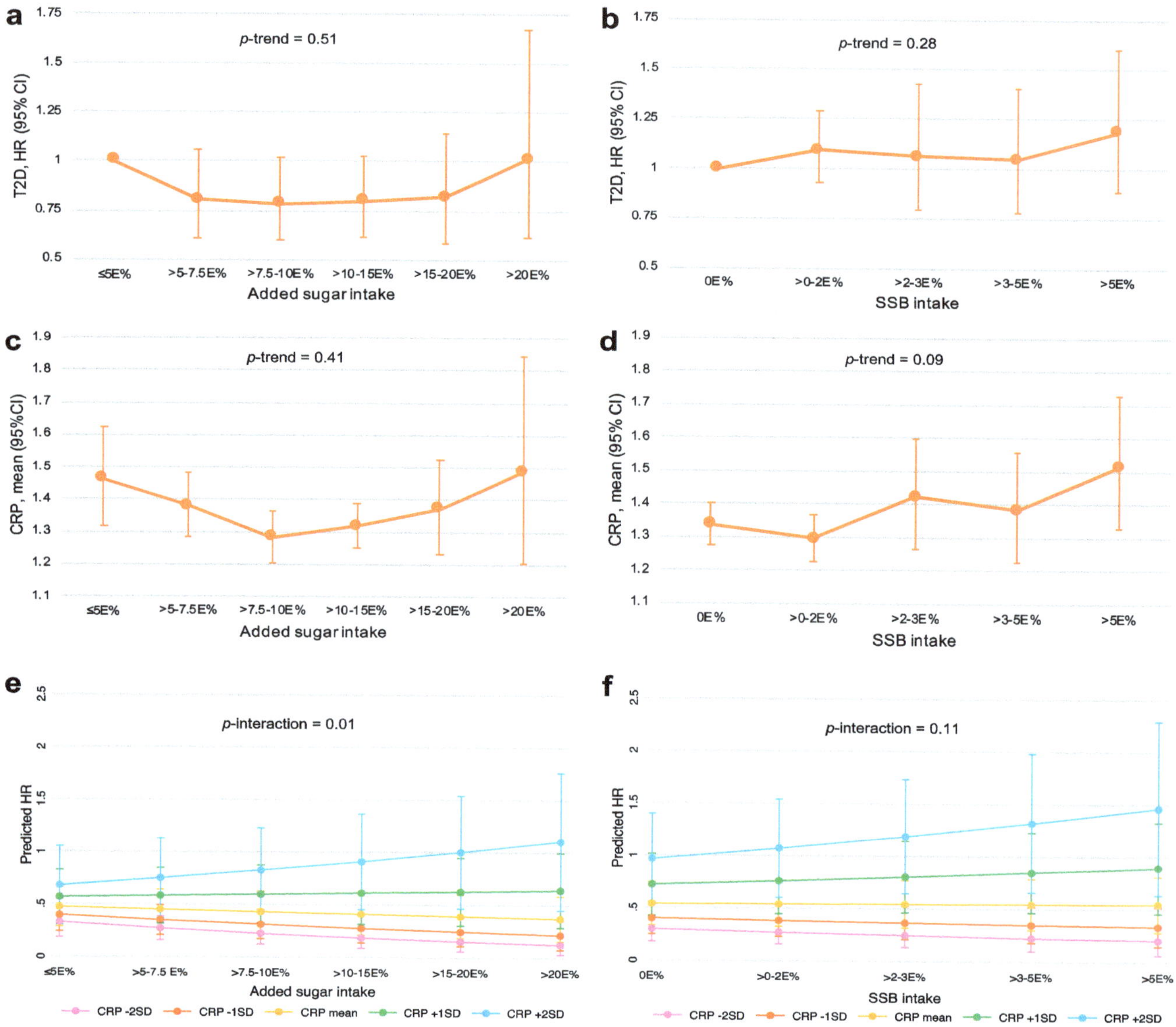

Figure 2. (**a**) Association between added sugar intake and T2D; (**b**) Association between SSB intake and T2D; (**c**) Association between added sugar intake and CRP; (**d**) Association between SSB intake and CRP; (**e**) Interaction between added sugar intake and CRP on T2D risk; (**f**) Interaction between SSB intake and CRP on T2D risk. Cox proportional hazards regressions and linear regressions were adjusted for age, sex, season, screening date, total energy intake, education, smoking, alcohol and LTPA. CRP was studied as log transformed and the predicted marginal means of CRP levels were exponentiated back for presentation. CRP, C-reactive protein; E%, percent of energy intake; HR, hazard ratio; LTPA, leisure time physical activity; SSB, sugar-sweetened beverage; T2D, type 2 diabetes.

4. Discussion

In the present study, we identified plasma proteins and proteomic signatures that cross-sectionally associated with added sugar and SSB intake. Most noteworthy is that we demonstrated that the SSB-associated proteins associated strongly with T2D incidence, indicating that SSB intake may be associated with a T2D-pathological proteomic signature, while such a signature was not observed for added sugar intake.

Using a TSIR approach, we identified nine plasma proteins that associated with added sugar intake after internal replication. Out of these, two proteins associated significantly with increased T2D incidence: CXCL13 and CD40L. We identified seven proteins that associated with SSB intake after internal replication and six of these were strongly associated with T2D incidence: HGF, tPA,

CHI3L1, IL1ra, PRSS8 and FUR. These six associations were much stronger than those of the two proteins that associated with added sugar intake. This indicates that SSB intake associates with a T2D-pathological proteomic profile, while this cannot be stated for added sugar intake. The associations between the identified proteins and T2D were not independent of baseline BMI and fasting glucose levels (of varying degree), but all six SSB-associated proteins remained strongly associated with T2D incidence after adjustment.

In brief, among all of the 16 internally replicated proteins, CXCL13, IL12, IL1ra, ICOSLG, HGF, CD40L, CHI3L1 and RETN are involved, one way or another, in inflammatory response signaling. TNFRSF4 is involved in atherosclerosis development and tPA is involved in thrombolysis, while PRSS8, FRalpha, MIA, FUR, CDH3 and HE4 are involved in various cancer processes [34,35]. The protein FUR has previously been studied in depth in MDC-CC and found to be strongly associated with diabetes incidence [36], and HGF plays a role in both hepatic glucose and lipid metabolism, and in the development of insulin resistance, fatty liver disease, cardiovascular diseases and cancers [37,38]. Nevertheless, among these proteins, some could potentially promote inflammation or disease, while other could be involved in negative feedback signaling. Hence, we cannot say whether the observed associations are causal or if the proteins only serve as potential markers of high SSB intake and T2D risk.

The finding that none of the 16 internally replicated proteins overlapped as being associated with both added sugar intake and SSB intake further emphasizes the notion that added sugar intake and SSB intake are rather different exposures and cannot be equated [39–41]. Although, this discrepancy may be due to the fact that self-reporting of SSB intake potentially could be more accurate, because SSBs generally are consumed in standardized portion sizes, i.e., in cans and bottles, as compared to the total intake of added sugar. Further, on average, SSB intake only contributed to 10% of the energy to the total intake of added sugar. However, it is reassuring that proteins such as PRSS8, IL12, IL1ra, FUR and CXCL1 were associated with both added sugar and SSB intake, although not exceeding the cutoff for internal replication for both.

The previous epidemiological literature on diet and inflammatory markers has mostly focused on CRP. Intake of SSBs have frequently been associated with higher CRP [42–47]. However, to our knowledge, the only published epidemiological study that has studied the association between sugar intake and CRP concluded that such an association could only be found when separately studying sugar from liquid sources, not total intake of free sugars [48]. We could similarly not find any significant linear association between added sugar intake and CRP, but neither could we observe any significant association between SSB intake and CRP, although a tendency for such an association could be observed (p-trend = 0.09).

Intervention trials that have studied inflammatory markers after high sugar interventions have focused on comparing effects between fructose and glucose, and only rarely sucrose. All such trials were summarized in a systematic review where only CRP was found sufficiently studied to perform a meta-analysis, and no differential effects between different sugars could be seen [49]. In addition, what is noteworthy in the previous literature on diet and inflammation is that the highly used Dietary Inflammatory Index, which estimates the inflammatory potential of a diet, does not incorporate intake of either added sugar or SSBs in its computation [50].

No significant linear associations were observed for either added sugar intake or SSB intake on T2D incidence. However, SSB intake has previously been found to associate with T2D incidence in a sample of 25,069 participants in the full MDC cohort [51]. Hence, the reduced power of the current study (n = 4382) is a probable reason for the lack of an association. Since no significant associations were found, it was not meaningful to perform mediation analysis of the internally replicated plasma proteins. Nevertheless, a significant positive interaction effect between added sugar intake and CRP on the risk of T2D was observed (p = 0.01), where increased T2D risk from high added sugar intake could only be observed at higher CRP levels. Baseline CRP has previously been shown to associate strongly with the incidence of diabetes mellitus in the MDC-CC [52].

Tendencies for a U-shaped association between added sugar intake and incident T2D were observed, while more linearly positive tendencies were observed with SSB intake. A U-shaped association was also observed between added sugar and CRP, while the association between SSB and CRP appeared more direct. Furthermore, the relatively large number of plasma proteins that associated inversely with added sugar intake but not with SSB intake, as displayed in Figure 1, indicates a potentially less healthy profile among those consuming the least amount of added sugar and could have contributed to the increased T2D risk in this group. In previous analyses of the full MDC cohort, the highest HR for T2D were observed in the lowest quintile of added sugar intake [53]. Furthermore, U-shaped associations have been observed between added sugar intake (studied in the same six categories as in the present study) and mortality in the full MDC cohort [30]. The reason for this U-shape is thought to at least partially be due to potential dietary misreporting and reversed causation, where those at high risk, e.g., overweight individuals, have reduced their sugar consumption or at least reported their dietary intakes as if they had. This is probably a source of bias in our analyses, and it may also apply to our plasma protein identification approach, which assumes linearity. However, the U-shaped nature of the associations between added sugar and T2D and CRP remained after exclusion of low and high energy reporters and past diet changers. Additionally, the dietary assessment method has been validated and shown relatively high Pearson's correlation coefficients regarding sugar intake (0.74 for women and 0.60 for men) [54].

A strength of this study is the use of the TSIR approach to identify plasma proteins. However, the main limitation is the lack of replication in external cohorts, which makes it difficult to make strong conclusions of any specific protein. Furthermore, the TSIR approach that was applied for internal replication has limitations, and it was modified to fit a more small-scale protein identification of 136 proteins rather than gene identification of millions of genes by lowering the α_1 criteria. In addition, our study may suffer from insufficient statistical power in some of its analyses, especially for analyses of interaction and in small intake categories of added sugar and SSBs. Furthermore, the skewness of the SSB variable certainly complicates the performed analyses. Due to the large proportion of zero consumers, log transformation (with a small added constant) marginally improved the distribution. Further, since this is a middle-aged population studied in the 1990's (born 1923–1950), the consumption habits may not be perfectly representative of a population of today. The large proportion of zero consumers of SSBs that were observed could be due to both underreporting and that consumption of SSBs might actually not have been very common in this population. This rather low overall SSB consumption (mean 1.2E%, median 0.07E%), as compared to what usually is observed in mainly American cohorts (and due to the skewness of the SSB variable), could have contributed to why we could not replicate an association between SSB intake and T2D, which so commonly is observed [9]. Finally, despite rigorous covariate adjustment, this is an epidemiological study where residual confounding cannot be ruled out and causality cannot be evaluated.

In conclusion, this is a hypothesis generating study that is the first of its kind to identify plasma proteins and proteomic signatures that are associated with added sugar and SSB intake. Turning to the proteome to elucidate the complex potential relationship between sugar intake and T2D incidence did not provide a clear enlightenment, but despite the fact that no significant associations were observed between added sugar and SSB intake with levels of CRP, the data suggests that SSB intake is related to a T2D-pathological proteomic signature, while this was not observed for added sugar intake. Replications in larger and more recent cohorts are necessary to verify our results.

Supplementary Materials:
Figure S1: Correlation matrix of internally replicated proteins that associates with added sugar intake and SSB intake, Figure S2: Pathways between internally replicated proteins according to the STRING database 11.0, Table S1: List of all 136 studied plasma proteins, Table S2: Proteins with a nominally significant ($p < 0.05$) interaction with added sugar or SSB intake on T2D risk from an exploratory analysis of 136 plasma proteins, Table S3: Sensitivity analyses excluding low and high energy reporters and diet changers in analyses of associations between added sugar and SSB intake and CRP and T2D risk.

Author Contributions: Conceptualization, S.R. and E.S.; methodology, S.R., E.S., G.E. and I.D.; Statistical analysis, S.R.; writing—original draft preparation, S.R.; writing—review and editing, I.D., U.E., J.N., M.O.-M., G.E. and E.S.; visualization, S.R.; supervision, E.S.; project administration, S.R.; funding acquisition, E.S., J.N., M.O.-M. and G.E. All authors have read and agreed to the published version of the manuscript.

Acknowledgments: We acknowledge all the participants and staff participating in the data collection of the Malmö Diet and Cancer–Cardiovascular Cohort.

References

1. Minihane, A.-M.; Vinoy, S.; Russell, W.R.; Baka, A.; Roche, H.M.; Tuohy, K.M.; Teeling, J.L.; Blaak, E.E.; Fenech, M.; Vauzour, D.; et al. Low-grade inflammation, diet composition and health: Current research evidence and its translation. *Br. J. Nutr.* **2015**, *114*, 999–1012. [CrossRef]
2. Lyons, C.L.; Kennedy, E.B.; Roche, H.M. Metabolic Inflammation-Differential Modulation by Dietary Constituents. *Nutrients* **2016**, *8*, 247. [CrossRef] [PubMed]
3. Herter-Aeberli, I.; Gerber, P.; Hochuli, M.; Kohler, S.; Haile, S.R.; Gouni-Berthold, I.; Berthold, H.K.; Spinas, G.A.; Berneis, K. Low to moderate sugar-sweetened beverage consumption impairs glucose and lipid metabolism and promotes inflammation in healthy young men: A randomized controlled trial. *Am. J. Clin. Nutr.* **2011**, *94*, 479–485. [CrossRef] [PubMed]
4. Sørensen, L.B.; Raben, A.; Stender, S.; Astrup, A. Effect of sucrose on inflammatory markers in overweight humans. *Am. J. Clin. Nutr.* **2005**, *82*, 421–427. [CrossRef]
5. Kuzma, J.N.; Cromer, G.; Hagman, D.; Breymeyer, K.L.; Roth, C.L.; Foster-Schubert, K.E.; Holte, S.E.; Weigle, D.S.; Kratz, M. No differential effect of beverages sweetened with fructose, high-fructose corn syrup, or glucose on systemic or adipose tissue inflammation in normal-weight to obese adults: A randomized controlled trial. *Am. J. Clin. Nutr.* **2016**, *104*, 306–314. [CrossRef] [PubMed]
6. Cox, C.L.; Stanhope, K.L.; Schwarz, J.M.; Graham, J.L.; Hatcher, B.; Griffen, S.C.; Bremer, A.A.; Berglund, L.; McGahan, J.P.; Keim, N.L.; et al. Circulating Concentrations of Monocyte Chemoattractant Protein-1, Plasminogen Activator Inhibitor-1, and Soluble Leukocyte Adhesion Molecule-1 in Overweight/Obese Men and Women Consuming Fructose- or Glucose-Sweetened Beverages for 10 Weeks. *J. Clin. Endocrinol. Metab.* **2011**, *96*, E2034–E2038. [CrossRef] [PubMed]
7. Silbernagel, G.; Machann, J.; Häring, H.-U.; Fritsche, A.; Péter, A. Plasminogen activator inhibitor-1, monocyte chemoattractant protein-1, e-selectin and C-reactive protein levels in response to 4-week very-high-fructose or -glucose diets. *Eur. J. Clin. Nutr.* **2013**, *68*, 97–100. [CrossRef]
8. Buyken, A.E.; Goletzke, J.; Joslowski, G.; Felbick, A.; Cheng, G.; Herder, C.; Brand-Miller, J.C. Association between carbohydrate quality and inflammatory markers: Systematic review of observational and interventional studies. *Am. J. Clin. Nutr.* **2014**, *99*, 813–833. [CrossRef]
9. Imamura, F.; O'Connor, L.; Ye, Z.; Mursu, J.; Hayashino, Y.; Bhupathiraju, S.N.; Forouhi, N.G. Consumption of sugar sweetened beverages, artificially sweetened beverages, and fruit juice and incidence of type 2 diabetes: Systematic review, meta-analysis, and estimation of population attributable fraction. *BMJ* **2015**, *351*, h3576. [CrossRef]
10. Malik, V.S.; Popkin, B.M.; Bray, G.A.; Després, J.-P.; Willett, W.C.; Hu, F.B. Sugar-Sweetened Beverages and Risk of Metabolic Syndrome and Type 2 Diabetes: A meta-analysis. *Diabetes Care* **2010**, *33*, 2477–2483. [CrossRef]
11. Schwingshackl, L.; Hoffmann, G.; Lampousi, A.-M.; Knüppel, S.; Iqbal, K.; Schwedhelm, C.; Bechthold, A.; Schlesinger, S.; Boeing, H. Food groups and risk of type 2 diabetes mellitus: A systematic review and meta-analysis of prospective studies. *Eur. J. Epidemiol.* **2017**, *32*, 363–375. [CrossRef] [PubMed]
12. Colditz, G.A.; Manson, J.E.; Stampfer, M.J.; Rosner, B.; Willett, W.C.; Speizer, F.E. Diet and risk of clinical diabetes in women. *Am. J. Clin. Nutr.* **1992**, *55*, 1018–1023. [CrossRef] [PubMed]
13. Feskens, E.J.; Virtanen, S.M.; Räsänen, L.; Tuomilehto, J.; Stengård, J.; Pekkanen, J.; Nissinen, A.; Kromhout, D. Dietary Factors Determining Diabetes and Impaired Glucose Tolerance: A 20-year follow-up of the Finnish and Dutch cohorts of the Seven Countries Study. *Diabetes Care* **1995**, *18*, 1104–1112. [CrossRef] [PubMed]
14. Janket, S.-J.; Manson, J.E.; Sesso, H.; Buring, J.E.; Liu, S. A prospective study of sugar intake and risk of type 2 diabetes in women. *Diabetes Care* **2003**, *26*, 1008–1015. [CrossRef]

15. Barclay, A.W.; Flood, V.M.; Rochtchina, E.; Mitchell, P.; Brand-Miller, J.C. Mappstat Glycemic Index, Dietary Fiber, and Risk of Type 2 Diabetes in a Cohort of Older Australians. *Diabetes Care* **2007**, *30*, 2811–2813. [CrossRef]
16. Montonen, J.; Järvinen, R.; Knekt, P.; Heliövaara, M.; Reunanen, A. Consumption of Sweetened Beverages and Intakes of Fructose and Glucose Predict Type 2 Diabetes Occurrence. *J. Nutr.* **2007**, *137*, 1447–1454. [CrossRef]
17. Boeing, H.; Schulz, M.; Heidemann, C.; Schienkiewitz, A.; Hoffmann, K.; Boeing, H. Carbohydrate intake and incidence of type 2 diabetes in the European Prospective Investigation into Cancer and Nutrition (EPIC)-Potsdam Study. *Br. J. Nutr.* **2008**, *99*, 1107–1116. [CrossRef]
18. Sluijs, I.; Van Der Schouw, Y.T.; van der Daphne, A.L.; Spijkerman, A.M.; Hu, F.B.; Grobbee, D.E.; Beulens, J.W. Carbohydrate quantity and quality and risk of type 2 diabetes in the European Prospective Investigation into Cancer and Nutrition–Netherlands (EPIC-NL) study. *Am. J. Clin. Nutr.* **2010**, *92*, 905–911. [CrossRef]
19. Heikkilä, H.M.; Schwab, U.; Krachler, B.; Männikkö, R.; Rauramaa, R. Dietary associations with prediabetic states—The DR's EXTRA Study (ISRCTN45977199). *Eur. J. Clin. Nutr.* **2012**, *66*, 819–824. [CrossRef]
20. Ahmadi-Abhari, S.; Luben, R.N.; Powell, N.; Bhaniani, A.; Chowdhury, R.; Wareham, N.J.; Forouhi, N.G.; Khaw, K.-T. Dietary intake of carbohydrates and risk of type 2 diabetes: The European Prospective Investigation into Cancer-Norfolk study. *Br. J. Nutr.* **2013**, *111*, 342–352. [CrossRef]
21. Biggelaar, L.J.C.J.D.; Eussen, S.J.; Sep, S.J.S.; Mari, A.; Ferrannini, E.; Van Dongen, M.C.J.M.; Denissen, K.F.M.; Wijckmans, N.E.G.; Schram, M.T.; Van Der Kallen, C.J.; et al. Associations of Dietary Glucose, Fructose, and Sucrose with β-Cell Function, Insulin Sensitivity, and Type 2 Diabetes in the Maastricht Study. *Nutrients* **2017**, *9*, 380. [CrossRef]
22. Tasevska, N.; Pettinger, M.; Kipnis, V.; Midthune, U.; Tinker, L.F.; Potischman, N.; Neuhouser, M.L.; Beasley, J.M.; Van Horn, L.; Howard, B.V.; et al. Associations of Biomarker-Calibrated Intake of Total Sugars with the Risk of Type 2 Diabetes and Cardiovascular Disease in the Women's Health Initiative Observational Study. *Am. J. Epidemiol.* **2018**, *187*, 2126–2135. [CrossRef]
23. Meyer, K.A.; Kushi, L.H.; Jacobs, D.R.; Slavin, J.; Sellers, T.A.; Folsom, A.R. Carbohydrates, dietary fiber, and incident type 2 diabetes in older women. *Am. J. Clin. Nutr.* **2000**, *71*, 921–930. [CrossRef] [PubMed]
24. Sartorelli, D.S.; Franco, L.; Gimeno, S.; Ferreira, S.R.G.; Cardoso, M.A. Dietary fructose, fruits, fruit juices and glucose tolerance status in Japanese–Brazilians. *Nutr. Metab. Cardiovasc. Dis.* **2009**, *19*, 77–83. [CrossRef] [PubMed]
25. Hodge, A.M.; English, D.R.; O'Dea, K.; Giles, G.G. Glycemic Index and Dietary Fiber and the Risk of Type 2 Diabetes. *Diabetes Care* **2004**, *27*, 2701–2706. [CrossRef] [PubMed]
26. Hotamisligil, G.S. Inflammation and metabolic disorders. *Nat. Cell Biol.* **2006**, *444*, 860–867. [CrossRef] [PubMed]
27. Donath, M.Y.; Shoelson, S.E. Type 2 diabetes as an inflammatory disease. *Nat. Rev. Immunol.* **2011**, *11*, 98–107. [CrossRef]
28. Wang, X.; Bao, W.; Liu, J.; Ouyang, Y.-Y.; Wang, D.; Rong, S.; Xiao, X.; Shan, Z.-L.; Zhang, Y.; Yao, P.; et al. Inflammatory Markers and Risk of Type 2 Diabetes: A systematic review and meta-analysis. *Diabetes Care* **2012**, *36*, 166–175. [CrossRef]
29. Liu, C.; Feng, X.; Li, Q.; Wang, Y.; Li, Q.; Hua, M. Adiponectin, TNF-α and inflammatory cytokines and risk of type 2 diabetes: A systematic review and meta-analysis. *Cytokine* **2016**, *86*, 100–109. [CrossRef]
30. Ramne, S.; Dias, J.A.; González-Padilla, E.; Olsson, K.; Lindahl, B.; Engström, G.; Ericson, U.; Johansson, I.; Sonestedt, E. Association between added sugar intake and mortality is nonlinear and dependent on sugar source in 2 Swedish population–based prospective cohorts. *Am. J. Clin. Nutr.* **2018**, *109*, 411–423. [CrossRef]
31. Mattisson, I.; Wirfält, E.; Aronsson, C.A.; Wallström, P.; Sonestedt, E.; Gullberg, B.; Berglund, G. Misreporting of energy: Prevalence, characteristics of misreporters and influence on observed risk estimates in the Malmö Diet and Cancer cohort. *Br. J. Nutr.* **2005**, *94*, 832–842. [CrossRef] [PubMed]
32. Enhörning, S.; Sjögren, M.; Hedblad, B.; Nilsson, P.M.; Struck, J.; Melander, O. Genetic vasopressin 1b receptor variance in overweight and diabetes mellitus. *Eur. J. Endocrinol.* **2016**, *174*, 69–75. [CrossRef] [PubMed]

33. Kang, G.; Liu, W.; Cheng, C.; Wilson, C.L.; Neale, G.; Yang, J.J.; Ness, K.K.; Robison, L.L.; Hudson, M.M.; Srivastava, D.K. Evaluation of a two-step iterative resampling procedure for internal validation of genome-wide association studies. *J. Hum. Genet.* **2015**, *60*, 729–738. [CrossRef] [PubMed]
34. Szklarczyk, D.; Gable, A.L.; Lyon, D.; Junge, A.; Wyder, S.; Huerta-Cepas, J.; Simonovic, M.; Doncheva, N.T.; Morris, J.H.; Bork, P.; et al. STRING v11: Protein–protein association networks with increased coverage, supporting functional discovery in genome-wide experimental datasets. *Nucleic Acids Res.* **2018**, *47*, D607–D613. [CrossRef] [PubMed]
35. Olink Proteomics. Complete Human Protein Biomarkers List. Available online: https://www.olink.com/products/complete-protein-biomarkers-list/ (accessed on 16 September 2020).
36. Fernandez, C.; Rysä, J.; Almgren, P.; Nilsson, J.; Engström, G.; Orho-Melander, M.; Ruskoaho, H.; Melander, O. Plasma levels of the proprotein convertase furin and incidence of diabetes and mortality. *J. Intern. Med.* **2018**, *284*, 377–387. [CrossRef]
37. Oliveira, A.G.; Araújo, T.G.; Carvalho, B.D.M.; Rocha, G.Z.; Dos Santos, A.; Saad, M.J.A. The Role of Hepatocyte Growth Factor (HGF) in Insulin Resistance and Diabetes. *Front. Endocrinol.* **2018**, *9*, 503. [CrossRef] [PubMed]
38. Madonna, R.; Cevik, C.; Nasser, M.; De Caterina, R. Hepatocyte growth factor: Molecular biomarker and player in cardioprotection and cardiovascular regeneration. *Thromb. Haemost.* **2012**, *107*, 656–661. [CrossRef]
39. Johnson, R.K.; Appel, L.J.; Brands, M.; Howard, B.V.; Lefevre, M.; Lustig, R.H.; Sacks, F.; Steffen, L.M.; Wylie-Rosett, J. Dietary Sugars Intake and Cardiovascular Health. *Circulation* **2009**, *120*, 1011–1020. [CrossRef]
40. Wang, J.; Light, K.; Henderson, M.; O'Loughlin, J.; Mathieu, M.-E.; Paradis, G.; Gray-Donald, K. Consumption of Added Sugars from Liquid but Not Solid Sources Predicts Impaired Glucose Homeostasis and Insulin Resistance among Youth at Risk of Obesity. *J. Nutr.* **2013**, *144*, 81–86. [CrossRef]
41. Welsh, J.A.; Wang, Y.; Figueroa, J.; Brumme, C. Sugar intake by type (added vs. naturally occurring) and physical form (liquid vs. solid) and its varying association with children's body weight, NHANES 2009-2014. *Pediatr. Obes.* **2018**, *13*, 213–221. [CrossRef]
42. De Koning, L.; Malik, V.S.; Kellogg, M.D.; Rimm, E.B.; Willett, W.C.; Hu, F.B. Sweetened Beverage Consumption, Incident Coronary Heart Disease, and Biomarkers of Risk in Men. *Circulation* **2012**, *125*, 1735–1741. [CrossRef]
43. Kosova, E.C.; Auinger, P.; Bremer, A.A. The Relationships between Sugar-Sweetened Beverage Intake and Cardiometabolic Markers in Young Children. *J. Acad. Nutr. Diet.* **2013**, *113*, 219–227. [CrossRef] [PubMed]
44. Hert, K.A.; Fisk, P.S.; Rhee, Y.S.; Brunt, A.R. Decreased consumption of sugar-sweetened beverages improved selected biomarkers of chronic disease risk among US adults: 1999 to 2010. *Nutr. Res.* **2014**, *34*, 58–65. [CrossRef] [PubMed]
45. Tamez, M.; Monge, A.; Lopez-Ridaura, R.; Fagherazzi, G.; Rinaldi, S.; Ortiz-Panozo, E.; Yunes, E.; Romieu, I.; Lajous, M. Soda Intake Is Directly Associated with Serum C-Reactive Protein Concentration in Mexican Women. *J. Nutr.* **2018**, *148*, 117–124. [CrossRef] [PubMed]
46. Yu, Z.; Ley, S.H.; Sun, Q.; Hu, F.B.; Malik, V.S. Cross-sectional association between sugar-sweetened beverage intake and cardiometabolic biomarkers in US women. *Br. J. Nutr.* **2018**, *119*, 570–580. [CrossRef]
47. Lin, W.-T.; Kao, Y.-H.; Sothern, M.S.; Seal, D.W.; Lee, C.-H.; Lin, H.-Y.; Chen, T.; Tseng, T.-S. The association between sugar-sweetened beverages intake, body mass index, and inflammation in US adults. *Int. J. Public Health* **2020**, *65*, 45–53. [CrossRef]
48. O'Connor, L.; Imamura, F.; Brage, S.; Griffin, S.J.; Wareham, N.J.; Forouhi, N.G. Intakes and sources of dietary sugars and their association with metabolic and inflammatory markers. *Clin. Nutr.* **2017**, *37*, 1313–1322. [CrossRef]
49. Della Corte, K.W.; Perrar, I.; Penczynski, K.J.; Schwingshackl, L.; Herder, C.; Buyken, A.E. Effect of Dietary Sugar Intake on Biomarkers of Subclinical Inflammation: A Systematic Review and Meta-Analysis of Intervention Studies. *Nutrients* **2018**, *10*, 606. [CrossRef]
50. Shivappa, N.; Steck, S.E.; Hurley, T.G.; Hussey, J.R.; Hebert, J.R. Designing and developing a literature-derived, population-based dietary inflammatory index. *Public Health Nutr.* **2013**, *17*, 1689–1696. [CrossRef]
51. Ericson, U.; Hindy, G.; Drake, I.; Schulz, C.-A.; Brunkwall, L.; Hellstrand, S.; Almgren, P.; Orho-Melander, M. Dietary and genetic risk scores and incidence of type 2 diabetes. *Genes Nutr.* **2018**, *13*, 13. [CrossRef]

52. Bao, X.; Borné, Y.; Johnson, L.S.; Muhammad, I.F.; Persson, M.; Niu, K.; Engström, G. Comparing the inflammatory profiles for incidence of diabetes mellitus and cardiovascular diseases: A prospective study exploring the 'common soil' hypothesis. *Cardiovasc. Diabetol.* **2018**, *17*, 87. [CrossRef] [PubMed]
53. Olsson, K.; Ramne, S.; Gonzàlez-Padilla, E.; Ericson, U.; Sonestedt, E. Associations of carbohydrates and carbohydrate-rich foods with incidence of type 2 diabetes. *Br. J. Nutr.* under review.
54. Riboli, E.; Elmståhl, S.; Saracci, R.; Gullberg, B.; Lindgärde, F. The Malmo Food Study: Validity of two dietary assessment methods for measuring nutrient intake. *Int. J. Epidemiol.* **1997**, *26*, 161S–173S. [CrossRef] [PubMed]

3

Combination of Aronia, Red Ginseng, Shiitake Mushroom and Nattokinase Potentiated Insulin Secretion and Reduced Insulin Resistance with Improving Gut Microbiome Dysbiosis in Insulin Deficient Type 2 Diabetic Rats

Hye Jeong Yang [1], Min Jung Kim [1], Dae Young Kwon [1], Da Sol Kim [2], Ting Zhang [2], Chulgyu Ha [3] and Sunmin Park [2,*]

1 Research Division of Food Functionality, Korean Food Research Institutes, Wanjoo 55365, Korea; yhj@kfri.re.kr (H.J.Y.); kmj@kfri.re.kr (M.J.K.); dykwon@kfri.re.kr (D.Y.K.)
2 Department of Food and Nutrition, Obesity/Diabetes Center, Hoseo University, Asan 31499, Korea; tpfptm14@daum.net (D.S.K.); zhangting92925@gmail.com (T.Z.)
3 Department of Bioprocess Technology, Bio Campus Korea Polytechnic, Nonsan 32943, Korea; hckue@kopo.ac.kr
* Correspondence: smpark@hoseo.edu

Abstract: The combination of freeze-dried aronia, red ginseng, ultraviolet-irradiated shiitake mushroom and nattokinase (AGM; 3.4:4.1:2.4:0.1) was examined to evaluate its effects on insulin resistance, insulin secretion and the gut microbiome in a non-obese type 2 diabetic animal model. Pancreatectomized (Px) rats were provided high fat diets supplemented with either (1) 0.5 g AGM (AGM-L), (2) 1 g AGM (AGM-H), (3) 1 g dextrin (control), or (4) 1 g dextrin with 120 mg metformin (positive-control) per kg body weight for 12 weeks. AGM (1 g) contained 6.22 mg cyanidin-3-galactose, 2.5 mg ginsenoside Rg3 and 244 mg β-glucan. Px rats had decreased bone mineral density in the lumbar spine and femur and lean body mass in the hip and leg compared to the normal-control and AGM-L and AGM-H prevented the decrease. Visceral fat mass was lower in the control group than the normal-control group and its decrease was smaller with AGM-L and AGM-H. HOMA-IR was lower in descending order of the control, positive-control, AGM-L, AGM-H and normal-control groups. Glucose tolerance deteriorated in the control group and was improved by AGM-L and AGM-H more than in the positive-control group. Glucose tolerance is associated with insulin resistance and insulin secretion. Insulin tolerance indicated insulin resistance was highly impaired in diabetic rats, but it was improved in the ascending order of the positive-control, AGM-L and AGM-H. Insulin secretion capacity, measured by hyperglycemic clamp, was much lower in the control group than the normal-control group and it was improved in the ascending order of the positive-control, AGM-L and AGM-H. Diabetes modulated the composition of the gut microbiome and AGM prevented the modulation of gut microbiome. In conclusion, AGM improved glucose metabolism by potentiating insulin secretion and reducing insulin resistance in insulin deficient type 2 diabetic rats. The improvement of diabetic status alleviated body composition changes and prevented changes of gut microbiome composition.

Keywords: aronia; ginseng; mushroom; pancreatectomy; type 2 diabetes; gut microbiome; insulin secretion

1. Introduction

The prevalence of type 2 diabetes is markedly increasing in Asian countries, including Korea and reached 8.7% of the Asian population by 2014; it is expected to reach 12–5% by 2025 [1]. This is associated with ethnic differences in the etiology of type 2 diabetes [1]. Type 2 diabetes generally develops as a consequence of the imbalance between insulin resistance and insulin secretion [2]. When insulin resistance increases due to obesity, inflammation, oxidative stress, aging, less physical activity, etc., insulin secretion is elevated to overcome insulin resistance and to maintain normoglycemia. Increased inflammation and oxidative stress may accelerate the development of type 2 diabetes especially in Asians. However, Asians are more susceptible to type 2 diabetes under the insulin resistant condition since their insulin secretory capacity and β-cell mass are low [3]. The Westernization of diets mostly elevate insulin resistance in Asians which that is not compensated due to low insulin secretion capacity. Thus, Westernization of diets can increase the prevalence of type 2 diabetes in many cases although obesity is much less in Asian than Caucasians.

Type 2 diabetes is prevented and treated by reducing insulin resistance and increasing insulin capacity in both Asians and non-Asians, although the disease has a somewhat different etiology in Asians than non-Asians. Asians with type 2 diabetes are usually not obese, although they are insulin resistant [3]. Thus, the proper animal model for Asian type 2 diabetes needs to be non-obese, have lower insulin secretion capacity, and higher insulin resistance than the non-diabetic rats. Partially pancreatectomized rats are an optimal model for studying Asian type 2 diabetes [4]. They have about 60% insulin secretion capacity and about 50% of the pancreatic mass of the rats with intact pancreas [4]. The Px rats gradually develop insulin resistance. A high fat diet accelerates the increase of insulin resistance in Px rats [5]. Anti-diabetic interventions for Asians can be examined for improvements in both insulin resistance and insulinotropic activity in Px rats fed with a high fat diet [6].

Previous studies have supported that the gut microbiome produces microbial metabolites including short-chain fatty acids (SCFAs), bile acids (BAs) and lipopolysaccharides (LPS) that modulate host glucose metabolism, mainly in the liver [7]. This is called the gut liver axis. These metabolites directly influence metabolic diseases including type 2 diabetes [7]. Low-grade peripheral inflammation also promotes the development of type 2 diabetes. Patients with a low bacterial α- diversity in the gut microbiome are at greater risk of metabolic diseases than are patients with high α-diversity [8]. Herbs rich in fiber, polyphenols and polysaccharides increase the abundance of the phylum *Bacteroidetes*, and genera *Akkermansia*, *Bifidobacteria*, *Lactobacillus*, *Bacteroides* and *Prevotella* [7]. However, it reduces the number of phylum *Firmicutes* and *Firmicutes/Bacteroidetes* ratio in the intestines. It is well known that some herbal compounds improve glucose metabolism by modulating insulin resistance and insulin secretion. The changes in some of the microbial metabolites from consuming plant compounds are correlated with changes to the gut microbiome that modulate glucose metabolism [9].

Aronia melanocarpa, red ginseng and shiitake mushroom have been reported to improve glucose metabolism. Aronia and its anthocyanins have anti-inflammatory and antioxidant properties that improve insulin sensitivity and prevent type 2 diabetes [10]. Red ginseng and ginsenoside Re, Rb1, and Rb2, its active ingredients, have demonstrated an antidiabetic action in in vitro, animal, and clinical studies [11–14]. Ultraviolet-irradiated shiitake mushroom (Lentinus edodes), polysaccharides, has antioxidant activity and it is a good source for vitamin D (V-D) in humans [5]. The dosage of 100–400 mg shiitake mushroom/kg bw is effective for anti-oxidant properties because it increases the content of the reduced form of glutathione, but at higher dosages it has an adverse effect on immunity [15]. Anti-diabetic effects of V-D are still controversial. V-D may exert anti-diabetic activity by improving insulin secretion and insulin sensitivity [5]. However, some placebo-controlled clinical studies of vitamin D administration have not shown that it improves insulin release and sensitivity [16]. Type 2 diabetes increases the thrombotic risk to develop cardiovascular diseases [17]. Although nattokinase has not been shown shown to possess anti-diabetic activity, it is reported to improve blood flow by inhibiting platelet aggregation and thrombosis to reduce cardiovascular events [18]. The water or ethanol extracts of aronia, red ginseng and shiitake mushroom have been well studied, but the whole foods, including dietary fiber, may be better for inducing changes to the gut microbiome that influence glucose metabolism.

Insulin resistance and β-cell function and mass are associated with increased oxidative stress and inflammation [1,10,19]. Aronia and shiitake mushrooms improve insulin resistance [5,10], red ginseng potentiates β-cell function and mass [11], and nattokinase prevents thrombosis [18]. The combination of aronia, red ginseng, shiitake mushroom and nattokinase, which have anti-oxidative and anti-inflammatory properties, may alleviate type 2 diabetic symptoms and its complications. However, its direct effects on anti-diabetic activity such as insulin resistance and insulin secretion have not been examined. The relationship between anti-diabetic activity and the gut microbiome is also not well characterized. We hypothesized that the combination of freeze-dried aronia, red ginseng, ultraviolet-irradiated shiitake mushroom and nattokinase would prevent or reverse insulin resistance, improve insulin secretion, and help normalize serum glucose levels, due to changes in the gut microbiome. We tested this hypothesis in Px rats, a non-obese type 2 diabetic animal model.

2. Materials and Methods

2.1. Preparation of the Product and Analysis of Ingredients

Each of aronia, red ginseng, and shiitake mushroom was washed, dried at room temperature, freeze-dried, and powdered. Freeze-dried Aronia, red ginseng, shitake mushroom and nattokinase were mixed with the ratio of (3.4:4.1:2.4:0.1) (Chakreis, AGM) and Chakreis was generously provided by YD Nutraceuticals Ltd. (Yongin-si, Korea). The dosages were determined by considering preliminary studies and previous studies [10,12,13,15,16,18]. The freeze-dried powder mixture was used for the animal study. The mixture was extracted with in distilled water at 95 °C for 12 h and the extracts were centrifuged at 10,000× *g* at 4 °C for 20 min. The supernatants were lyophilized in a freeze-dryer.

For measuring indicative components in the mixture, it was extracted with methanol and lysophilized. The extracts were dissolved in methanol, and a syringe filter was used to remove undissolved contents. The contents of ginsenoside Rg, cyanidin-galactoside, cyanidin-glucoside and cyanidin-arabinoside in the extract were measured were analyzed by high performance liquid chromatography using a Luna C18 column (4.6 mm × 250 mm; ID, 5 μm). The mobile phase solvents were acetonitrile and 0.1% formic acid in water (6:4, vol:vol) with isocratic elution at a flow rate of 1 mL/min, 40 °C in-column temperature, and UV detection at 270 nm. We used ginsenoside Rg, cyanidin-galactose, cyanidin-glucose and cyanidin-arabinoside as standards to quantify the sample.

The β-glucan contents of shitake mushroom were sequentially digested with digestion enzymes by incubating in lower temperature for 2 h. The enzymes used to digest the shitake mushroom were amylase (20 units, pH 6.9) at 20 °C, cellulase (50 units, pH 5.0) at 37 °C, protease (10 units, pH 7.5) at 37 °C, and amyloglucosidase (70 units, pH 4.8) at 60 °C. The digested shiitake mushroom was mixed with 95% ethanol and the mixture was left at 4 °C for 12 h. The mixture was centrifuged at 10,000 rpm for 10 min and water was added into the precipitates. Sulfuric acid was added (1:5) into the diluted precipitate. The mixture was left at room temperature for 20 min and the optical density was measured at 470 nm. Glucose solution was used as a standard.

2.2. Animals and Ethics

Eight-week-old male Sprague–Dawley rats (weight, 218 ± 23 g) were housed individually in stainless steel cages in a controlled environment (23 °C; 12-h light/dark cycle). All surgical and experimental procedures were performed according to the guidelines of the Animal Care and Use Review Committee of Hoseo University, Korea (HUACUC-17-57). The rats underwent a 90% pancreatectomy using the Hosokawa technique [20] or received a sham pancreatectomy (sham) under anesthesia induced by intramuscular injection of a mixture of ketamine and xylazine (100 and 10 mg/kg body weight, respectively). The pancreatectomized (Px) rats exhibited characteristics of type 2 diabetes (random glucose levels >180 mg/dL), whereas the sham rats did not [20,21].

2.3. Experimental Design

A total of 40 Px rats were assigned randomly to the following four groups, which differed according to diet: (1) 1 g dextrin/kg bw (negative-control) (2) 0.5 g AGM/kg bw, (3) 1 g AGM/kg bw, and (4) 120 mg/kg bw metformin (positive-control). Each group included 10 Px rats. The sham-operated rats were given 1 g dextrin/kg bw for normal-control ($n = 10$). All experimental animals were given free access to water and a high-fat diet containing either the assigned extracts or dextrin for 12 weeks. The high-fat diet was a modified semi-purified AIN-93 formulation for experimental animals [22] that consisted of 42% carbohydrate, 15% protein, and 43% fat. The major carbohydrate, protein, and fat sources were starch and sugar, casein (milk protein), and lard (CJ Co., Seoul, Korea), respectively.

2.4. Body Composition Measurement

After calibrating a dual-energy X-ray Absorptiometer (DEXA; Norland pDEXA Sabre; Norland Medical Systems Inc., Fort Atkinson, WI, USA) with a phantom supplied by the manufacturer, the body compositions of the rats were measured at the 7th week of the experimental period. The animals were anesthetized with ketamine and xylazine (100 and 10 mg/kg bw, respectively), and laid in a prone position, with the posterior legs maintained in external rotation with tape. The hip, knee, and ankle articulations were in 90° flexion. Upon the completion of scanning, lean mass was determined in the leg and hip using the DEXA instrument equipped with the appropriate software for the assessment of bone density in small animals [22]. Similarly, the fat mass was measured in the leg and abdominal areas using the DEXA instrument.

2.5. Glucose Homeostasis

Overnight fasted serum glucose levels, food intake, and body weights were measured every week. An oral glucose tolerance test (OGTT) was performed at the 7th week in overnight-fasted animals by orally administering 2 g glucose/kg body weight [23]. Blood samples were taken by tail bleeding at 0, 10, 20, 30, 40, 50, 60, 70, 80, 90, and 120 min after glucose loading. The serum insulin levels were determined at 0, 20, 40, 90, and 120 min. The averages of the total areas under the curves for the serum glucose and insulin concentrations were calculated using the trapezoidal rule. At 3 days after OGTT, an intraperitoneal insulin tolerance test (IPITT) was conducted after the food was removed for 6 h. The serum glucose levels were measured every 15 min for 90 min after an intraperitoneal injection of insulin (0.75 U/kg body weight). Serum glucose and insulin levels were analyzed with a Glucose Analyzer II (Beckman Coulter, Palo Alto, CA, USA) and rat Ultrasensitive insulin kit (Crystal Chem, Elk Grove Village, IL, USA), respectively.

2.6. Hyperglycemic Clamp and Cerebral Blood Flow

Catheters were surgically implanted into the right carotid artery and left jugular vein in all rats after 7 weeks of treatment and anesthetization with ketamine and xylazine. A hyperglycemic clamp was performed in 10 free-moving and overnight-fasted rats/group after 5–6 days of implantation to determine insulin secretion capacity, as described previously [20,24,25]. During the clamp, glucose was infused to maintain a serum glucose level of 5.5 mM above baseline, and serum insulin level was measured at designated times. After the clamp, the rats were freely provided food and water for 2 days and then deprived of food for 16 h the next day. After anesthesia with a mixture of ketamine and xylazine, the rats were placed in a stereotaxic device with a midline incision of the scalp exposing the periosteum. A small pore was made with a drill in the right lateral ventricle with stereotaxic coordinates: 1.0 mm posterior, 6 mm lateral, 3.7 mm ventral to bregma. A Doppler flow probe was placed on the cerebral vein and blood flow was measured continuously with Laser Doppler Flowmetry (LDF100C-1, BIOPAC Systems, Inc., Goleta, CA, USA) for 10 min.

After measuring cerebral blood flow regular human insulin (5 U/kg body weight; Humulin; Eli Lilly, Indianapolis, IN, USA) was injected through the inferior vena cava. The rats were euthanized by decapitation 10 min later, and tissues were collected rapidly, frozen in liquid nitrogen, and stored at −70 °C for further experiments. Insulin resistance was determined using the homeostasis model assessment estimate of insulin resistance (HOMA-IR) and calculated using the following equation: HOMA-IR = fasting insulin (μIU/mL) × fasting glucose (mM)/22.5. Lipid profiles in the circulation were measured using colorimetry kits from Asan Pharmaceutical (Seoul, Korea).

2.7. Immunohistochemistry

Five rats from each group were injected with BrdU (100 μg/kg body weight) after 6 weeks of treatment. The rats were anesthetized intraperitoneally 6 h post-injection with a mixture of ketamine and xylazine, and the brain and pancreas were dissected immediately, perfused with saline and a 4% paraformaldehyde solution (pH 7.2) sequentially, and post-fixed with the same fixative overnight at room temperature [24].

Two serial 5-μm paraffin-embedded tissue sections were selected from the seventh or eighth sections to avoid counting the same islets twice when measuring β-cell area, BrdU incorporation, and apoptosis, were determined as described previously using an immunohistochemistry method [24]. Endocrine β-cells were identified by applying guinea pig anti-insulin and rabbit anti-glucagon antibodies to the sections. Pancreatic β-cell area was measured by examining all non-overlapping images in two insulin-stained sections from each rat at 10× magnification with a Zeiss Axiovert microscope (Carl Zeiss Microimaging, Thornwood, NY, USA). Pancreatic β-cell mass, individual β-cell size, β-cell proliferation by BrdU incorporation, and apoptotic β-cell were measured as described previously [24].

2.8. Next Generation Sequencing of the Gut Microbiome

The gut microbiome composition was measured from feces of each rat by analyzing metagenome sequencing using next-generation sequencing [26]. Bacterial DNA was extracted from the samples of each rat using a Power Water DNA Isolation Kit (MoBio, Carlsbad, CA, USA) according to the manufacturer's instructions. Each library was prepared using polymerase chain reaction (PCR) products according to the GS FLX plus library prep guide. The emPCR, corresponding to clonal amplification of the purified library, was carried out using the GS-FLX plus emPCR Kit (454 Life Sciences, Branford, CT, USA). Libraries were immobilized onto DNA capture beads. The library-beads were added to the amplification mix and oil, and the mixture was vigorously shaken on a Tissue Lyser II (Qiagen, Valencia, CA, USA) to create "micro-reactors" containing both amplification mix and a single bead. The emulsion was dispensed into a 96-well plate and the PCR amplification program was run with 16S universal primers in the FastStart High Fidelity PCR System (Roche, Basel, Switzerland) according to the manufacturer's recommendations. Sequencing of bacterial DNA in the feces was performed by the Macrogen Ltd. (Seoul, Korea) by a Genome Sequencer FLX plus (454 Life Sciences) as previously reported.

2.9. Statistical Analyses

All data are expressed as means ± standard deviations, and all statistical analyses were performed using SAS ver. 9.1 (SAS Institute, Cary, NC, USA). Significant differences among the control, AGM-L, AGM-H, positive-control and normal-control animal groups were identified with one-way analyses of variance. Significant differences in the main effects among the groups were detected using post-hoc Tukey's tests. A p-value <0.05 was considered significant.

3. Results

3.1. Contents of Anthocyanins and Ginsenoide Rg3

Aronia mainly contained cyanidin-galactoside, but also and cyanidin-glucoside, and cyanidin-arabinoside, whereas red ginseng had mostly ginsenoside Rg3 (2.5 mg/g sample). Shiitake mushroom contained 244 mg β-glucans/g sample (Table 1).

3.2. Body Composition

Body weight gains for 11 weeks were higher in the normal-control group than the control group whereas the positive-control and AGM-H increased body weight more than the control group but less than the normal-control ($p < 0.05$). Unlike body weight gain, food intake was not significantly different among the groups. Food efficiency decreased in the control group compared to the normal-control group and its reduction was prevented by AGM-H the most ($p < 0.05$). Epididymal and retroperitoneal fat contents and visceral fat mass, were much lower in the control group than the normal-control group (Table 2). The visceral fat mass was higher in the AGM-L and AGM-H groups than the positive-control group ($p < 0.05$), but it was not significantly different between the control and positive-control groups (Table 2). Thus, less increase of body weight and fat mass might be associated with urinary glucose loss.

Table 1. The contents of ingredients in the mixture.

	Contents (mg/g Powder)
C3-Galactoside	6.22
C3-Glucoside	0.33
C3-Arabinoside	1.53
Total Anthocyanin	8.08
Ginsenoside Rg3	2.5
β-glucan	244

Table 2. Energy metabolism and visceral fat mass.

	Normal-Control (n = 10)	Control (n = 10)	Positive-Control (n = 10)	AGM-L (n = 10)	AGM-H (n = 10)
Body weight gain for 10 week (g)	283 ± 10.5 ^{a}	144 ± 10.7 ^{b}	169 ± 11.8 ^{b}	156 ± 19.1 ^{b}	155 ± 13.0 ^{b}
Food intake (g/day)	14.4 ± 1.0 ^{a}	15.1 ± 0.8 ^{a}	15.0 ± 1.0 ^{a}	13.4 ± 1.5 ^{b}	12.3 ± 1.5 ^{b}
Food efficiency	0.30 ± 0.01 ^{a}	0.15 ± 0.01 ^{d}	0.18 ± 0.12 ^{c}	0.19 ± 0.03 ^{c}	0.22 ± 0.02 ^{b}
Epididymal fat pads (g)	6.7 ± 0.7 ^{a}	3.0 ± 0.4 ^{c}	2.9 ± 0.3 ^{c}	3.8 ± 0.5 ^{b}	3.3 ± 0.4 ^{c}
Retroperitoneal fat mass (g)	8.1 ± 0.8 ^{a}	3.6 ± 0.5 ^{c}	3.8 ± 0.5 ^{c}	4.3 ± 0.6 ^{b,c}	5.0 ± 0.7 ^{b}
Visceral fat (g)	14.8 ± 1.6 ^{a}	6.7 ± 0.9 ^{c}	6.7 ± 0.8 ^{c}	8.1 ± 1.0 ^{b}	8.3 ± 1.0 ^{b}

Food efficiency: daily energy intake/daily weight gain × 100. Values are means ± standard deviation. The test product was the mixture of free-dried aronia, red ginseng, mushroom and nattokinase. Px rats fed a high fat diet supplemented with (1) 0.5 g mixture/kg bw/day (AGM-L), (2) 1 g mixture/kg bw/day (AGM-H), (3) 1 g dextrin/kg bw/day (control), or (4) metformin (120 mg/kg body weight; positive-control) for 12 weeks. Sham-operated rats (normal-control) fed the same diet of control. ^{a,b,c,d} Values on the same row with different superscripts were significantly different at $p < 0.05$.

BMD in the lumbar spine and femur was much lower in the control group than the normal-control group whereas AGM-L and AGM-H prevented the decrease of BMD as much as the positive-control group ($p < 0.05$; Figure 1A). LBM showed a similar pattern of BMD. LBM exhibited a lower value in the control group than the normal-control and AGM-L and AGM-H protected against the decrease of LBM as much as the positive-control group ($p < 0.05$; Figure 1B). Fat mass also showed the similar tendency to LBM (Figure 1C).

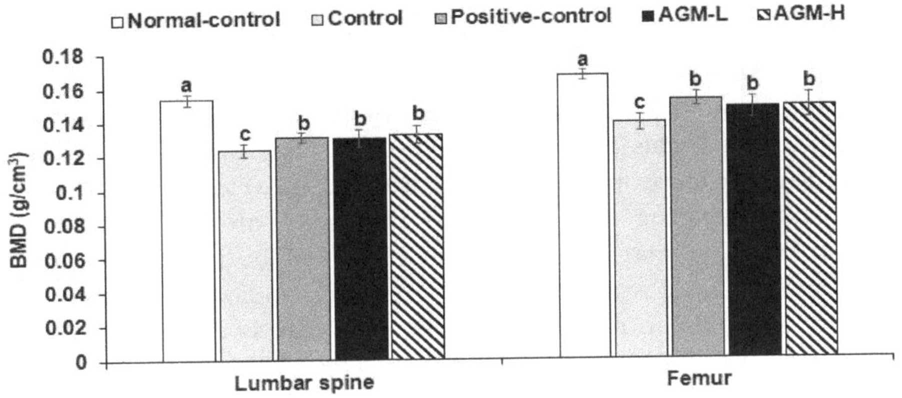

(A)

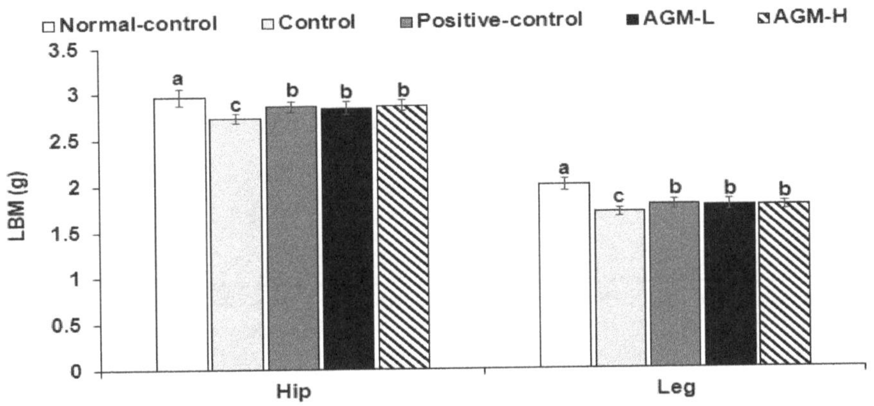

(B)

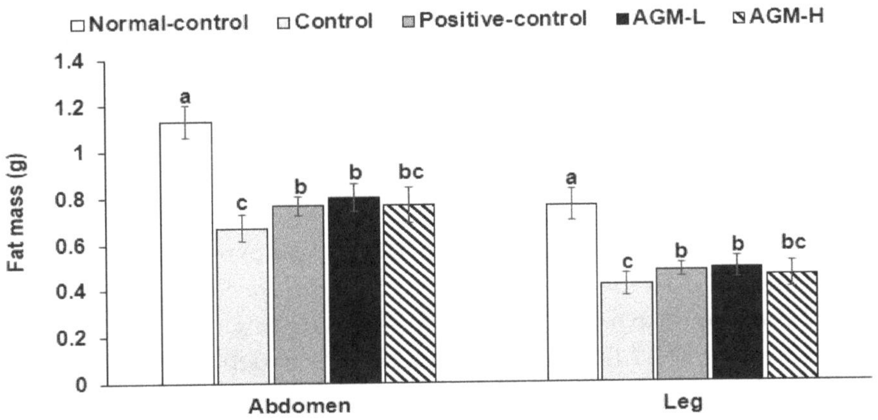

(C)

Figure 1. Bone mineral density (BMD), lean body mass (LMB) and fat mass (FM) at the end of experiment. Px rats were fed a high fat diet supplemented with aronia, red ginseng, shiitake mushroom, and nattokinase powders (1) 0.5 g mixture/kg bw/day (AGM-L), (2) 1 g mixture/kg bw/day (AGM-H), (3) 1 g dextrin/kg bw/day (control), or (4) metformin (120 mg/kg body weight; positive-control) for 12 weeks. Sham rats fed the same diet of control. BMD (**A**) in the lumbar spine and femurs, LBM (**B**) of the hip and legs and FM of the abdomen and legs (**C**) were measured by DEXA. Each bar and error bar represents the mean ± SD (n = 10 of each group). [a,b,c] Different superscripts on the bars represent significant differences at $p < 0.05$.

3.3. Glucose Metabolism

Overnight-fasting serum glucose levels in the control group were higher than those in the normal-control group indicating the diabetic conditions of the control group, and AGM-L and AGM-H decreased the serum glucose levels at fating states ($p < 0.05$; Table 3). Overnight serum insulin levels were lower in the control group than in the normal-control group. As calculated from serum glucose and insulin levels at fasting state, HOMA-IR, an index of insulin resistance, was higher in the control group than in the normal-control (Table 3). AGM-L and positive-control group showed a similar HOMA-IR, and AGM-H was lowered the most ($p < 0.05$). Mean cerebral blood flow was lower in the control than normal-control and it was not significantly different between the control and positive-control. However, AGM-L and AGM-H protected against the decrease in cerebral blood flow in Px rats and the levels in AGM-L were similar to normal-control.

Table 3. Serum glucose and insulin levels at fasting states and insulin resistance.

	Normal-Control (n = 10)	Control (n = 10)	Positive-Control (n = 10)	AGM-L (n = 10)	AGM-H (n = 10)
Serum glucose at fasting state (mM)	5.4 ± 0.5 [d]	9.8 ± 0.6 [a]	8.4 ± 0.6 [b]	8.1 ± 0.7 [b]	7.2 ± 0.5 [c]
Serum insulin at fasting state (ng/mL)	3.78 ± 0.36 [a]	2.83 ± 0.32 [c]	3.55 ± 0.35 [a,b]	3.27 ± 0.34 [b]	3.23 ± 0.36 [b]
HOMA-IR	5.4 ± 0.6 [d]	9.8 ± 1.0 [a]	8.4 ± 0.9 [b]	8.1 ± 0.8 [b]	7.2 ± 0.8 [c]
Urinary glucose	-	++++	+++	++	+
Mean cerebral blood flow (mm/s)	657 ± 45 [a]	405 ± 42 [c]	424 ± 45 [c]	643 ± 65 [a]	571 ± 67 [b]

+, ++, +++, ++++ higher amount of urinary glucose detection with more +. [-] No detection of urinary glucose. Values are means ± standard deviation. The test product was the mixture of free-dried aronia, red ginseng, mushroom and nattokinase. Px rats fed a high fat diet supplemented with (1) 0.5 g mixture/kg bw/day (AGM-L), (2) 1 g mixture/kg bw/day (AGM-H), (3) 1 g dextrin/kg bw/day (control), or (4) metformin (120 mg/kg body weight; positive-control) for 12 weeks. Sham-operated rats (normal-control) fed the same diet of control. [a,b,c,d] Values on the same row with different superscripts were significantly different at $p < 0.05$.

Cerebral blood flow was much lower in the control group than the normal-control group and positive-control did not improve blood flow compared to the control. However, AGM-L and AGM-H prevented the decrease and the level in the AGM-L group was similar to the normal-control group.

The OGTT revealed that glucose tolerance was highly impaired in the control group compared to the normal-control group and it was improved by metformin in the positive-control group (Figure 2A). AGM-L and AGM-H improved the glucose tolerance better than the positive-control but the improvement did not return it to normal-control group values ($p < 0.05$; Figure 2A). AUC of serum glucose levels during OGTT in the first phase was much higher in the control group than the normal-control group whereas AGM-L and AGM-H decreased the AUC of serum glucose levels ($p < 0.05$; Figure 2B). In the second phase of OGTT, AUC of serum glucose concentrations were much higher in the control group than in the normal-control group and AGM-L prevented the increase (Figure 2B). AGM-H increased the 2nd part of the serum insulin levels in comparison to the control but it was not significantly different (Figure 2C).

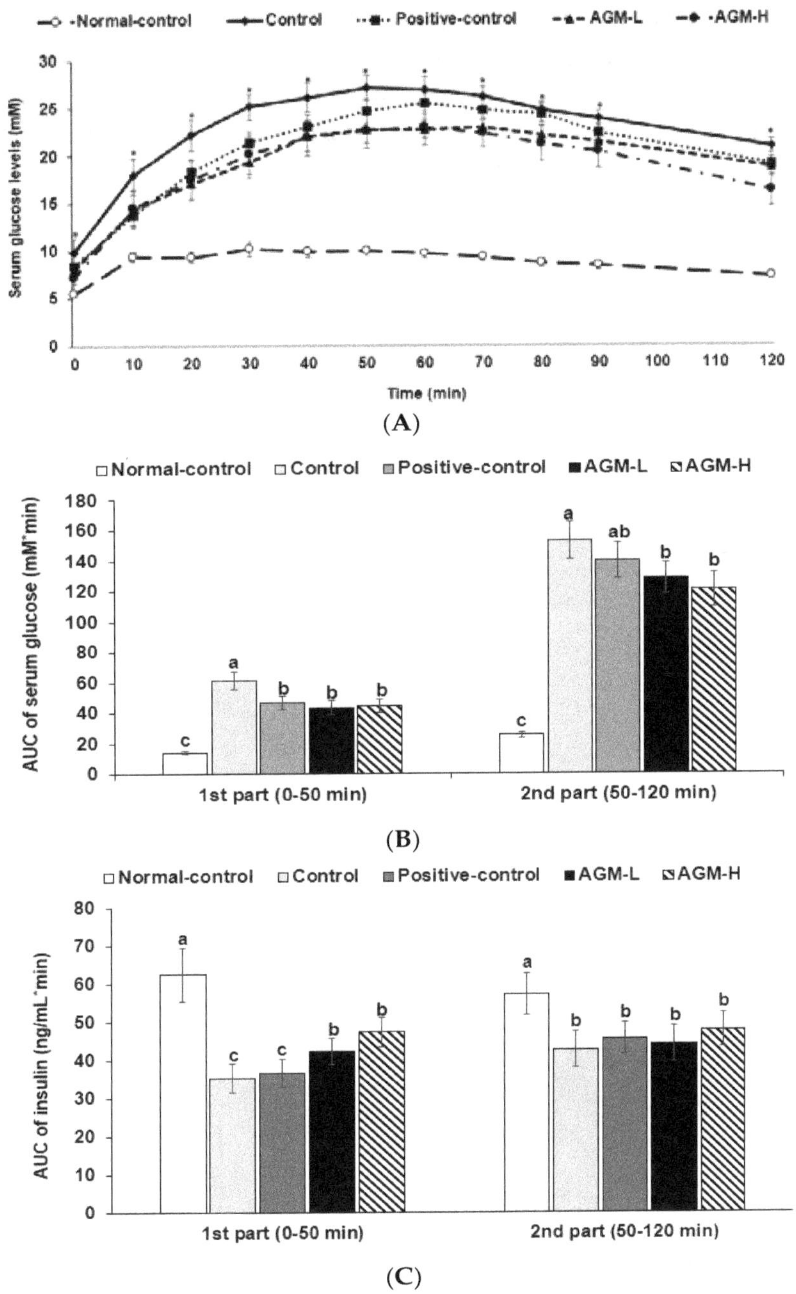

Figure 2. Serum glucose and insulin levels and area under the curve (AUC) of serum glucose and insulin during oral glucose tolerance test (OGTT). Px rats were fed a high fat diet supplemented with aronia, red ginseng, shiitake mushroom, and nattokinase powders (1) 0.5 g mixture/kg bw/day (AGM-L), (2) 1 g mixture/kg bw/day (AGM-H), (3) 1 g dextrin /kg bw/day (control), or (4) metformin (120 mg/kg body weight; positive-control) for 12 weeks. Sham rats fed the same diet of control. Changes of serum glucose levels (**A**) were measured after orally giving 2 g of glucose/kg body weight. The average of the area under the curve (AUC) of glucose (**B**) and insulin (**C**) during the first part (0–40 min) and second part (40–120 min) of OGTT. Each dot and bar and error bar represent the mean ± SD (n = 10 of each group). * Significantly different among the groups at each time point at $p < 0.05$. ^{a,b,c} Different superscripts on the bars represent significant differences at $S < 0.05$.

3.4. Insulin Tolerance

At 6 h after food deprivation, serum glucose levels were much higher in the control group than the normal-control group and the levels were lowered in the descending order of the control, positive-control, AGM-L and AGM-H ($p < 0.05$; Figure 3A). After insulin injection, serum glucose levels decreased until 60 min in all groups and the levels were almost maintained in all groups except the control group. The AUC of serum glucose concentrations were much higher in the control than in the normal-control in the 1st and 2nd phase (Figure 3B). AGM-L and AGM-H markedly decreased serum glucose levels during the 1st phase and the levels at the 2nd phase was similar to the normal-control group ($p < 0.05$; Figure 3B). Thus, AGM-L and AGM-H improved insulin tolerance in comparison to the control.

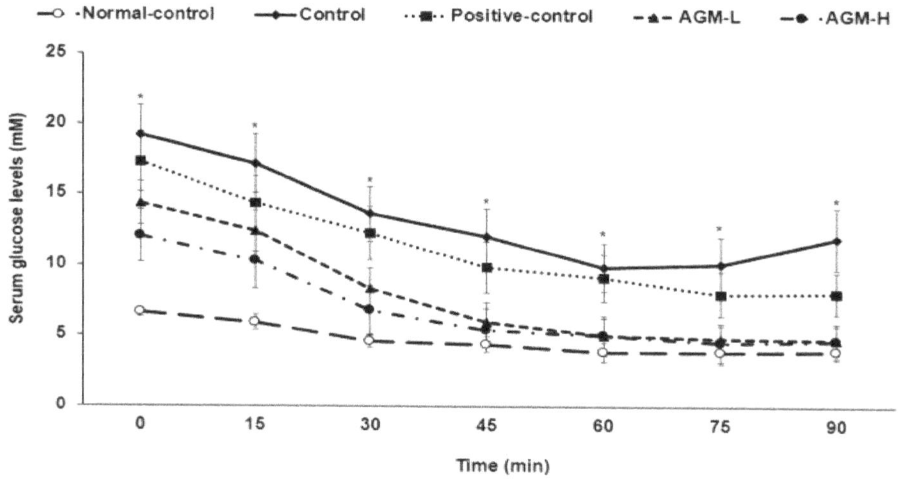

(A)

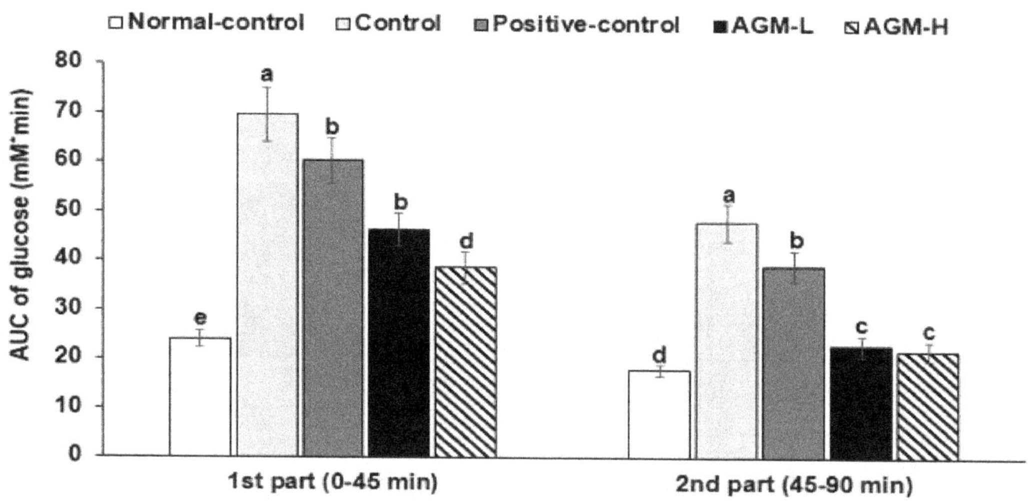

(B)

Figure 3. Changes of serum glucose concentrations during the intraperitoneal insulin tolerance test (IPITT). Px rats were fed a high fat diet supplemented with aronia, red ginseng, shiitake mushroom, and nattokinase powders (1) 0.5 g mixture/kg bw/day (AGM-L), (2) 1 g mixture/kg bw/day (AGM-H), (3) 1 g dextrin /kg bw/day (control), or (4) metformin (120 mg/kg body weight; positive-control) for 12 weeks. Sham rats fed the same diet of the control. IPITT was conducted with intraperitoneal injection of 0.75 IU insulin/kg body weight and measured serum glucose concentrations in blood collected from the tail every 15 min for 90 min. Changes of serum glucose levels were measured during IPITT (**A**). The average of the area under the curve (AUC) of glucose (**B**) during the first part (0–45 min) and second part (45–120 min) of IPITT. Each dot and bar and error bar represents the mean ± SD ($n = 10$ of each group). * Significantly different among the groups at each time point at $p < 0.05$. [a,b,c,d] Different superscripts on the bars represent significant differences at $p < 0.05$.

3.5. Hyperglycemic Clamp

Serum insulin levels were much lower in the control group than normal-control group for 90 min after glucose challenge ($p < 0.05$; Figure 4A). Serum insulin levels exhibited the 1st (0–10 min) and 2nd (60–90 min) phases in all groups. The AUC of 1st and 2nd phases of serum insulin levels increased in AGM-L the most whereas AGM-H elevated the AUC 1st and 2nd phases more than the control but less than the AGM-L ($p < 0.05$; Figure 4B). Glucose infusion rates during hyperglycemic clamp were much lower in the control group than the normal-control group whereas AGM-H prevented the decrease in Px rats, but the levels were less than the normal-control ($p < 0.05$; Table 4). AGM-H showed a higher glucose infusion rates and the levels were higher than the positive-control group ($p < 0.05$). Insulin sensitivity in the hyperglycemic state markedly decreased in the control group compared to the normal-control group and it was higher in the ascending order of control, AGM-H, positive-control and AGM-L ($p < 0.05$; Table 4).

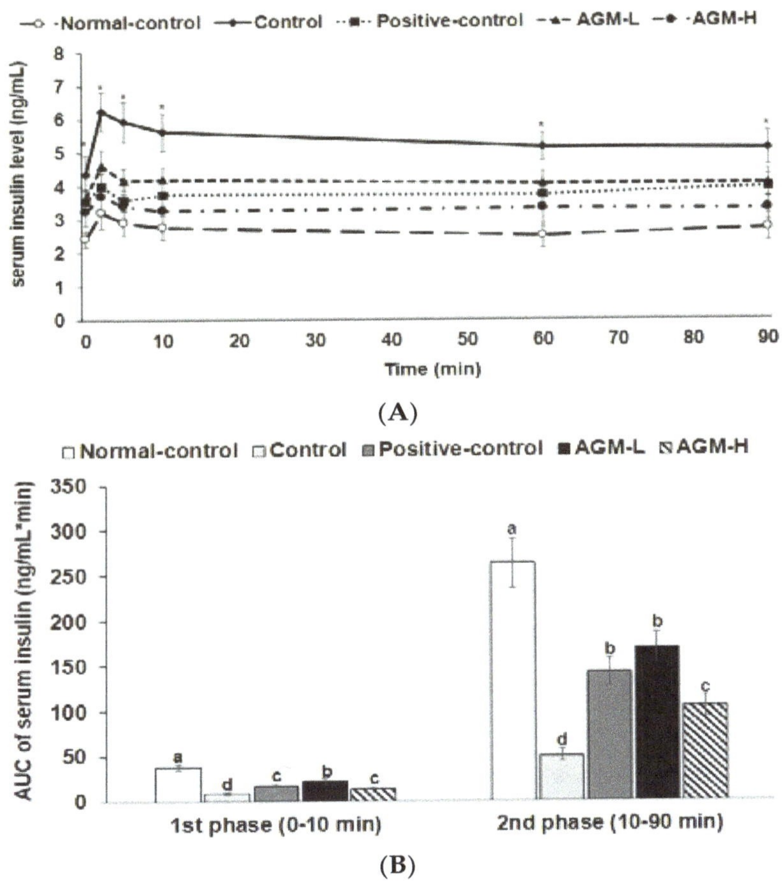

Figure 4. Insulin secretion during hyperglycemic clamp. Px rats were fed a high fat diet supplemented with aronia, red ginseng, shiitake mushroom, and nattokinase powders (1) 0.5 g mixture/kg bw/day (AGM-L), (2) 1 g mixture/kg bw/day (AGM-H), (3) 1 g dextrin /kg bw/day (control), or (4) metformin [illegible] weight; positive-control) for 12 weeks. Sham rats fed the same diet of the control. [illegible] as conducted in conscious, free moving, and overnight fasted rats to measure [illegible] lin secretion. As exogenous glucose was infused into jugular vein to make [illegible] above overnight fasted serum glucose levels, serum insulin levels were [illegible] 30, 60, 90 and 120 min (**A**). The average of the area under the curve (AUC) [illegible] (**B**) during the first part (0–10 min) and second part (10–90 min) during [illegible] **B**). Each dot and bar and error bar represents the mean ± SD ($n = 10$ of each [illegible] different among the groups at each time point at $p < 0.05$. [a,b,c,d] Different [illegible] s represent significant differences at $p < 0.05$.

Table 4. Glucose metabolism during hyperglycemic clamp.

	Normal-Control (n = 10)	Control (n = 10)	Positive-Control (n = 10)	AGM-L (n = 10)	AGM-H (n = 10)
Serum glucose levels at 60 min (mM)	9.8 ± 0.9 [c]	17.7 ± 1.4 [a]	14.6 ± 1.7 [b]	15.1 ± 1.6 [b]	15.1 ± 1.1 [b]
Serum glucose levels at 90 min (mM)	9.9 ± 0.9 [c]	18.3 ± 1.7 [a]	15.6 ± 1.7 [b]	15.2 ± 1.3 [b]	14.6 ± 1.2 [b]
Serum insulin levels at 2 min (ng/mL)	6.2 ± 0.6 [a]	3.2 ± 0.5 [d]	4.0 ± 0.4 [c]	4.6 ± 0.5 [b]	3.7 ± 0.4 [c]
Serum insulin levels at 60 min (ng/mL)	5.1 ± 0.4 [a]	2.5 ± 0.4 [d]	3.7 ± 0.3 [b,c]	4.1 ± 0.5 [b]	3.3 ± 0.6 [c]
Glucose infusion rates (umol/kg bw/min)	59.4 ± 3.9 [a]	26.1 ± 2.8 [d]	35.6 ± 3.9 [c]	32.8 ± 4.4 [c]	43.9 ± 3.9 [b]
Insulin sensitivity at hyperglycemic state (μmol glucose min−1 100 g−1 per μmol insulin/L)	33.3 ± 3.9 [a]	19.8 ± 2.4 [d]	25.8 ± 2.9 [c]	23.4 ± 2.6 [c]	28.9 ± 3.3 [b]

Values are means ± standard deviation (n = 10 of each group). The test product was the mixture of free-dried aronia, red ginseng, mushroom and nattokinase. Px rats fed a high fat diet supplemented with (1) 0.5 g mixture/kg bw/day (AGM-L), (2) 1 g mixture/kg bw/day (AGM-H), (3) 1 g dextrin /kg bw/day (control), or (4) metformin (120 mg/kg body weight; positive-control) for 12 weeks. Sham-operated rats (normal-control) fed the same diet of the control. [a,b,c,d] Values on the same row with different superscripts were significantly different at $p < 0.05$.

3.6. Pancreatic β-cell Mass, Proliferation, and Apoptosis

Pancreatic β-cell area is calculated by the number and individual size of β-cells. The increased number of β-cells improves diabetic status. However, individual β-cell size increases with β-cell hypertrophy that is associated with increased insulin resistance. Pancreatic β-cell area was higher in the control group than the normal-control group, but individual β-cell size was higher in the control group than in the normal-control group ($p < 0.05$; Table 5). AGM-H increased pancreatic β-cell area with smaller individual sized beta-cells, demonstrating that AGM-H increased β-cell number (Table 5). Pancreatic β-cell mass, calculated by multiplying β-cell area by pancreatic weight, was much lower in the control group than the normal-control group. Pancreatic β-cell mass increased in the ascending order of the control, positive-control, AGM-L, and AGM-H ($p < 0.05$; Table 5).

Table 5. The modulation of islet morphometry in the pancreas section.

	Normal-Control (n = 5)	Control (n = 5)	Positive-Control (n = 5)	AGM-L (n = 5)	AGM-H (n = 5)
β-cell area (%)	5.5 ± 0.7 [c]	6.3 ± 0.8 [b]	6.8 ± 0.8 [a,b]	6.9 ± 0.8 [a,b]	7.6 ± 0.9 [a]
Individual β-cell size (μm^2)	185 ± 23 [c]	239 ± 26 [a]	209 ± 23 [b]	206 ± 25 [b]	189 ± 22 [b,c]
Absolute β-cell mass (mg)	33.4 ± 2.9 [a]	17.9 ± 1.9 [d]	22.4 ± 2.6 [c]	23.7 ± 2.9 [c]	28.8 ± 3.5 [b]
BrdU$^+$ cells (% BrdU$^+$ cells of islets)	0.72 ± 0.09 [c]	0.84 ± 0.09 [b]	0.89 ± 0.11 [b]	0.90 ± 0.12 [b]	1.04 ± 0.12 [a]
Apoptosis (% apoptotic bodies of islets)	0.64 ± 0.07 [a,b]	0.70 ± 0.09 [a]	0.66 ± 0.07 [a,b]	0.65 ± 0.07 [a,b]	0.59 ± 0.07 [b]

Values are means ± standard deviation. The test product was the mixture of free-dried aronia, red ginseng, mushroom and nattokinase. Px rats fed a high fat diet supplemented with (1) 0.5 g mixture/kg bw/day (AGM-L), (2) 1 g mixture/kg bw/day (AGM-H), (3) 1 g dextrin /kg bw/day (control), or (4) metformin (120 mg/kg body weight; positive-control) for 12 weeks. Sham-operated rats (normal-control) fed the same diet of the control. [a,b,c,d] Values on the same row with different superscripts were significantly different at $p < 0.05$.

The β-cell number is balanced by β-cell proliferation and β-cell apoptosis. The control rats exhibited a higher β-cell apoptosis than the positive-control rats and AGM-H decreased β-cell apoptosis ($p < 0.05$; Table 5). The β-cell proliferation was lower in the control group than the normal-control group. AGM-H increased the β-cell proliferation ($p < 0.05$; Table 5). Therefore, AGM-H increased β-cell mass by elevating β-cell proliferation and decreasing β-cell apoptosis.

3.7. Gut Microbiome

Community composition of the gut microbiota was compared with both total and sha operational taxonomic units among the groups by analysis of molecular variance (AM The AMOVA test revealed significant differences between the fecal bacterial communitie the groups ($p < 0.01$). Principal coordinate analysis (PCoA) illustrates the clustering of g community (Figure 5A). Normal-control and control showed a significant separation of g AGM-L and AGM-H also had separate gut microbiota clustering from control but t with the normal-control. However, positive-control exhibited a similar pattern to that of the control group (Figure 5A). These results indicated that diabetes modulated the composition of gut microbiome and AGM prevented the modulation of gut microbiome.

The bacterial distribution was different among the groups at the phylum and order levels (Figure 5B,C). The major bacteria were *Firmicutes*, *Bacteriodetes*, *Proteobacteria*, *Actinobacteria*, and *Deferribacteres* at the phylum level. The percentage of *Firmicutes* was higher in the control group than the normal-control group and AGM-L and AGM-H reduced its percentage (Figure 5B). In contrast to *Firmicutes*, the percentage of *Bacteroidetes* was lower in the control than the normal-control and it increased with AGM-L and AGM-H ($p < 0.05$; Figure 5B). The percentages of *Proteobacteria*, *Actinobacteria*, and *Deferribacteres* were not altered by diabetic status and AGM supplementation (Figure 5B). The bacteria community was different among the groups in order level more than the phylum level. The percentage of *Bacteroidales* was much lower in the control than the normal-control and it was increased by AGM-L and AGM-H (Figure 5C). The percentages of *Erysipelotrichales* and *Clostridiales* were higher in the control than the normal-control and they were decreased by AGM-L and AGM-H. AGM-L increased the percentage of *Desulfovibrionales* ($p < 0.05$; Figure 5C). Thus, AGM-L modulated gut microbiome to make it similar to the normal-control.

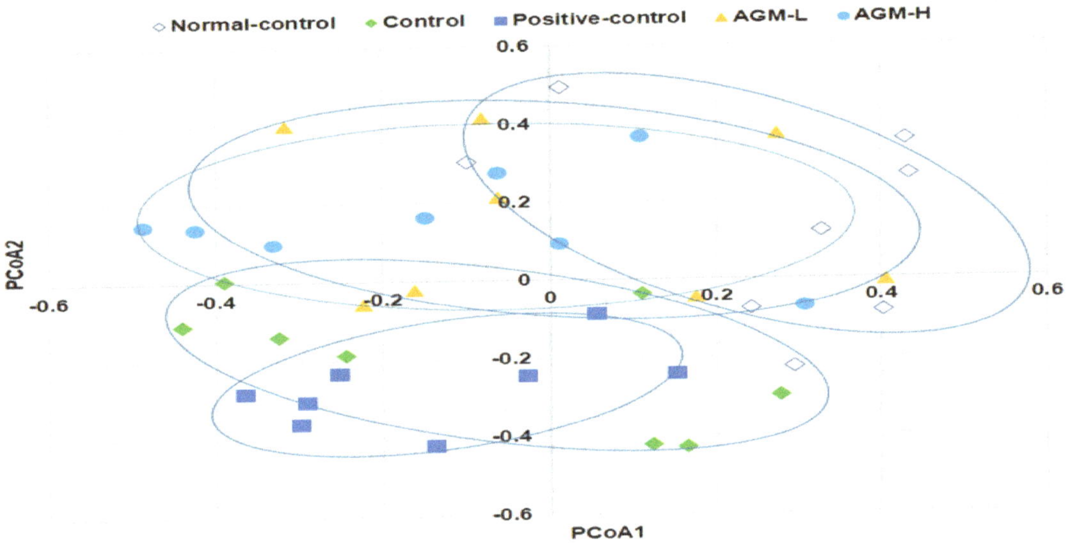

(A)

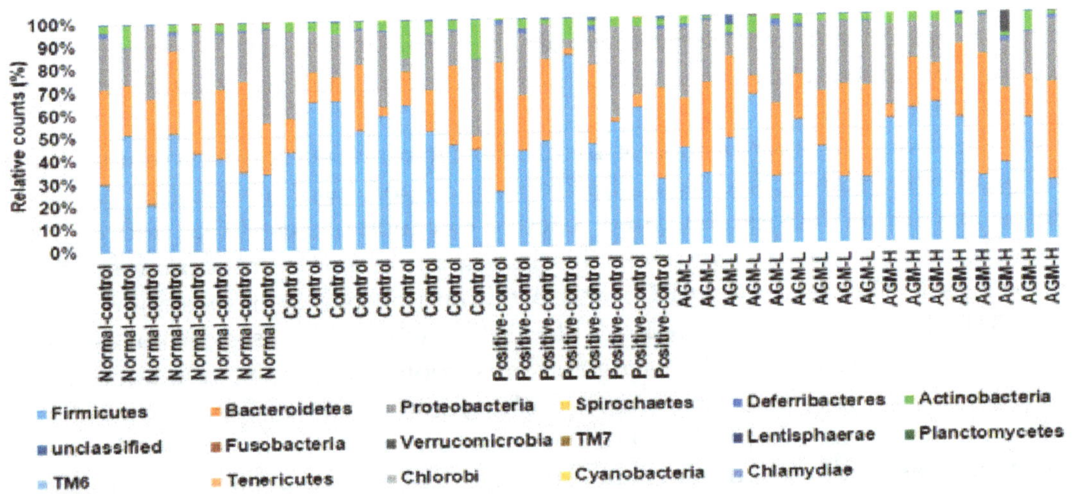

(B)

Figure 5. *Cont.*

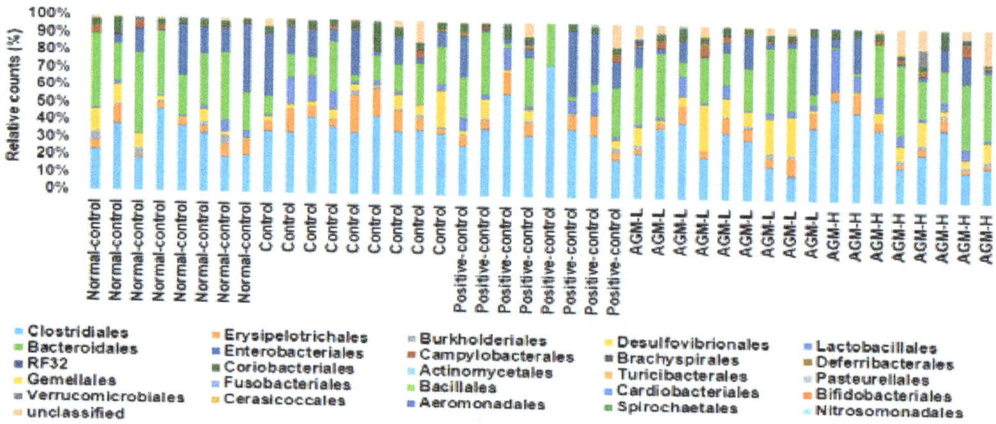

(C)

Figure 5. The profiles of gut microbiomes Px rats were fed a high fat diet supplemented with aronia, red ginseng, shiitake mushroom, and nattokinase powders (1) 0.5 g mixture/kg bw/day (AGM-L; $n = 8$), (2) 1 g mixture/kg bw/day (AGM-H; $n = 8$), (3) 1 g dextrin/kg bw/day (control; $n = 8$), or (4) metformin (120 mg/kg body weight; positive-control; $n = 8$) for 12 weeks. Sham rats were fed the same diet as the control ($n = 8$). At the end of experimental periods feces were collected and the bacterial DNA was analyzed. The fecal bacterial community was shown in principal coordinate analysis (PCoA) (**A**). Proportion of taxonomic assignments [Phylum (**B**) and Order (**C**)] for gut microbiomes was analyzed.

4. Discussion

Aronia, red ginseng and ultraviolet-irradiated shiitake mushroom have been reported to influence glucose metabolism. Based on a previous study, freeze-dried aronia, red ginseng, ultraviolet-irradiated shiitake mushroom and nattokinase were mixed at the ratio of 3.4:4.1:2.5:0.1 and the anti-diabetic activity was examined by assessing its efficacy for improving insulin sensitivity and potentiating insulin secretion in non-obese type 2 diabetic rats (Px rats). Px rats fed high fat diets, a well-established model of Asians type 2 diabetes, were used as the animal model for investigating the efficacy of the mixture in the present study. The Px rats had hyperglycemia due to increased insulin resistance and decreased insulin secretion. We used whole food not extracts since the gut microbiome is influenced by dietary fiber in the ingredients and anthocyanins can be easily degraded due to high temperature during extraction. Aronia, red ginseng, ultraviolet-irradiated shiitake mushroom and nattokinase contain different effective components such as anthocyanins, ginsenoside and β-glucan with vitamin D [27–29]. The major ingredients are known to be beneficial for alleviating type 2 diabetic symptoms and they are not overlapped between the plants. Thus, the efficacy of the mixture was examined for anti-diabetic activity in the present study.

Hyperglycemia develops when there is insufficient insulin secretion to compensate for insulin resistance. Insulin resistance is due to the impairment of insulin signaling by inflammation, oxidative stress and other factors. Elevated reactive oxygen species (ROS) and proinflammatory cytokines are also associated with impaired insulin signaling and β-cell function, with increasing β-cell apoptosis [30]. The decrease in ROS and proinflammatory cytokines alleviates the diabetic symptoms [29,31]. Hyperglycemia also reduces blood flow, which increases cardiovascular events [32]. The mixture of *Aronia melanocarpa*, red ginseng and mushroom is a good combination for anti-diabetic activity. *Aronia melanocarpa* extracts are rich in anthocyanins that suppress the production of ROS and proinflammatory cytokines [33,34]. Furthermore, aronia extracts prevent hyperglycemia by inhibiting α-glucosidase activity in the small intestines, by their ROS scavenging in humans and animal models [35,36]. Red ginseng can complement the anti-diabetic activity of aronia. Ginsenosides in red ginseng are known to prevent insulin resistance by activating insulin signaling in cells, animals and humans [11–13,28]. Red ginseng enhances insulin secretion and increases the pancreatic β-cell mass, which has hypoglycemic effects [14]. A systematic review and meta-analysis of randomized controlled clinical trials demonstrates that ginseng modestly, but significantly, improved fasting blood glucose in non-diabetic and diabetic patients but it does not change hemoglobin A1c and plasma insulin levels [37]. However, Reeds et al. [28] reported that ginseng and ginsenoside Re do not improve insulin sensitivity and β-cell function in obese type 2 diabetic patients. The ginsenosides are not detected in the blood after ginseng and ginsenoside Re treatment due to poor systemic bioavailability of ginsenosides [28]. Shiitake mushroom, which is rich in β-glucans and vitamin D, also has anti-diabetic activities [5,38,39]. β-glucan changes the gut microbiome and may be associated with improving insulin sensitivity. β-glucan mainly reduces insulin resistance to improve glucose metabolism [39]. Koreans have low levels of 25-OH-cholecalciferol in the blood, indicating vitamin D insufficiency that may affect glucose homeostasis with decreasing lean body mass [40,41]. Hyperglycemia increases platelet aggregation and thrombose formation that elevate the susceptibility to cardiovascular events [32]. Nattokinase is reported to suppress thrombosis [17,18]. The present study showed that AGM improved cerebral blood flow to as much as the normal-control. Since serum glucose levels in AGM were higher than the normal-control, the improvement of cerebral blood flow was associated with the factors beyond serum glucose levels. Nattokinase might be involved in the increase of cerebral blood flow in AGM. Therefore, the combination of aronia, red ginseng, shiitake mushroom and nattokinase may have a potent ant-diabetic activity and reduce the diabetic complications such as cardiovascular events. We decided to investigate the anti-diabetic activity of the combination treatment in Px rats. The present study showed that AGM-L and AGM-H improved glucose tolerance by improving insulin sensitivity in a dose-dependent manner, but AGM-L potentiated glucose-stimulated insulin secretion more than AGM-H. Thus, the combination supplementation alleviated the diabetic symptoms in Px rats.

The present study also showed that Px changed the body composition in comparison to the normal-control rats: Body weight and body fat were lower in Px rats compared to the normal-control rats due to increased urinary glucose loss. Fat mass was lower in the Px rats than the normal-control rats and both AGM-L and AGM-H suppressed the decrease in fat mass, but the fat mass of the AGM-L and AGM-H groups was still much lower than that of the normal-control. The suppression of fat mass loss was associated with the reduction of urinary glucose loss. The decrease of fat mass was not prevented as much as the urinary glucose loss. That may be associated with the properties of aronia and ginseng to suppress body fat synthesis and to increase skeletal muscle mass [42–44]. Furthermore, Px rats had lower BMD in the lumbar spine and femur and lower LBM in the hip and leg in comparison to the normal-control. These results suggested that the decrease of BMD is associated with lower insulin sensitivity and insulin secretion in diabetic rats. Sufficient insulin release promotes osteoblast activity by binding to insulin receptors in insulin insufficient states [45]. When osteoblasts are activated, osteocalcin is released from the bone and it binds to osteocalcin receptors that are highly expressed in pancreatic β-cells [45]. V-D is weakly correlated with osteocalcin [46] and it may not be involved in osteocalcin activity in insulin signaling. The activation of osterocalcin receptor by binding with osteocalcin promotes β-cell proliferation to improve β-cell function when glucose levels are elevated [47,48]. However, the osteocalcin effect on insulin resistance is still controversial [49,50]. In addition, BMD is associated with peroxisome proliferator-activated receptor (PPAR)-γ activation [41]. Skeletal muscle mass is reduced by decreasing anabolic signaling in the myocytes [51]. Ginsenosides in ginseng are reported to activate the PPAR-γ pathway to improve insulin sensitivity in various tissues [52,53]. The AGM-L inhibited the decrease of BMD and LBM, indicating that the inhibition by AGM was associated with the improvement of insulin sensitivity and potentiating insulin secretion. A potential limitation of the study is stress induced by multiple invasive procedures. However, the stress effects were mitigated by separating invasive procedures by at least one week to allow recovery from the stress. A unique aspect of this study was the use whole herbs instead of their extracts since the gut microbiome plays an important role in host metabolism of energy, glucose and lipids [54]. Dietary fiber works as food for gut microbes which produce short-chain fatty acids [54]. Dietary fibers in lyophilized aronia, red ginseng and shiitake mushroom may improve the composition and richness of the gut microbiome to establish eubiosis. However, another limitation of this study was not to include an AGM extract group in this study. The involvement of the gut microbiome in the development and progression of metabolic diseases is well recognized. Qin et al. has reported that several *Clostridium* species are increased in type 2 diabetes, and butyrate-producing bacteria are decreased [55]. Our preliminary study demonstrated that metabolism of β-glucan produced propionate and butyrate more than dextrin by 3.5 and 2 folds in vitro. However, the effects of dietary fiber in aronia and red ginseng on the microbiome were not examined. The present study also showed that *Clostridales* and *Erysipelorichales*, which are included in the *Fircumicultes*. was higher in the control than the normal-control but AGM decreased them. These changes in the gut microbiome might be associated with modulating the production of propionate and butyrate to influence gut-brain axis [56]. However, metformin treatment, the positive-control, did not alter the *Fircumicutes* although it improved glucose tolerance in the present study. Previous studies have shown that metformin modulates the gut microbiota composition by increasing the growth of some bacteria, such as *Akkermansia muciniphila*, *Escherichia* spp. or *Lactobacillus* and by decreasing the levels of some other bacteria such as *Intestinibacter* [57]. However, metformin treatment has adverse effects such as diarrhea, nausea, heartburn and gas and it may negatively influence the gut microbiome. Further study is needed to elucidate the metformin effect on gut dysbiosis. The present study showed that AGM had a beneficial effect on gut dysbiosis caused by type 2 diabetes: AGM inhibited the increase of *Clostridales* and increased *Bacterioidales* in the type 2 diabetic rats. Therefore, AGM improved glucose metabolism and prevented gut dysbiosis.

5. Conclusions

Hyperglycemia caused gut dysbiosis by increasing *Fircumicultes*, and AGM protected against gut dysbiosis. AGM improved glucose metabolism and lipid profiles in insulin insufficient type 2 diabetic rats, with Asian type 2 diabetes. The improved glucose metabolism protected against the decrease in BMD. Thus, AGM may be useful for preventing type 2 diabetes in Asians.

Author Contributions: S.P.; M.J.K.; D.Y.K. participated in designing the study and writing the manuscript. M.J.K.; H.J.Y., T.Z. and C.H. conducted biochemical experiments. M.J.K. and H.J.Y. quantified individual components of herbs. D.S.K. participated by conducting the animal study.

References

1. Yuan, H.; Li, X.; Wan, G.; Sun, L.; Zhu, X.; Che, F.; Yang, Z. Type 2 diabetes epidemic in East Asia: A 35-year systematic trend analysis. *Oncotarget* **2018**, *9*, 6718–6727. [CrossRef] [PubMed]
2. DeFronzo, R.A.; Ferrannini, E.; Groop, L.; Henry, R.R.; Herman, W.H.; Holst, J.J.; Hu, F.B.; Kahn, C.R.; Raz, I.; Shulman, G.I.; et al. Type 2 diabetes mellitus. *Nat. Rev. Dis. Primers* **2015**, *1*, 15019. [CrossRef] [PubMed]
3. Kim, D.S.; Kim, B.C.; Daily, J.W.; Park, S. High genetic risk scores for impaired insulin secretory capacity doubles the risk for type 2 diabetes in asians and is exacerbated by western-type diets. *Diabetes Metab. Res. Rev.* **2018**, *34*. [CrossRef] [PubMed]
4. Yang, H.J.; Kim, M.J.; Kwon, D.Y.; Kim, D.S.; Lee, Y.H.; Kim, J.E.; Park, S. Anti-diabetic activities of *Gastrodia elata* blume water extracts are mediated mainly by potentiating glucose-stimulated insulin secretion and increasing beta-cell mass in non-obese type 2 diabetic animals. *Nutrients* **2016**, *8*, 161. [CrossRef] [PubMed]
5. Park, S.; Kim, D.S.; Kang, S. Vitamin D deficiency impairs glucose-stimulated insulin secretion and increases insulin resistance by reducing PPAR-gamma expression in nonobese type 2 diabetic rats. *J. Nutr. Biochem.* **2016**, *27*, 257–265. [CrossRef] [PubMed]
6. Park, S.; Kim, D.S.; Kang, S.; Moon, B.R. Fermented soybeans, Chungkookjang, prevent hippocampal cell death and beta-cell apoptosis by decreasing pro-inflammatory cytokines in gerbils with transient artery occlusion. *Exp. Biol. Med.* **2016**, *241*, 296–307. [CrossRef] [PubMed]
7. Lyu, M.; Wang, Y.F.; Fan, G.W.; Wang, X.Y.; Xu, S.Y.; Zhu, Y. Balancing herbal medicine and functional food for prevention and treatment of cardiometabolic diseases through modulating gut microbiota. *Front. Microbiol.* **2017**, *8*, 2146. [CrossRef] [PubMed]

8. Wen, L.; Duffy, A. Factors influencing the gut microbiota, inflammation, and type 2 diabetes. *J. Nutr.* **2017**, *147*, 1468s–1475s. [CrossRef] [PubMed]
9. Brunkwall, L.; Orho-Melander, M. The gut microbiome as a target for prevention and treatment of hyperglycaemia in type 2 diabetes: From current human evidence to future possibilities. *Diabetologia* **2017**, *60*, 943–951. [CrossRef] [PubMed]
10. Wedick, N.M.; Pan, A.; Cassidy, A.; Rimm, E.B.; Sampson, L.; Rosner, B.; Willett, W.; Hu, F.B.; Sun, Q.; van Dam, R.M. Dietary flavonoid intakes and risk of type 2 diabetes in US men and women. *Am. J. Clin. Nutr.* **2012**, *95*, 925–933. [CrossRef] [PubMed]
11. Park, S.; Ahn, I.S.; Kwon, D.Y.; Ko, B.S.; Jun, W.K. Ginsenosides Rb1 and Rg1 suppress triglyceride accumulation in 3T3-L1 adipocytes and enhance beta-cell insulin secretion and viability in min6 cells via pka-dependent pathways. *Biosci. Biotechnol. Biochem.* **2008**, *72*, 2815–2823. [CrossRef] [PubMed]
12. Lee, H.J.; Lee, Y.H.; Park, S.K.; Kang, E.S.; Kim, H.J.; Lee, Y.C.; Choi, C.S.; Park, S.E.; Ahn, C.W.; Cha, B.S.; et al. Korean red ginseng (*Panax ginseng*) improves insulin sensitivity and attenuates the development of diabetes in Otsuka Long-Evans Tokushima fatty rats. *Metabolism* **2009**, *58*, 1170–1177. [CrossRef] [PubMed]
13. Park, S.H.; Oh, M.R.; Choi, E.K.; Kim, M.G.; Ha, K.C.; Lee, S.K.; Kim, Y.G.; Park, B.H.; Kim, D.S.; Chae, S.W. An 8-wk, randomized, double-blind, placebo-controlled clinical trial for the antidiabetic effects of hydrolyzed ginseng extract. *J. Ginseng Res.* **2014**, *38*, 239–243. [CrossRef] [PubMed]
14. Kim, H.Y.; Kim, K. Regulation of signaling molecules associated with insulin action, insulin secretion and pancreatic beta-cell mass in the hypoglycemic effects of Korean red ginseng in Goto-Kakizaki rats. *J. Ethnopharmacol.* **2012**, *142*, 53–58. [CrossRef] [PubMed]
15. Grotto, D.; Bueno, D.C.; Ramos, G.K.; da Costa, S.R.; Spim, S.R.; Gerenutti, M. Assessment of the safety of the shiitake culinary-medicinal mushroom, lentinus edodes (agaricomycetes), in rats: Biochemical, hematological, and antioxidative parameters. *Int. J. Med. Mushrooms* **2016**, *18*, 861–870. [CrossRef] [PubMed]
16. Wagner, H.; Alvarsson, M.; Mannheimer, B.; Degerblad, M.; Östenson, C.G. No Effect of high-dose vitamin D treatment on β-cell function, insulin sensitivity, or glucose homeostasis in subjects with abnormal glucose tolerance: A randomized clinical trial. *Diabetes Care* **2016**, *39*, 345–352. [CrossRef] [PubMed]
17. Westein, E.; Hoefer, T.; Calkin, A.C. Thrombosis in diabetes: A shear flow effect? *Clin. Sci.* **2017**, *131*, 1245–1260. [CrossRef] [PubMed]
18. Fujita, M.; Hong, K.; Ito, Y.; Fujii, R.; Kariya, K.; Nishimuro, S. Thrombolytic effect of nattokinase on a chemically induced thrombosis model in rat. *Biol. Pharm. Bull.* **1995**, *18*, 1387–1391. [CrossRef] [PubMed]
19. O'Keefe, J.H.; Gheewala, N.M.; O'Keefe, J.O. Dietary strategies for improving post-prandial glucose, lipids, inflammation, and cardiovascular health. *J. Am. Coll. Cardiol.* **2008**, *51*, 249–255. [CrossRef] [PubMed]
20. Hosokawa, Y.A.; Hosokawa, H.; Chen, C.; Leahy, J.L. Mechanism of impaired glucose-potentiated insulin secretion in diabetic 90% pancreatectomy rats. Study using glucagonlike peptide-1 (7-37). *J. Clin. Investig.* **1996**, *97*, 180–186. [CrossRef] [PubMed]
21. Islam, M.S.; Wilson, R.D. Experimentally induced rodent models of type 2 diabetes. *Methods Mol. Biol.* **2012**, *933*, 161–174. [PubMed]
22. Reeves, P.G.; Nielsen, F.H.; Fahey, G.C., Jr. Ain-93 purified diets for laboratory rodents: Final report of the american institute of nutrition ad hoc writing committee on the reformulation of the ain-76a rodent diet. *J. Nutr.* **1993**, *123*, 1939–1951. [CrossRef] [PubMed]
23. Park, S.; da Kim, S.; Kang, S. *Gastrodia elata* blume water extracts improve insulin resistance by decreasing body fat in diet-induced obese rats: Vanillin and 4-hydroxybenzaldehyde are the bioactive candidates. *Eur. J. Nutr.* **2011**, *50*, 107–118. [CrossRef] [PubMed]
24. Choi, S.B.; Jang, J.S.; Park, S. Estrogen and exercise may enhance beta-cell function and mass via insulin receptor substrate 2 induction in ovariectomized diabetic rats. *Endocrinology* **2005**, *146*, 4786–4794. [CrossRef] [PubMed]
25. Dobbins, R.L.; Szczepaniak, L.S.; Myhill, J.; Tamura, Y.; Uchino, H.; Giacca, A.; McGarry, J.D. The composition of dietary fat directly influences glucose-stimulated insulin secretion in rats. *Diabetes* **2002**, *51*, 1825–1833. [CrossRef] [PubMed]
26. Park, S.; Kim, D.S.; Kang, E.S.; Kim, D.B.; Kang, S. Low dose brain estrogen prevents menopausal syndrome while maintaining the diversity of the gut microbiomes in estrogen-deficient rats. *Am. J. Physiol. Endocrinol. Metab.* **2018**, *315*, E99–E109. [CrossRef] [PubMed]

27. Kamweru, P.K.; Tindibale, E.L. Vitamin d and vitamin d from ultraviolet-irradiated mushrooms (review). *Int. J. Med. Mushrooms* **2016**, *18*, 205–214. [CrossRef] [PubMed]
28. Reeds, D.N.; Patterson, B.W.; Okunade, A.; Holloszy, J.O.; Polonsky, K.S.; Klein, S. Ginseng and ginsenoside re do not improve beta-cell function or insulin sensitivity in overweight and obese subjects with impaired glucose tolerance or diabetes. *Diabetes Care* **2011**, *34*, 1071–1076. [CrossRef] [PubMed]
29. Banjari, I.; Misir, A.; Savikin, K.; Jokic, S.; Molnar, M.; De Zoysa, H.K.S.; Waisundara, V.Y. Antidiabetic effects of *Aronia melanocarpa* and its other therapeutic properties. *Front. Nutr.* **2017**, *4*, 53. [CrossRef] [PubMed]
30. Newsholme, P.; Cruzat, V.F.; Keane, K.N.; Carlessi, R.; de Bittencourt, P.I., Jr. Molecular mechanisms of ROS production and oxidative stress in diabetes. *Biochem. J.* **2016**, *473*, 4527–4550. [CrossRef] [PubMed]
31. Pahwa, R.; Jialal, I. Hyperglycemia induces toll-like receptor activity through increased oxidative stress. *Metab. Syndr. Relat. Disord.* **2016**, *14*, 239–241. [CrossRef] [PubMed]
32. Tang, W.H.; Stitham, J.; Gleim, S.; Di Febbo, C.; Porreca, E.; Fava, C.; Tacconelli, S.; Capone, M.; Evangelista, V.; Levantesi, G.; et al. Glucose and collagen regulate human platelet activity through aldose reductase induction of thromboxane. *J. Clin. Investig.* **2011**, *121*, 4462–4476. [CrossRef] [PubMed]
33. Rugina, D.; Diaconeasa, Z.; Coman, C.; Bunea, A.; Socaciu, C.; Pintea, A. Chokeberry anthocyanin extract as pancreatic beta-cell protectors in two models of induced oxidative stress. *Oxid. Med. Cell. Longev.* **2015**, *2015*, 429075. [CrossRef] [PubMed]
34. Zhu, W.; Jia, Q.; Wang, Y.; Zhang, Y.; Xia, M. The anthocyanin cyanidin-3-*O*-beta-glucoside, a flavonoid, increases hepatic glutathione synthesis and protects hepatocytes against reactive oxygen species during hyperglycemia: Involvement of a cAMP-PKA-dependent signaling pathway. *Free Radic. Biol. Med.* **2012**, *52*, 314–327. [CrossRef] [PubMed]
35. Yamane, T.; Kozuka, M.; Konda, D.; Nakano, Y.; Nakagaki, T.; Ohkubo, I.; Ariga, H. Improvement of blood glucose levels and obesity in mice given aronia juice by inhibition of dipeptidyl peptidase iv and alpha-glucosidase. *J. Nutr. Biochem.* **2016**, *31*, 106–112. [CrossRef] [PubMed]
36. Simeonov, S.B.; Botushanov, N.P.; Karahanian, E.B.; Pavlova, M.B.; Husianitis, H.K.; Troev, D.M. Effects of aronia melanocarpa juice as part of the dietary regimen in patients with diabetes mellitus. *Folia Med.* **2002**, *44*, 20–23.
37. Shishtar, E.; Sievenpiper, J.L.; Djedovic, V.; Cozma, A.I.; Ha, V.; Jayalath, V.H.; Jenkins, D.J.; Meija, S.B.; de Souza, R.J.; Jovanovski, E.; et al. The effect of ginseng (the *Genus panax*) on glycemic control: A systematic review and meta-analysis of randomized controlled clinical trials. *PLoS ONE* **2014**, *9*, e107391. [CrossRef] [PubMed]
38. Maschio, B.H.; Gentil, B.C.; Caetano, E.L.A.; Rodrigues, L.S.; Laurino, L.F.; Spim, S.R.V.; Jozala, A.F.; Dos Santos, C.A.; Grotto, D.; Gerenutti, M. Characterization of the effects of the shiitake culinary-medicinal mushroom, lentinus edodes (agaricomycetes), on severe gestational diabetes mellitus in rats. *Int. J. Med. Mushrooms* **2017**, *19*, 991–1000. [CrossRef] [PubMed]
39. Jeong, S.Y.; Kang, S.; Hua, C.S.; Ting, Z.; Park, S. Synbiotic effects of beta-glucans from cauliflower mushroom and *Lactobacillus fermentum* on metabolic changes and gut microbiome in estrogen-deficient rats. *Genes Nutr.* **2017**, *12*, 31. [CrossRef] [PubMed]
40. Lee, B.K.; Park, S.; Kim, Y. Age- and gender-specific associations between low serum 25-hydroxyvitamin d level and type 2 diabetes in the Korean general population: Analysis of 2008–2009 Korean national health and nutrition examination survey data. *Asia Pac. J. Clin. Nutr.* **2012**, *21*, 536–546. [PubMed]
41. Park, S.; Ham, J.O.; Lee, B.K. A positive association of vitamin d deficiency and sarcopenia in 50 year old women, but not men. *Clin. Nutr.* **2014**, *33*, 900–905. [CrossRef] [PubMed]
42. Lee, H.M.; Lee, O.H.; Kim, K.J.; Lee, B.Y. Ginsenoside Rg1 promotes glucose uptake through activated AMPK pathway in insulin-resistant muscle cells. *Phytother. Res.* **2012**, *26*, 1017–1022. [CrossRef] [PubMed]
43. Shin, S.S.; Yoon, M. Korean red ginseng (*Panax ginseng*) inhibits obesity and improves lipid metabolism in high fat diet-fed castrated mice. *J. Ethnopharmacol.* **2018**, *210*, 80–87. [CrossRef] [PubMed]
44. Sikora, J.; Broncel, M.; Markowicz, M.; Chalubinski, M.; Wojdan, K.; Mikiciuk-Olasik, E. Short-term supplementation with *Aronia melanocarpa* extract improves platelet aggregation, clotting, and fibrinolysis in patients with metabolic syndrome. *Eur. J. Nutr.* **2012**, *51*, 549–556. [CrossRef] [PubMed]
45. Liang, J.; Lian, S.; Qian, X.; Wang, N.; Huang, H.; Yao, J.; Tang, K.; Chen, L.; Li, L.; Lin, W.; et al. Association between bone mineral density and pancreatic beta-cell function in elderly men and postmenopausal women. *J. Endocr. Soc.* **2017**, *1*, 1085–1094. [CrossRef] [PubMed]

46. Buranasinsup, S.; Bunyaratavej, N. The Intriguing Correlation between Undercarboxylated Osteocalcin and Vitamin D. *J. Med. Assoc. Thail.* **2015**, *98*, S16–S20.
47. Sabek, O.M.; Nishimoto, S.K.; Fraga, D.; Tejpal, N.; Ricordi, C.; Gaber, A.O. Osteocalcin Effect on Human β-Cells Mass and Function. *Endocrinology* **2015**, *156*, 3137–3146. [CrossRef] [PubMed]
48. Kover, K.; Yan, Y.; Tong, P.Y.; Watkins, D.; Li, X.; Tasch, J.; Hager, M.; Clements, M.; Moore, W.V. Osteocalcin protects pancreatic beta cell function and survival under high glucose conditions. *Biochem. Biophys. Res. Commun.* **2015**, *462*, 21–26. [CrossRef] [PubMed]
49. Gower, B.A.; Pollock, N.K.; Casazza, K.; Clemens, T.L.; Goree, L.L.; Granger, W.M. Associations of total and undercarboxylated osteocalcin with peripheral and hepatic insulin sensitivity and β-cell function in overweight adults. *J. Clin. Endocrinol. Metab.* **2013**, *98*, E1173–E1180. [CrossRef] [PubMed]
50. Choi, H.J.; Yu, J.; Choi, H.; An, J.H.; Kim, S.W.; Park, K.S.; Jang, H.C.; Kim, S.Y.; Shin, C.S. Vitamin K2 supplementation improves insulin sensitivity via osteocalcin metabolism: A placebo-controlled trial. *Diabetes Care* **2011**, *34*, e147. [CrossRef] [PubMed]
51. Lecka-Czernik, B. Diabetes, bone and glucose-lowering agents: Basic biology. *Diabetologia* **2017**, *60*, 1163–1169. [CrossRef] [PubMed]
52. Gao, Y.; Yang, M.F.; Su, Y.P.; Jiang, H.M.; You, X.J.; Yang, Y.J.; Zhang, H.L. Ginsenoside Re reduces insulin resistance through activation of PPAR-gamma pathway and inhibition of TNF-alpha production. *J. Ethnopharmacol.* **2013**, *147*, 509–516. [CrossRef] [PubMed]
53. Mollah, M.L.; Kim, G.S.; Moon, H.K.; Chung, S.K.; Cheon, Y.P.; Kim, J.K.; Kim, K.S. Antiobesity effects of wild ginseng (*Panax ginseng* C.A. Meyer) mediated by PPAR-gamma, GLUT4 and LPL in ob/ob mice. *Phytother. Res.* **2009**, *23*, 220–225. [CrossRef] [PubMed]
54. Zhao, L.; Zhang, F.; Ding, X.; Wu, G.; Lam, Y.Y.; Wang, X.; Fu, H.; Xue, X.; Lu, C.; Ma, J.; et al. Gut bacteria selectively promoted by dietary fibers alleviate type 2 diabetes. *Science* **2018**, *359*, 1151–1156. [CrossRef] [PubMed]
55. Forslund, K.; Hildebrand, F.; Nielsen, T.; Falony, G.; Le Chatelier, E.; Sunagawa, S.; Prifti, E.; Vieira-Silva, S.; Gudmundsdottir, V.; Pedersen, H.K.; et al. Disentangling type 2 diabetes and metformin treatment signatures in the human gut microbiota. *Nature* **2015**, *528*, 262–266. [CrossRef] [PubMed]
56. Perry, R.J.; Peng, L.; Barry, N.A.; Cline, G.W.; Zhang, D.; Cardone, R.L.; Petersen, K.F.; Kibbey, R.G.; Goodman, A.L.; Shulman, G.I. Acetate mediates a microbiome-brain-β-cell axis to promote metabolic syndrome. *Nature* **2016**, *534*, 213–217. [CrossRef] [PubMed]
57. Rodriguez, J.; Hiel, S.; Delzenne, N.M. Metformin: Old friend, new ways of action-implication of the gut microbiome? *Curr. Opin. Clin. Nutr. Metab. Care* **2018**, *21*, 294–301. [CrossRef] [PubMed]

4

Effects of Ketogenic Diets on Cardiovascular Risk Factors: Evidence from Animal and Human Studies

Christophe Kosinski [1] and François R. Jornayvaz [2,*]

[1] Service of Endocrinology, Diabetes and Metabolism, Lausanne University Hospital (CHUV), Avenue de la Sallaz 8, 1011 Lausanne, Switzerland; christophe.kosinski@chuv.ch

[2] Service of Endocrinology, Diabetes, Hypertension and Nutrition, Geneva University Hospitals, Rue Gabrielle-Perret-Gentil 4, 1205 Geneva, Switzerland

* Correspondence: françois.jornayvaz@hcuge.ch

Abstract: The treatment of obesity and cardiovascular diseases is one of the most difficult and important challenges nowadays. Weight loss is frequently offered as a therapy and is aimed at improving some of the components of the metabolic syndrome. Among various diets, ketogenic diets, which are very low in carbohydrates and usually high in fats and/or proteins, have gained in popularity. Results regarding the impact of such diets on cardiovascular risk factors are controversial, both in animals and humans, but some improvements notably in obesity and type 2 diabetes have been described. Unfortunately, these effects seem to be limited in time. Moreover, these diets are not totally safe and can be associated with some adverse events. Notably, in rodents, development of nonalcoholic fatty liver disease (NAFLD) and insulin resistance have been described. The aim of this review is to discuss the role of ketogenic diets on different cardiovascular risk factors in both animals and humans based on available evidence.

Keywords: ketogenic diets; obesity; NAFLD; fibroblast growth factor (FGF21); insulin resistance; type 2 diabetes; cardiovascular risk factors

1. Introduction

As a consequence of the rising obesity prevalence in industrialized countries, the incidence of cardiovascular diseases also increases [1]. Obesity is also a major risk factor for insulin resistance and type 2 diabetes [2]. This state of insulin resistance is frequently associated with ectopic lipid accumulation, notably in the liver and skeletal muscle. This can lead to the development of nonalcoholic fatty liver disease (NAFLD), which is an independent predictor of cardiovascular disease [3,4]. NAFLD is defined as steatosis which is not due to excess consumption of alcohol, viral or autoimmune causes, and iron overload [5,6]. No evidence-based pharmacological treatment for NAFLD exists so far. NAFLD is an important risk factor for the development of insulin resistance and type 2 diabetes, which may be associated with other cardiovascular risk factors such as dyslipidemia and high blood pressure. As NAFLD is present in almost 90% of obese patients [7], weight loss represents one of the pillars of the treatments among others, such as physical activity.

In the literature, diets rich in carbohydrates, and notably rich in refined sugars and fructose, are associated with the metabolic syndrome [8,9]. Therefore, to lose weight, different diets have been suggested. Among them, carbohydrate restriction has been proposed to be the single most effective intervention for reducing all features of the metabolic syndrome [10–12]. Since the publication of Atkins's book in the early 1970s [13], low-carbohydrate diets have become increasingly popular, particularly ketogenic diets (KD). These diets are known for being very low in carbohydrates, but usually high in fats and/or proteins. In practice, KD are characterized by a reduction in carbohydrates (usually less than 50 g/day) and a relative increase in the proportions of proteins and fats [14]. Some variations exist, like very-low-carbohydrate KD, which are even more restrictive, with less than 30 g/day (Table 1).

Table 1. Standard composition of ketogenic diets in adults * (calculated for a 2000 kcal diet/day).

Classical KD	Defined as <130 g carbohydrate per day or <26% of caloric intake by the American Diabetes Association
Modified Atkins Diet	65% caloric intake from fat, 30% protein, 6% carbohydrates
Very low-carbohydrate KD	Carbohydrates < 30 g/day

KD, Ketogenic Diet. * Adapted from Kossoff et al. [15], Feinman et al. [16], Accurso et al. [17].

After a few days of such diets, glucose reserves (i.e., glycogen stored in liver and skeletal muscle) become insufficient to provide body energy needs. This leads to the production of ketone bodies by the liver, which will be used as an alternative energy source notably by the central nervous system [18].

KD are known to be efficient in the treatment of seizures and can be used as an alternative treatment [19], but this aspect will not be discussed in this review. Nevertheless, for about forty years, the potential use of KD has also been investigated in the prevention and treatment of cardiovascular risk factors. The aim of this review is to discuss the available evidence in animal and human studies, and the role of KD on different cardiovascular risk factors, namely obesity, NAFLD, insulin resistance and type 2 diabetes, dyslipidemia and high blood pressure. To our knowledge, this is the first review comparing the effects of KD on cardiovascular risk factors in animals and humans.

2. Method

This article is neither a systematic review nor a meta-analysis. We searched Medline (PubMed) for trials in animals and humans, reviews or meta-analyses, using the query "ketogenic diet" + "weight loss", "obesity", "fibroblast growth factor (FGF21)", "NAFLD", "diabetes", "insulin resistance", "dyslipidemia" or "blood pressure". Then, we selected the most recent papers (less than 15 years) and publications with potential practical usefulness. Finally, we only kept studies of adults, not children.

3. Results

3.1. KD and Obesity

Studies in rodents (obese or non obese) show that KD are efficient for weight loss [20,21]. Nevertheless, it is important to assess body composition changes, as it is always better to lose fat mass than lean mass. Indeed, in a study by Garbow et al., after 12 weeks KD led to a significantly lower weight gain compared to chow-fed and high-simple-carbohydrate high-fat Western diet fed mice, but lean mass was significantly reduced in KD-fed mice compared to chow-fed mice [22]. In another study, accumulation of visceral fat mass was significantly higher (at least 30%) in rats fed a KD (two compositions of KD were tested: a high-protein "Atkins-style" or a low-protein diet, both with a low-carbohydrate and high-fat content), compared with chow-fed controls, after 4 weeks of diet [23]. Finally, Jornayvaz et al. showed that KD-fed mice during 5 weeks gained significantly less weight than regular-chow fed mice. Nevertheless, KD-fed mice had an increased fat mass percentage than regular-chow fed mice, without differences in the percentage of lean body mass between diets [24].

It is also important to assess whether weight loss can be maintained. Long-term studies reveal an absence of weight loss after 22 weeks of KD in mice, despite an initial weight loss during the first week of diet [25]. Moreover, another study showed that mice fed a KD for 80 weeks initially lost weight, but after 18 weeks, their weight returned to baseline and then increased gradually [26]. Nevertheless, they gained less weight than chow-fed mice, and, with body composition analysis, the authors showed that this difference resulted from both a lower lean mass and a lower fat mass. Moreover, the survival curves were the same between the two diets. Finally, KD-fed mice also had an increased energy expenditure and a loss of the diurnal pattern of the respiratory exchange ratio, which indicated continuous use of fatty acids as an energy substrate [26]. This rise in energy expenditure was analyzed in another study which showed that KD promotes weight loss (20% of total body weight) through an increased energy expenditure and this correlated with a rise in plasma fibroblast growth factor 21 (FGF21) levels [27]. The role of FGF21 in KD will be further discussed later. In another study, compared to non-KD, rats fed a low protein (10% of total content) KD had a waste of energy in urine. [28]. Indeed, KD-fed rats had a lower urine nitrogen excretion due to a lower protein intake and a urine energy-to-nitrogen ratio almost twice as high as the other diets.

Overall, an increase in energy expenditure in mice fed a KD compared to mice fed a chow diet could be the mechanism responsible for decreased weight gain or weight loss seen in rodents, despite a similar caloric intake [24]. As a potential component of the increased energy expenditure, other authors performed microarrays in the liver of KD-fed mice and described an increased expression of genes involved in fatty acid oxidation and a reduced expression in genes involved in lipid synthesis [20].

A recent study analyzed the effects of KD on exercising rats and sedentary rats [29]. Compared to other diets (Western diet, standard chow), after 6 weeks, sedentary KD-fed rats had an approximately 25% lower body mass, a lower size of adipocytes from omental adipose tissue, 80% lower levels of serum insulin, 50% lower levels of glucose, 55% lower levels of triglycerides and 20% lower levels of total cholesterol. Activity did not confer a benefit, as KD-fed exercising rats did not show better results than the sedentary rats. Nevertheless, exercising rats had 40% lower serum β-hydroxybutyrate levels than sedentary rats, independent of diet, while they had more favorable adipose tissue characteristics. These results suggest that body fat regulation (e.g., reduced adipose tissue mass and cell size) under a KD (with or without exercise) could rather be due to lower insulin levels. Therefore, increased serum ketones may have a smaller role.

In humans, KD are known to be an effective weight-loss therapy [30–33] (in average up to 5% of body weight at 6 months), but the mechanisms are not clearly established. Some authors suggest that it results simply from reduced caloric intake and an increased satiety effect of proteins [34]. Other studies suggest a metabolic effect of KD: possibly, the use of energy from proteins in KD is an expensive process and therefore increases weight loss [35–37]. Also, there is the suggestion that gluconeogenesis, which is increased with carbohydrate restriction, is energy demanding [35,38]. Another hypothesis of KD-induced weight loss is decreased appetite induced by ketosis [39]. Some authors also suggest digestive metabolic changes: with ketogenic very-low energy diets, ghrelin levels and subjective appetite (usually increased in a hypocaloric diet) were reduced when patients were in a ketotic state [39]. Surprisingly, leptin levels were lower under ketosis. A study in 132 severely obese patients (mean body mass index (BMI) 43 kg/m^2) with a high prevalence of type 2 diabetes or metabolic syndrome showed that participants using a low-carbohydrate diet lost more weight than those using other diets, suggesting a greater reduction in overall caloric intake, rather than a direct effect of macronutrient composition [32].

As discussed in rodents, the problem is that a lot of studies are of short duration. For example, a small study [40] of 17 obese men, randomized to two different high-protein diets (one low-carbohydrate, "ketogenic"; one medium-carbohydrate, "non-ketogenic") with a cross-over design, eating ad libitum during 4 weeks each, revealed that KD reduced hunger and was associated with a lower food intake. Weight loss was also significantly greater with the ketogenic diet than with the non-ketogenic diet, and weight loss was equally comprised of fat mass and fat-free mass. Only 35% of the difference in total weight loss between the two diets was due to water depletion; the remainder was attributed to fat mass and lean mass loss [40]. In a bigger study of 311 participants [41], a very low-carbohydrate KD followed by a period of slow re-insertion of a Mediterranean diet and alimentary education was associated with an overall improvement (mean total body weight loss of 14 ± 10 kg, BMI 5 ± 3 kg/m^2, waist circumference 13 ± 7 cm) at 1–4 months, which remained stable after 1 year [41]. The limitations were the composition of the diet (low-carbohydrate, but also low-fat) and the fact that it was an observational study. Other authors [42] compared different diets in the same group of patients eating alternatively a KD (two different periods of 20 days), a low-carbohydrate non-KD (two different periods of 20 days), and a normal Mediterranean diet (4 months during the rotation of the two other diets, then 6 months) during 1 year. Significant weight loss and reduction of body fat percentages were observed only during ketogenic periods compared to the two other diets. Moreover, if the patients were compliant to the prescribed Mediterranean diet (which was relatively strict: 1800 kcal/day) during the maintenance period, no weight regain was observed at 12 months [42]. In an older study in obese non-diabetic participants, a low-carbohydrate diet led to a greater weight loss after 6 months, but no significant difference at 1 year [33]. The authors suggested that weight loss was probably due to a greater energy deficit, but the mechanisms remain unknown, and no relation between weight loss and ketosis was found at any time during the study. Finally, in a study with obese type 2 diabetes patients [43], the authors compared a low-carbohydrate high unsaturated fat diet to a high-carbohydrate low-fat diet, in adjunction with structured exercise: weight loss was similar in both groups (−9.1%), but a trend toward regaining more weight was observed in the low-carbohydrate diet group at 52 weeks. Weight loss is usually related to a high intensity of lifestyle interventions. Thus, it would be interesting to know the evolution on the next months/years of follow-up, and if the weight loss would be maintained without structured exercise. Exercise has an impact on body weight, but also on body composition as described in a study that analyzed the association of KD or regular diet in combination with exercise (resistance training) in overweight women [44]. The KD group lost fat mass without experiencing a significant alteration in lean mass, while the other group gained lean mass without a significant change in fat mass [44].

To summarize, in rodents and humans, KD seem to have a benefit on weight loss, notably by increased energy expenditure in animals and decreasing food intake in humans. In humans, weight loss affects both fat mass and lean mass. Greater weight loss is also associated with structured professional support, which may be difficult and expensive to maintain over time. Long-term studies are nevertheless needed to assess the evolution of weight loss.

3.2. KD and NAFLD

In mice, KD induce hepatic inflammation and lipid accumulation [22], while inflammation is reduced in white adipose tissue [27]. KD also lead to hepatic steatosis in both short-term [24,25] and long-term feeding in mice [26]. Biological markers such as aspartate aminotransferase (AST) and alanine aminotransferase (ALT) are increased at least twofold in parallel with increased intrahepatic triglyceride content [24,25]. On the contrary, a study described that compared to other diets (Western diet, standard chow), KD-fed mice display reduced ALT levels, hepatic triglyceride accumulation and markers of liver inflammation [29]. The authors explained that these results, different from previous studies, could be due to the protein content of the diet (they used a KD with 20% protein, versus <10% in other studies) and differences in animal models (rat in this study, versus mice in others). Thus, this shows the importance of the diet's composition. Another study reported an increase in hepatic triglyceride content in KD-fed mice after 12 weeks, and this correlated with an elevation in ALT levels, suggesting that chronic KD feeding causes an injury pattern similar to a NAFLD phenotype [22]. Another interesting marker of NAFLD is FGF21. In humans, FGF21 levels are increased in NAFLD and correlate with hepatic triglyceride content [45–47]. Nevertheless, the role of FGF21 in NAFLD induced by a KD has mostly been studied in rodents [26,27,48,49]. Notably, a study in mice showed that FGF21 plasma levels and liver expression are increased by 5 weeks of KD feeding, and this was accompanied by an increased hepatic fat content as revealed by increased hepatic triglycerides, diacylglycerols and ceramides levels [24]. Moreover, KD-fed mice developed hepatic insulin resistance and this was due to increased hepatic diacylglycerol content, as diacylglycerols are known to activate protein kinase Cε [50]. In this study [24], the authors suggested that increased plasma FGF21 levels and hepatic expression in KD-fed mice was probably secondary to hepatic fat accumulation and may represent a compensatory mechanism to counteract hepatic insulin resistance, suggesting that FGF21 may be beneficial in reversing hepatic insulin resistance. This has been further verified in high-fat diet fed mice treated with exogenous FGF21. In a study in wild-type mice, FGF21 decreased hepatic fat content, notably hepatic diacylglycerol content, and improved hepatic insulin sensitivity [51]. The beneficial role of FGF21 on hepatic insulin sensitivity was also shown by other authors [52]. Moreover, mice lacking FGF21 gain weight, have an increased fat mass and develop glucose intolerance. Moreover, when the chow diet was changed for a KD, these mice not only gained weight and developed glucose intolerance, but also developed NAFLD [53]. Finally, another study revealed that FGF21 knock-out mice fed a KD develop NAFLD and severe hepatic insulin resistance as assessed by the gold-standard technique, the hyperinsulinemic-euglycemic clamp [54]. Finally, FGF21 has been shown to act as an endocrine signal of protein restriction [55]. In summary, these studies suggest an important role of FGF21 in the pathophysiology of NAFLD.

In humans, liver fat content was shown to be increased during an isocaloric high-fat low-carbohydrate diet [56]. This result should be analyzed with caution, as with 31% of carbohydrates the diet is not a "real" KD. Caloric restriction also had an impact: compared to the high-carbohydrate ("standard") hypocaloric diet, reduction of liver fat content was significantly higher with the hypocaloric low-carbohydrate diet [57,58]. This effect was limited in time, with no significant difference at 11 weeks [57]. KD have also been associated with a higher decrease in liver volume compared with a standard hypocaloric diet, probably due to the depletion of liver glycogen [59]. Finally, the response to KD may be influenced by genetic predisposition to NAFLD, as shown by two studies with a better response to KD for patients with variants of the PNPLA3 gene [60,61]. When fed a KD, subjects with PNPLA3 variants had a lower liver fat content than controls.

To summarize, the effect of KD on the liver was mostly investigated in rodents. The results are rather negative, with induction of hepatic inflammation and NAFLD, but these findings have not been reported in humans. An alteration of FGF21 expression could be a potential cause or consequence. More studies are warranted in humans to assess whether KD could induce or improve NAFLD.

3.3. *KD and Insulin Resistance / Type 2 Diabetes*

Obesity is often associated with the development of NAFLD, insulin resistance and type 2 diabetes. Notably, as already discussed, KD can lead to decreased weight gain in mice but with concomitant development of NAFLD and associated hepatic insulin resistance [24]. In the latter study, mice fed a KD for 5 weeks developed whole body insulin resistance despite reduced basal plasma glucose and insulin levels. In this case, the use of indices of insulin sensitivity, such as the homeostatic model assessment for insulin resistance (HOMA-IR) and quantitative insulin-sensitivity check index (QUICKI) indices, would lead to the conclusion that insulin sensitivity is improved in KD fed mice [62]. However, using the hyperinsulinemic-euglycemic clamp, glucose infusion rates were 47% lower in KD-fed mice than in chow-fed mice, demonstrating whole body insulin resistance in KD-fed mice [24]. KD-fed mice also had an impaired insulin ability to suppress endogenous glucose production confirming insulin resistance at the level of the liver. In this case, KD induced severe hepatic insulin resistance in mice despite lower body weight gain, and this was attributed to an increased hepatic diacylglycerol content. Finally, insulin resistance was also attributed to a decreased insulin-stimulated whole body glucose disposal, which was notably due to decreased glucose uptake in brown adipose tissue and the heart [24].

In another study, mice fed a KD during 12 weeks remained euglycemic, but had reduced mean serum insulin levels and HOMA-IR indices, and exhibited glucose intolerance as assessed by intra-peritoneal glucose tolerance tests [22]. However, despite mild hepatic steatosis, systemic response to insulin was preserved, unlike in other studies. The authors explained this discrepancy by a relatively reduced lean body mass in KD-fed mice, resulting in higher insulin dose in insulin-tolerance tests. Also, hepatic insulin resistance may confer a smaller contribution to overall glucose homeostasis than peripheral glucose disposal [22]. In studies using rats, KD also induced glucose intolerance and insulin resistance [23,63], despite reduced glucose and insulin levels [23]. In the latter study, the authors showed that these effects were not due to energy overconsumption. Moreover, as KD-fed rats had a significant accumulation of visceral fat, the effects on glucose homeostasis were not dependent upon visceral fat mass. In the same study, short term KD feeding in rats was also associated with decreased β-cell mass, but this effect could be due to a lower lean body mass of KD fed rats [23]. Nevertheless, these findings were corroborated by another study where long term KD feeding in mice led to glucose intolerance that was associated with insufficient insulin secretion from β-cells, potentially due to a decrease in β-cell mass [25]. Interestingly, after only 6 days of KD feeding, mice showed impairments in glucose tolerance and insulin sensitivity, and this was attributed to a possible adaptation to maintain blood glucose levels against insufficient amounts of carbohydrates [48]. In this case, insulin signaling was impaired only in white adipose tissue, but not in liver and muscle. The authors suggested that this impairment in white adipose tissue could not be the only culprit for whole body glucose intolerance in KD fed mice. Indeed, a low-carbohydrate diet might account for an impaired nutritional state compared to a chow diet. These results were explained by a lower lean mass and a proportionally higher insulin dose in insulin tolerance tests. The possible role of KD in inducing insulin resistance is nevertheless controversial. Indeed, several authors reported that long term KD fed mice had normal glucose tolerance, lower baseline insulin levels and improved insulin sensitivity [26,29].

In humans, the effect of KD on glucose homeostasis is more controversial, and notably depends on the presence of type 2 diabetes or not at baseline. A study showed that a high-fat, low-carbohydrate intake reduces the ability of insulin to suppress endogenous glucose production in healthy men, by using the gold standard method, the hyperinsulinemic-euglycemic clamp [64]. The limitation is the small number of participants (only 6). Other studies described the opposite: with a KD, obese non-diabetic participants had a significant lower HOMA-IR and fasting glucose after a KD than at baseline [40], and an improvement in insulin sensitivity using the QUICKI [32]. Finally, another trial also described a better insulin sensitivity by consuming a KD [33], but this improvement does not seem to be permanent. Indeed, Forster et al. found a significant improvement in insulin sensitivity at 6 months, but not at 1 year [33]. This reduction in insulin levels could be explained by the satietogenic effect of this diet [65].

In type 2 diabetic patients, KD could be an interesting approach, as most patients have glycemic variability due to food carbohydrate content. A lot of studies have been designed around this purpose. KD are frequently associated with a diminution of blood glucose levels (up to 0.5 mmol/L) [41,66–68], glycosylated hemoglobin (HbA1c (up to 0.3%) [41,66,68,69], glycemic variability [70] and improvement in insulin sensitivity [32,68], sometimes without weight loss [67]. Low-carbohydrate diets can lead to a reduction in medications in type 2 diabetic patients [69–74]. An important aspect is to assess the long-term effect of a KD on these outcomes. In studies in obese type 2 diabetic patients fed a KD, a significant improvement in fasting glucose levels was seen after 12 weeks and continued after 56 weeks [75]. Nevertheless, in another study, a short-term decrease in HbA1c was observed at 6 months, but was not sustained at 24 months [76]. The latter study is probably more relevant to daily clinical practice because it was a low-intensity intervention. A recent study in obese type 2 diabetic patients compared a hypocaloric high-unsaturated/low-saturated fat very-low-carbohydrate diet to a high-carbohydrate low-fat diet [43]. After 52 weeks, the low-carbohydrate diet group showed a decrease in glycemic variability two times greater that the low-fat diet group, which indicates a greater diurnal blood glucose stability. However, improvement in HbA1c was similar in both diets (−1%). Nevertheless, the low-carbohydrate diet led to a greater reduction in antidiabetic medications, which could overall be helpful to optimize glycemic control [43]. Still, long-term effects of such dietary changes need to be evaluated.

In a prospective cohort of non-diabetic men, health professionals younger than 65 years old followed during 20 years, a low-carbohydrate diet high in animal proteins and fats was associated with a twofold increased risk of type 2 diabetes [77]. On the other hand, a low-carbohydrate diet high in vegetal proteins and fats was associated with a decreased risk of type 2 diabetes [77]. These findings suggest that a low-carbohydrate diet should contain proteins and fats from foods other than red and processed meat. However, these results were found from non-ketogenic diets. Therefore, further studies with "vegetal versus animal protein and fat content" KD are necessary to assess if these assumptions are validated. In another trial [32], a greater decrease of mean fasting glucose levels (−9%) was observed in all subjects of the low-carbohydrate group, but was significant only in diabetic patients (−15%), with more reduction of oral hypoglycemic agents or insulin in the low-carbohydrate group. Interestingly, in a study in obese non diabetic patients, after 8 weeks, a very-low-energy KD led to a rise in postprandial glucose levels, but not in fasting glucose levels [39]. The authors postulated that KD reduces insulin ability to suppress endogenous glucose production and impairs insulin-stimulated glucose oxidation, suggesting that there may be a different effect of ketosis on glucose homeostasis between diabetic and non-diabetic patients. For example, in obese type 2 diabetic patients, a strong inverse correlation between circulating ketones and hepatic glucose output has been described [78], suggesting that higher levels of ketones are associated with more favorable effects on glycemic control in these subjects.

An interesting study using biology systems approaches found a strong relationship between the insulin resistance pathway and the ketosis main pathway, providing a possible explanation for the improvement in glucose homeostasis found in clinical trials using low-carbohydrate diets. Notably, maps analyses suggest a direct implication of glucose transporters and inflammatory processes [79].

In summary, in rodents, KD mostly induces insulin resistance and glucose intolerance, while in type 2 diabetic humans KD is associated with a better control in glucose homeostasis and a reduction in antidiabetic medications. Nevertheless, these improvements seem to be limited in time. Further studies should evaluate if a higher weight loss correlates with a better glucose control or with higher ketones levels.

3.4. KD and Dyslipidemia

Dyslipidemia is a well-known risk factor for cardiovascular diseases. As KD are usually high in fats, it is necessary to assess their potential effect on the lipid profile.

In rodents, short term (14 days) studies showed no change in fatty acids and triglycerides levels in mice fed a KD [48]. The duration and the composition of KD feeding are very important. In a study of 4 weeks, Bielohuby et al. compared the effects on rats of chow diet and two different KD: one with 78.7% fat, 19.1% protein, 2.2% carbohydrates, and the other with 92.8% fat, 5.5% protein, 1.7% carbohydrates. The very high-fat KD-fed group had a reduction in high-density lipoproteins (HDL) cholesterol levels and higher triglycerides levels. No significant difference in total cholesterol levels was found between the three groups [23]. It should be noticed that the authors did not mention the effect on low-density lipoproteins (LDL) cholesterol levels. In another study, Jornayvaz et al. showed that mice fed a KD during 5 weeks had similar levels of LDL cholesterol than mice fed a chow diet [24]. In longer term (28–80 weeks) studies, KD fed mice displayed a twofold increase in plasma total cholesterol and triglyceride levels [25,26]. On the opposite, a recent study reported that mice fed a KD during 6 weeks had lower total cholesterol and triglycerides levels than with other diets [29]. The authors suggested that there was a KD-induced reduction in insulin levels, which further decreased liver fatty acids and cholesterol biosynthesis pathways [20,29]. Overall, most studies in animals used KD rich in saturated fats, which may have detrimental effects on the lipid profile compared to KD rich in unsaturated fats, and therefore limits definitive conclusions on the role of KD on dyslipidemia.

In humans, KD have been associated with significant reductions in total cholesterol [75], increases in HDL cholesterol levels [33,70,75,80–83], decreases in triglycerides levels [32,33,70,75,82,83] and reductions in LDL cholesterol levels [75]. These results were obtained in non epileptic obese participants with [32,70,75,83] or without [33,82] at least one risk factor of the metabolic syndrome, but also in healthy normal weight participants [80]. This is of importance as the effects of KD on the lipid profile may differ in epileptic subjects [84]. KD have also been associated with an increase in size and volume of LDL cholesterol particles, which is considered to reduce cardiovascular risk by decreasing atherogenicity [81]. Nevertheless, several studies showed an increase in LDL cholesterol levels [82,83,85,86], but not significantly in the trial by Westman et al. [85]; in these cases, KD were mostly composed of saturated fats. In other studies, total and LDL cholesterol were significantly more reduced with a high-protein medium-carbohydrate diet than with a KD [40]. Another study [33] reported no significant difference in total and LDL cholesterol levels after 12 months of a KD compared to a conventional diet, except at 3 months, where LDL cholesterol levels were lower in the conventional diet group. The absence of improvement suggests that weight loss with a low-carbohydrate diet is not associated with a decrease in LDL cholesterol usually observed with moderate weight loss [33]. Interestingly, the effect of a KD on lipid profile may be associated with ethnicity: in a study, white subjects lost more weight and had a bigger decrease in triglycerides levels than black subjects [32]. However, in this study, there was no significant change in total cholesterol, HDL cholesterol and LDL cholesterol levels.

As discussed for other cardiovascular risk factors, the composition of the diet used is very important. For example, in a study that reported a benefit of a KD on triglycerides and HDL cholesterol levels [70], the authors decided to use a low-carbohydrate diet rich in unsaturated but low in saturated fatty acids, which may greatly influence the lipid profile, but also the development of other metabolic complications such as NAFLD, insulin resistance and type 2 diabetes, as discussed earlier.

The impact of KD on the lipid profile differs between rodents and humans. In rodents, KD seem to be associated with worsened levels of total, HDL and LDL cholesterol, and triglycerides. In humans, the opposite is reported. These differences are mostly explained by differences in the composition of the diets, which are usually higher in total fat, but also in saturated fat in animal studies. Both in rodents and humans, comparison between saturated fat and unsaturated fat KD in long-term studies would be necessary. Later in this review, we will discuss whether saturated fat diets are as harmful as once thought.

3.5. KD and Blood Pressure

Studies reporting a potential effect of KD on blood pressure are scarce. We could not find studies in animals. In humans, KD are usually associated with a slight but not significant reduction in systolic and/or diastolic blood pressure [32]. Moreover, no change in antihypertensive therapy was observed [32,33]. Nevertheless, a study described an improvement in both systolic and diastolic blood pressure in obese participants when fed a KD during 48 weeks compared to a low-fat diet plus orlistat [69]. Weight loss was not a confounding factor as weight loss was similar in both arms. Finally, a reduction in systolic blood pressure was found in a study using a KD, but only after 3 months, without change after 1 year of observation [41].

Overall, there is a clear lack of conclusive data on the potential beneficial effect of KD on arterial blood pressure and further studies are therefore needed.

4. Discussion

Both in rodents and humans, controversies remain regarding the effect of KD on metabolic risk factors such as NAFLD, insulin resistance, type 2 diabetes and dyslipidemia. The potential beneficial and adverse effects of KD are summarized in Figure 1, and the effects of KD on different biomolecular markers in Figure 2.

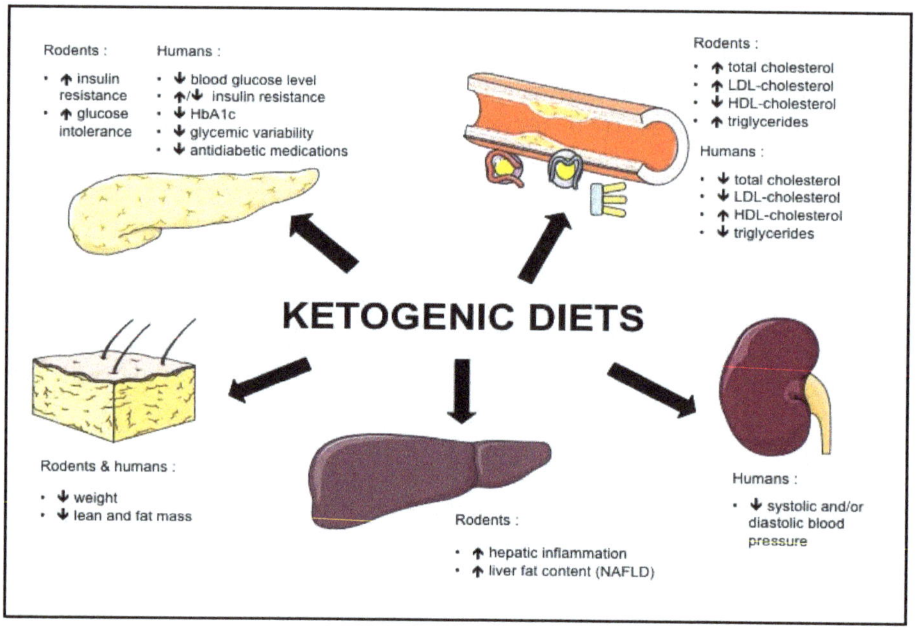

Figure 1. Effects of ketogenic diets in rodents and humans.

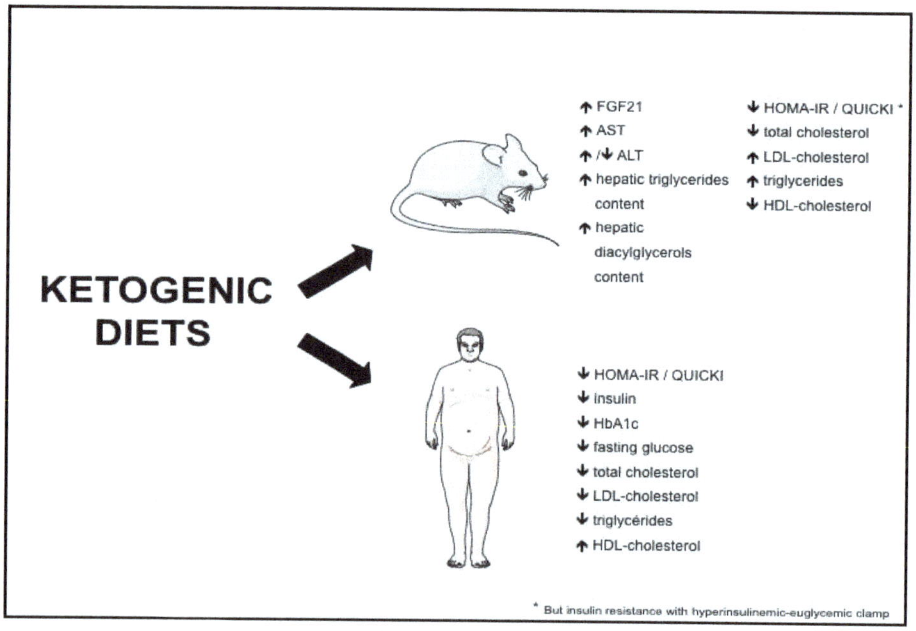

Figure 2. Effects of ketogenic diets on biomolecular markers. FGF21: fibroblast growth factor-21; ALT: alanine aminotransferase; AST: aspartate aminotransferase; QUICKI: quantitative insulin-sensitivity check index; HOMA-IR: homeostasis model assessment of insulin resistance.

Overall, KD composition greatly differs between studies. KD used in rodents are usually not similar to KD used in humans (almost no carbohydrates and low protein content in rodent KD). Moreover, low-carbohydrate diets can be different in macronutrient composition, i.e., high-fat versus high-protein content, which may account for some of the differences between the studies. Moreover, as previously mentioned, fat composition can substantially differ between studies, some using KD rich in unsaturated fatty acids and others rich in saturated fatty acids. Nevertheless, a recent systematic review and meta-analysis revealed that saturated fat intake was not associated with all-cause and cardiovascular mortality, coronary heart disease, ischemic stroke or type 2 diabetes, but with heterogenous evidence [87]. The authors conclude that trans fats were associated with all-cause and cardiovascular mortality and also with coronary heart disease. Moreover, it is well known that different ratios of some unsaturated and saturated fatty acids in diet compositions can alter metabolic parameters such as insulin sensitivity [9]. Therefore, it is a real challenge for physicians to advise patients with different metabolic diseases about the best diet composition to use. If a KD has to be prescribed, maybe it could be better to favor a vegetable-based KD, as vegetable-based low-carbohydrate diets have been correlated with a decrease in all-cause and cardiovascular-related mortality [88]. In the latter study, two US cohorts (121,700 females, 51,529 males) were followed during 26 and 20 years, respectively. Both in men and women, animal-based low-carbohydrate diets were found to be associated with higher all-cause (especially cardiovascular mortality) and cancer mortality, compared to vegetable-based low-carbohydrate diets. Nevertheless, similar studies with "real" KD need to be performed to confirm this assumption, as a low-carbohdyrate diet is not necessarily inducing ketosis and is therefore not a ketogenic diet per se. Another problem when using a KD is the long-term effect and sustainability of effects, notably due to a lack of long-term studies in metabolic diseases such as type 2 diabetes. Restrictive diets are often associated with poor long-term adherence [89]. Nevertheless, some evidence suggests that adherence to low-carbohydrate diets is better than to low-fat diets, because of the allowance to unlimited access to food as long as carbohydrates are reduced, given that proteins and fats are known to induce satiety [16].

Three meta-analyses about the effect of KD on cardiovascular risk factors were published recently [90–92]. Their conclusions are unanimous about general positive effects, but not unanimous about each single variable. Santos et al. concluded in 2012 that low-carbohydrate diets lead to a significant decrease in body weight, BMI, abdominal circumference, both systolic and diastolic blood pressure, triglycerides levels, fasting plasma glucose and HbA1c, an increase in HDL cholesterol levels, and no change in LDL cholesterol levels. As we mentioned before, the authors suggested a possible duration effect, specifically for body weight and blood pressure, where benefits seem to decrease over time [90]. Bezerra Bueno et al. compared very-low carbohydrate diets to low-fat diets and their effects after a follow-up of at least 12 months. Very-low carbohydrate diets confer a greater weight loss, reduction in triglycerides and diastolic blood pressure, and increase in HDL and LDL cholesterol levels. There was however no difference in systolic blood pressure. There was no significant difference between diets for fasting blood glucose and insulin levels, and HbA1c. It is interesting to note that in the studies (only 4) with 24 months of follow-up, only the change in HDL cholesterol levels remained significant [91]. The latest meta-analysis on KD by Naude et al. included 19 randomized controlled trials (RCT) and revealed that there is probably little or no difference in changes in weight or cardiovascular risk factors when comparing low-carbohydrate diets to isoenergetic diets (both showed weight loss) after two years of follow-up. These results were found in overweight and obese patients, with or without type 2 diabetes. This meta-analysis showed that strict adherence failed and declined with follow-up in most trials [92].

It is also important to keep in mind that KD could have some adverse side effects when chronically used. Indeed, studies in children using KD to treat epilepsy and other neurological disorders show an increase in kidney stones, osteoporosis, hyperlipidemia and impaired growth [93,94]. While several authors found that a low-carbohydrate high-protein diet was not associated with higher mortality after 12 years of follow-up [95], others described a weak statistically significant higher mortality rate after 10 years [96]. However, they did not evaluate sources of proteins and fats.

Finally, it should be mentioned that it is difficult to really know in studies if low-carbohydrate diets were "real" KD. Indeed, most of the time there is no report about a potential induction of ketosis, by for example reporting measurements of plasma ketone bodies.

5. Conclusions

Based on the available literature, KD may be associated with some improvements in some cardiovascular risk factors, such as obesity, type 2 diabetes and HDL cholesterol levels, but these effects are usually limited in time. As KD are often rich in fats, some negative effects could happen. Mainly in rodents, developments of NAFLD and insulin resistance were described. In humans, insulin resistance is also a potential negative effect, but some studies have shown improvements in insulin sensitivity. Nevertheless, many subjects contemplating such diets are overweight or obese at baseline, and even a moderate weight loss could be metabolically beneficial for them. However, it is mandatory to maintain body weight after weight loss, which is usually a major problem. More studies are therefore warranted to better assess the effects of long term use of KD on metabolic diseases and cardiovascular risk factors, but also to better define which dietary macronutrient composition is optimal.

Acknowledgments: F.R.J. is supported by a grant from the Gottfried und Julia Bangerter-Rhyner-Stiftung and from the Fondation de l'Association Suisse du Diabète.

Author Contributions: C.K. and F.R.J. wrote the paper and contributed equally.

References

1. Ng, M.; Fleming, T.; Robinson, M.; Thomson, B.; Graetz, N.; Margono, C.; Mullany, E.C.; Biryukov, S.; Abbafati, C.; Abera, S.F.; et al. Global, regional, and national prevalence of overweight and obesity in children and adults during 1980–2013: A systematic analysis for the Global Burden of Disease Study 2013. *Lancet* **2014**, *384*, 766–781. [CrossRef]
2. Koh-Banerjee, P.; Wang, Y.; Hu, F.B.; Spiegelman, D.; Willett, W.C.; Rimm, E.B. Changes in body weight and body fat distribution as risk factors for clinical diabetes in US men. *Am. J. Epidemiol.* **2004**, *159*, 1150–1159. [CrossRef] [PubMed]
3. Fabbrini, E.; Magkos, F.; Mohammed, B.S.; Pietka, T.; Abumrad, N.A.; Patterson, B.W.; Okunade, A.; Klein, S. Intrahepatic fat, not visceral fat, is linked with metabolic complications of obesity. *Proc. Natl. Acad. Sci. USA* **2009**, *106*, 15430–15435. [CrossRef] [PubMed]
4. Fabbrini, E.; Sullivan, S.; Klein, S. Obesity and nonalcoholic fatty liver disease: Biochemical, metabolic, and clinical implications. *Hepatology* **2010**, *51*, 679–689. [CrossRef] [PubMed]
5. Chalasani, N.; Younossi, Z.; Lavine, J.E.; Diehl, A.M.; Brunt, E.M.; Cusi, K.; Charlton, M.; Sanyal, A.J. The diagnosis and management of non-alcoholic fatty liver disease: Practice guideline by the American Gastroenterological Association, American Association for the Study of Liver Diseases, and American College of Gastroenterology. *Gastroenterology* **2012**, *142*, 1592–1609. [CrossRef] [PubMed]
6. Gariani, K.; Philippe, J.; Jornayvaz, F.R. Non-alcoholic fatty liver disease and insulin resistance: From bench to bedside. *Diabetes Metab.* **2013**, *39*, 16–26. [CrossRef] [PubMed]
7. Machado, M.; Marques-Vidal, P.; Cortez-Pinto, H. Hepatic histology in obese patients undergoing bariatric surgery. *J. Hepatol.* **2006**, *45*, 600–606. [CrossRef] [PubMed]
8. McKeown, N.M.; Meigs, J.B.; Liu, S.; Saltzman, E.; Wilson, P.W.F.; Jacques, P.F. Carbohydrate nutrition, insulin resistance, and the prevalence of the metabolic syndrome in the Framingham Offspring Cohort. *Diabetes Care* **2004**, *27*, 538–546. [CrossRef] [PubMed]
9. Asrih, M.; Jornayvaz, F.R. Diets and nonalcoholic fatty liver disease: The good and the bad. *Clin. Nutr.* **2014**, *33*, 186–190. [CrossRef] [PubMed]
10. Volek, J.S.; Fernandez, M.L.; Feinman, R.D.; Phinney, S.D. Dietary carbohydrate restriction induces a unique metabolic state positively affecting atherogenic dyslipidemia, fatty acid partitioning, and metabolic syndrome. *Prog. Lipid Res.* **2008**, *47*, 307–318. [CrossRef] [PubMed]
11. Volek, J.S.; Phinney, S.D.; Forsythe, C.E.; Quann, E.E.; Wood, R.J.; Puglisi, M.J.; Kraemer, W.J.; Bibus, D.M.; Fernandez, M.L.; Feinman, R.D. Carbohydrate restriction has a more favorable impact on the metabolic syndrome than a low fat diet. *Lipids* **2009**, *44*, 297–309. [CrossRef] [PubMed]
12. Volek, J.S.; Feinman, R.D. Carbohydrate restriction improves the features of Metabolic Syndrome. Metabolic Syndrome may be defined by the response to carbohydrate restriction. *Nutr. Metab.* **2005**, *2*, 31. [CrossRef] [PubMed]
13. Atkins, R.C. *Dr Atkins' Diet Revolution: The High Calorie Way to Stay Thin Forever*; D. McKay Co.: New York, NY, USA, 1972.

14. Veech, R.L. The therapeutic implications of ketone bodies: The effects of ketone bodies in pathological conditions: Ketosis, ketogenic diet, redox states, insulin resistance, and mitochondrial metabolism. *Prostaglandins Leukot. Essent. Fat. Acids* **2004**, *70*, 309–319. [CrossRef] [PubMed]
15. Kossoff, E.H.; Cervenka, M.C.; Henry, B.J.; Haney, C.A.; Turner, Z. A decade of the modified Atkins diet (2003–2013): Results, insights, and future directions. *Epilepsy Behav.* **2013**, *29*, 437–442. [CrossRef] [PubMed]
16. Feinman, R.D.; Pogozelski, W.K.; Astrup, A.; Bernstein, R.K.; Fine, E.J.; Westman, E.C.; Westman, E.C.; Accurso, A.; Frassetto, L.; Gower, B.A.; et al. Dietary carbohydrate restriction as the first approach in diabetes management: Critical review and evidence base. *Nutrition* **2015**, *31*, 1–13. [CrossRef] [PubMed]
17. Accurso, A.; Bernstein, R.K.; Dahlqvist, A.; Draznin, B.; Feinman, R.D.; Fine, E.J.; Gleed, A.; Jacobs, D.B.; Larson, G.; Lustig, R.H.; et al. Dietary carbohydrate restriction in type 2 diabetes mellitus and metabolic syndrome: Time for a critical appraisal. *Nutr. Metab.* **2008**, *5*, 9. [CrossRef] [PubMed]
18. Owen, O.E.; Morgan, A.P.; Kemp, H.G.; Sullivan, J.M.; Herrera, M.G.; Cahill, G.F. Brain metabolism during fasting. *J. Clin. Invest.* **1967**, *46*, 1589–1595. [CrossRef] [PubMed]
19. Kessler, S.K.; Neal, E.G.; Camfield, C.S.; Kossoff, E.H. Dietary therapies for epilepsy: Future research. *Epilepsy Behav.* **2011**, *22*, 17–22. [CrossRef] [PubMed]
20. Kennedy, A.R.; Pissios, P.; Otu, H.; Roberson, R.; Xue, B.; Asakura, K.; Furukawa, N.; Marino, F.E.; Liu, F.F.; Kahn, B.B.; et al. A high-fat, ketogenic diet induces a unique metabolic state in mice. *Am. J. Physiol. Endocrinol. Metab.* **2007**, *292*, E1724–E1739. [CrossRef] [PubMed]
21. Badman, M.K.; Kennedy, A.R.; Adams, A.C.; Pissios, P.; Maratos-Flier, E. A very low carbohydrate ketogenic diet improves glucose tolerance in ob/ob mice independently of weight loss. *Am. J. Physiol. Endocrinol. Metab.* **2009**, *297*, E1197–E1204. [CrossRef] [PubMed]
22. Garbow, J.R.; Doherty, J.M.; Schugar, R.C.; Travers, S.; Weber, M.L.; Wentz, A.E.; Ezenwajiaku, N.; Cotter, D.G.; Brunt, E.M.; Crawford, P.A. Hepatic steatosis, inflammation, and ER stress in mice maintained long term on a very low-carbohydrate ketogenic diet. *Am. J. Physiol. Gastrointest. Liver Physiol.* **2011**, *300*, G956–G967. [CrossRef] [PubMed]
23. Bielohuby, M.; Sisley, S.; Sandoval, D.; Herbach, N.; Zengin, A.; Fischereder, M.; Menhofer, D.; Stoehr, B.J.M.; Stemmer, K.; Wanke, R.; et al. Impaired glucose tolerance in rats fed low-carbohydrate, high-fat diets. *Am. J. Physiol. Endocrinol. Metab.* **2013**, *305*, E1059–E1070. [CrossRef] [PubMed]
24. Jornayvaz, F.R.; Jurczak, M.J.; Lee, H.-Y.; Birkenfeld, A.L.; Frederick, D.W.; Zhang, D.; Zhang, X.M.; Samuel, V.T.; Shulman, G.I. A high-fat, ketogenic diet causes hepatic insulin resistance in mice, despite increasing energy expenditure and preventing weight gain. *Am. J. Physiol. Endocrinol. Metab.* **2010**, *299*, E808–E815. [CrossRef] [PubMed]
25. Ellenbroek, J.H.; van Dijck, L.; Tons, H.A.; Rabelink, T.J.; Carlotti, F.; Ballieux, B.E.; de Koning, E.J.P. Long-term ketogenic diet causes glucose intolerance and reduced B- and a-cell mass but no weight loss in mice. *Am. J. Physiol. Endocrinol. Metab.* **2014**, *306*, E552–E558. [CrossRef] [PubMed]
26. Douris, N.; Melman, T.; Pecherer, J.M.; Pissios, P.; Flier, J.S.; Cantley, L.C.; Locasale, J.W.; Maratos-Flier, E. Adaptive changes in amino acid metabolism permit normal longevity in mice consuming a low-carbohydrate ketogenic diet. *Biochim. Biophys. Acta* **2015**, *1852*, 2056–2065. [CrossRef] [PubMed]
27. Asrih, M.; Altirriba, J.; Rohner-Jeanrenaud, F.; Jornayvaz, F.R. Ketogenic Diet Impairs FGF21 Signaling and Promotes Differential Inflammatory Responses in the Liver and White Adipose Tissue. *PLoS ONE* **2015**, *10*, e0126364. [CrossRef] [PubMed]
28. Frommelt, L.; Bielohuby, M.; Menhofer, D.; Stoehr, B.J.M.; Bidlingmaier, M.; Kienzle, E. Effects of low carbohydrate diets on energy and nitrogen balance and body composition in rats depend on dietary protein-to-energy ratio. *Nutrition* **2014**, *30*, 863–868. [CrossRef] [PubMed]
29. Holland, A.M.; Kephart, W.C.; Mumford, P.W.; Mobley, C.B.; Lowery, R.P.; Shake, J.J.; Patel, R.K.; Healy, J.C.; McCullough, D.J.; Kluess, H.A.; et al. Effects of a ketogenic diet on adipose tissue, liver, and serum biomarkers in sedentary rats and rats that exercised via resisted voluntary wheel running. *Am. J. Physiol. Regul. Integr. Comp. Physiol.* **2016**, *311*, R337–R351. [CrossRef] [PubMed]
30. Partsalaki, I.; Karvela, A.; Spiliotis, B.E. Metabolic impact of a ketogenic diet compared to a hypocaloric diet in obese children and adolescents. *J. Pediatr. Endocrinol. Metab.* **2012**, *25*, 697–704. [CrossRef] [PubMed]
31. Saisho, Y.; Butler, A.E.; Manesso, E.; Elashoff, D.; Rizza, R.A.; Butler, P.C. β-cell mass and turnover in humans: Effects of obesity and aging. *Diabetes Care* **2013**, *36*, 111–117. [CrossRef] [PubMed]

32. Samaha, F.F.; Iqbal, N.; Seshadri, P.; Chicano, K.L.; Daily, D.A.; McGrory, J.; Williams, T.; Williams, M.; Gracely, E.J.; Stem, L. A Low-Carbohydrate as Compared with a Low-Fat Diet in Severe Obesity. *N. Engl. J. Med.* **2003**, *348*, 2074–2081. [CrossRef] [PubMed]
33. Foster, G.D.; Wyatt, H.R.; Hill, J.O.; McGuckin, B.G.; Brill, C.; Mohammed, B.S.; Szapary, P.O.; Rader, D.J.; Edman, J.S.; Klein, S. A Randomized Trial of a Low-Carbohydrate Diet for Obesity. *N. Engl. J. Med.* **2003**, *348*, 2082–2090. [CrossRef] [PubMed]
34. Westerterp-Plantenga, M.S.; Nieuwenhuizen, A.; Tomé, D.; Soenen, S.; Westerterp, K.R. Dietary protein, weight loss, and weight maintenance. *Annu. Rev. Nutr.* **2009**, *29*, 21–41. [CrossRef] [PubMed]
35. Fine, E.J.; Feinman, R.D. Thermodynamics of weight loss diets. *Nutr. Metab.* **2004**, *1*, 15. [CrossRef] [PubMed]
36. Feinman, R.D.; Fine, E.J. Nonequilibrium thermodynamics and energy efficiency in weight loss diets. *Theor. Biol. Med. Model.* **2007**, *4*, 27. [CrossRef] [PubMed]
37. Halton, T.L.; Hu, F.B. The effects of high protein diets on thermogenesis, satiety and weight loss: A critical review. *J. Am. Coll. Nutr.* **2004**, *23*, 373–385. [CrossRef] [PubMed]
38. Veldhorst, M.A.B.; Westerterp-Plantenga, M.S.; Westerterp, K.R. Gluconeogenesis and energy expenditure after a high-protein, carbohydrate-free diet. *Am. J. Clin. Nutr.* **2009**, *90*, 519–526. [CrossRef] [PubMed]
39. Sumithran, P.; Prendergast, L.A.; Delbridge, E.; Purcell, K.; Shulkes, A.; Kriketos, A.; Proietto, J. Ketosis and appetite-mediating nutrients and hormones after weight loss. *Eur. J. Clin. Nutr.* **2013**, *67*, 759–764. [CrossRef] [PubMed]
40. Johnstone, A.M.; Horgan, G.W.; Murison, S.D.; Bremner, D.M.; Lobley, G.E. Effects of a high-protein ketogenic diet on hunger, appetite, and weight loss in obese men feeding ad libitum. *Am. J. Clin. Nutr.* **2008**, *87*, 44–55. [PubMed]
41. Cicero, A.F.G.; Benelli, M.; Brancaleoni, M.; Dainelli, G.; Merlini, D.; Negri, R. Middle and Long-Term Impact of a Very Low-Carbohydrate Ketogenic Diet on Cardiometabolic Factors: A Multi-Center, Cross-Sectional, Clinical Study. *High Blood Press. Cardiovasc. Prev.* **2015**, *22*, 389–394. [CrossRef] [PubMed]
42. Paoli, A.; Bianco, A.; Grimaldi, K.A.; Lodi, A.; Bosco, G. Long term successful weight loss with a combination biphasic ketogenic Mediterranean diet and Mediterranean diet maintenance protocol. *Nutrients* **2013**, *5*, 5205–5217. [CrossRef] [PubMed]
43. Tay, J.; Luscombe-Marsh, N.D.; Thompson, C.H.; Noakes, M.; Buckley, J.D.; Wittert, G.A.; Yancy, W.S.; Brinkworth, G.D. Comparison of low- and high-carbohydrate diets for type 2 diabetes management: A randomized trial. *Am. J. Clin. Nutr.* **2015**, *102*, 780–790. [CrossRef] [PubMed]
44. Jabekk, P.T.; Moe, I.A.; Meen, H.D.; Tomten, S.E.; Høstmark, A.T. Resistance training in overweight women on a ketogenic diet conserved lean body mass while reducing body fat. *Nutr. Metab.* **2010**, *7*, 17. [CrossRef] [PubMed]
45. Morris-Stiff, G.; Feldstein, A.E. Fibroblast growth factor 21 as a biomarker for NAFLD: Integrating pathobiology into clinical practice. *J. Hepatol.* **2010**, *53*, 795–796. [CrossRef] [PubMed]
46. Dushay, J.; Chui, P.C.; Gopalakrishnan, G.S.; Varela-Rey, M.; Crawley, M.; Fisher, F.M.; Badman, M.K.; Martinez-Chantar, M.L.; Maratos-Flier, E. Increased fibroblast growth factor 21 in obesity and nonalcoholic fatty liver disease. *Gastroenterology* **2010**, *139*, 456–463. [CrossRef] [PubMed]
47. Li, H.; Fang, Q.; Gao, F.; Fan, J.; Zhou, J.; Wang, X.; Zhang, H.; Pan, X.; Bao, Y.; Xiang, K.; et al. Fibroblast growth factor 21 levels are increased in nonalcoholic fatty liver disease patients and are correlated with hepatic triglyceride. *J. Hepatol.* **2010**, *53*, 934–940. [CrossRef] [PubMed]
48. Murata, Y.; Nishio, K.; Mochiyama, T.; Konishi, M.; Shimada, M.; Ohta, H.; Itoh, N. Fgf21 Impairs Adipocyte Insulin Sensitivity in Mice Fed a Low-Carbohydrate, High-Fat Ketogenic Diet. *PLoS ONE* **2013**, *8*, e69330. [CrossRef] [PubMed]
49. Badman, M.K.; Pissios, P.; Kennedy, A.R.; Koukos, G.; Flier, J.S.; Maratos-Flier, E. Hepatic fibroblast growth factor 21 is regulated by PPARalpha and is a key mediator of hepatic lipid metabolism in ketotic states. *Cell Metab.* **2007**, *5*, 426–437. [CrossRef] [PubMed]
50. Jornayvaz, F.R.; Shulman, G.I. Diacylglycerol activation of protein kinase Cε and hepatic insulin resistance. *Cell Metab.* **2012**, *15*, 574–584. [CrossRef] [PubMed]
51. Camporez, J.P.G.; Jornayvaz, F.R.; Petersen, M.C.; Pesta, D.; Guigni, B.A.; Serr, J.; Zhang, D.; Kahn, M.; Samuel, V.T.; Jurczak, M.J.; et al. Cellular mechanisms by which FGF21 improves insulin sensitivity in male mice. *Endocrinology* **2013**, *154*, 3099–3109. [CrossRef] [PubMed]

52. Xu, J.; Lloyd, D.J.; Hale, C.; Stanislaus, S.; Chen, M.; Sivits, G.; Vonderfecht, S.; Hecht, R.; Li, Y.S.; Lindberg, R.A.; et al. Fibroblast growth factor 21 reverses hepatic steatosis, increases energy expenditure, and improves insulin sensitivity in diet-induced obese mice. *Diabetes* **2009**, *58*, 250–259. [CrossRef] [PubMed]
53. Badman, M.K.; Koester, A.; Flier, J.S.; Kharitonenkov, A.; Maratos-Flier, E. Fibroblast growth factor 21-deficient mice demonstrate impaired adaptation to ketosis. *Endocrinology* **2009**, *150*, 4931–4940. [CrossRef] [PubMed]
54. Camporez, J.P.G.; Asrih, M.; Zhang, D.; Kahn, M.; Samuel, V.T.; Jurczak, M.J.; Jornayvaz, F.R. Hepatic insulin resistance and increased hepatic glucose production in mice lacking Fgf21. *J. Endocrinol.* **2015**, *226*, 207–217. [CrossRef] [PubMed]
55. Laeger, T.; Henagan, T.M.; Albarado, D.C.; Redman, L.M.; Bray, G.A.; Noland, R.C.; Münzberg, H.; Hutson, S.M.; Gettys, T.W.; Schwartz, M.W.; et al. FGF21 is an endocrine signal of protein restriction. *J. Clin. Investig.* **2014**, *124*, 3913–3922. [CrossRef] [PubMed]
56. Westerbacka, J.; Lammi, K.; Häkkinen, A.-M.; Rissanen, A.; Salminen, I.; Aro, A.; Yki-Järvinen, H. Dietary fat content modifies liver fat in overweight nondiabetic subjects. *J. Clin. Endocrinol. Metab.* **2005**, *90*, 2804–2809. [CrossRef] [PubMed]
57. Kirk, E.; Reeds, D.N.; Finck, B.N.; Mayurranjan, S.M.; Mayurranjan, M.S.; Patterson, B.W.; Klein, S. Dietary fat and carbohydrates differentially alter insulin sensitivity during caloric restriction. *Gastroenterology* **2009**, *136*, 1552–1560. [CrossRef] [PubMed]
58. Browning, J.D.; Baker, J.A.; Rogers, T.; Davis, J.; Satapati, S.; Burgess, S.C. Short-term weight loss and hepatic triglyceride reduction: Evidence of a metabolic advantage with dietary carbohydrate restriction. *Am. J. Clin. Nutr.* **2011**, *93*, 1048–1052. [CrossRef] [PubMed]
59. Bian, H.; Hakkarainen, A.; Lundbom, N.; Yki-Järvinen, H. Effects of dietary interventions on liver volume in humans. *Obesity* **2014**, *22*, 989–995. [CrossRef] [PubMed]
60. Sevastianova, K.; Kotronen, A.; Gastaldelli, A.; Perttilä, J.; Hakkarainen, A.; Lundbom, J.; Orho-Melander, M.; Lundbom, N.; Ferrannini, E.; Rissanen, A.; et al. Genetic variation in PNPLA3 (adiponutrin) confers sensitivity to weight loss-induced decrease in liver fat in humans. *Am. J. Clin. Nutr.* **2011**, *94*, 104–111. [CrossRef] [PubMed]
61. Shen, J.; Wong, G.L.-H.; Chan, H.L.-Y.; Chan, R.S.-M.; Chan, H.-Y.; Chu, W.C.-W.; Cheung, B.H.-K.; Yeung, D.K.-W.; Li, L.S.; Sea, M.M.-M.; et al. PNPLA3 gene polymorphism and response to lifestyle modification in patients with nonalcoholic fatty liver disease. *J. Gastroenterol. Hepatol.* **2015**, *30*, 139–146. [CrossRef] [PubMed]
62. Jornayvaz, F.R. Fibroblast growth factor 21, ketogenic diets, and insulin resistance. *Am. J. Clin. Nutr.* **2011**, *94*, 955. [CrossRef] [PubMed]
63. Kinzig, K.P.; Honors, M.A.; Hargrave, S.L. Insulin sensitivity and glucose tolerance are altered by maintenance on a ketogenic diet. *Endocrinology* **2010**, *151*, 3105–3114. [CrossRef] [PubMed]
64. Bisschop, P.H.; de Metz, J.; Ackermans, M.T.; Endert, E.; Pijl, H.; Kuipers, F.; Meijer, A.J.; Sauerwein, H.P.; Romijn, J.A. Dietary fat content alters insulin-mediated glucose metabolism in healthy men. *Am. J. Clin. Nutr.* **2001**, *73*, 554–559. [PubMed]
65. Westman, E.C.; Feinman, R.D.; Mavropoulos, J.C.; Vernon, M.C.; Volek, J.S.; Wortman, J.A.; Yancy, W.S.; Phinney, S.D. Low-carbohydrate nutrition and metabolism. *Am. J. Clin. Nutr.* **2007**, *86*, 276–284. [PubMed]
66. Hussain, T.A.; Mathew, T.C.; Dashti, A.A.; Asfar, S.; Al-Zaid, N.; Dashti, H.M. Effect of low-calorie versus low-carbohydrate ketogenic diet in type 2 diabetes. *Nutrition* **2012**, *28*, 1016–1021. [CrossRef] [PubMed]
67. Gannon, M.C.; Nuttall, F.Q. Control of blood glucose in type 2 diabetes without weight loss by modification of diet composition. *Nutr. Metab.* **2006**, *3*, 16. [CrossRef] [PubMed]
68. Boden, G.; Sargrad, K.; Homko, C.; Mozzoli, M.; Stein, T.P. Effect of a low-carbohydrate diet on appetite, blood glucose levels, and insulin resistance in obese patients with type 2 diabetes. *Ann. Intern. Med.* **2005**, *142*, 403–411. [CrossRef] [PubMed]
69. Mayer, S.B.; Jeffreys, A.S.; Olsen, M.K.; McDuffie, J.R.; Feinglos, M.N.; Yancy, W.S. Two diets with different haemoglobin A1c and antiglycaemic medication effects despite similar weight loss in type 2 diabetes. *Diabetes Obes. Metab.* **2014**, *16*, 90–93. [CrossRef] [PubMed]
70. Tay, J.; Luscombe-Marsh, N.D.; Thompson, C.H.; Noakes, M.; Buckley, J.D.; Wittert, G.A.; Yancy, W.S.; Brinkworth, G.D. A Very Low-Carbohydrate, Low–Saturated Fat Diet for Type 2 Diabetes Management: A Randomized Trial. *Diabetes Care* **2014**, *37*, 2909–2918. [CrossRef] [PubMed]

71. Gannon, M.C.; Nuttall, F.Q. Effect of a high-protein, low-carbohydrate diet on blood glucose control in people with type 2 diabetes. *Diabetes* **2004**, *53*, 2375–2382. [CrossRef] [PubMed]
72. Halton, T.L.; Liu, S.; Manson, J.E.; Hu, F.B. Low-carbohydrate-diet score and risk of type 2 diabetes in women. *Am. J. Clin. Nutr.* **2008**, *87*, 339–346. [PubMed]
73. Yancy, W.S.; Foy, M.; Chalecki, A.M.; Vernon, M.C.; Westman, E.C. A low-carbohydrate, ketogenic diet to treat type 2 diabetes. *Nutr. Metab.* **2005**, *2*, 34. [CrossRef] [PubMed]
74. Saslow, L.R.; Kim, S.; Daubenmier, J.J.; Moskowitz, J.T.; Phinney, S.D.; Goldman, V.; Murphy, E.J.; Cox, R.M.; Moran, P.; Hecht, F.M. A randomized pilot trial of a moderate carbohydrate diet compared to a very low carbohydrate diet in overweight or obese individuals with type 2 diabetes mellitus or prediabetes. *PLoS ONE* **2014**, *9*, e91027. [CrossRef] [PubMed]
75. Dashti, H.M.; Al-Zaid, N.S.; Mathew, T.C.; Al-Mousawi, M.; Talib, H.; Asfar, S.K.; Behbahani, A.I. Long term effects of ketogenic diet in obese subjects with high cholesterol level. *Mol. Cell. Biochem.* **2006**, *286*, 1–9. [CrossRef] [PubMed]
76. Iqbal, N.; Vetter, M.L.; Moore, R.H.; Chittams, J.L.; Dalton-Bakes, C.V.; Dowd, M.; Williams-Smith, C.; Cardillo, S.; Wadden, T.A. Effects of a low-intensity intervention that prescribed a low-carbohydrate vs. a low-fat diet in obese, diabetic participants. *Obesity* **2010**, *18*, 1733–1738. [CrossRef] [PubMed]
77. De Koning, L.; Fung, T.T.; Liao, X.; Chiuve, S.E.; Rimm, E.B.; Willett, W.C.; Spiegelman, D.; Hu, F.B. Low-carbohydrate diet scores and risk of type 2 diabetes in men. *Am. J. Clin. Nutr.* **2011**, *93*, 844–850. [CrossRef] [PubMed]
78. Gumbiner, B.; Wendel, J.A.; McDermott, M.P. Effects of diet composition and ketosis on glycemia during very-low-energy-diet therapy in obese patients with non-insulin-dependent diabetes mellitus. *Am. J. Clin. Nutr.* **1996**, *63*, 110–115. [PubMed]
79. Farrés, J.; Pujol, A.; Coma, M.; Ruiz, J.; Naval, J.; Mas, J.; Molins, A.; Fondevila, J.; Aloy, P. Revealing the molecular relationship between type 2 diabetes and the metabolic changes induced by a very-low-carbohydrate low-fat ketogenic diet. *Nutr. Metab.* **2010**, *7*, 88. [CrossRef] [PubMed]
80. Sharman, M.J.; Kraemer, W.J.; Love, D.M.; Avery, N.G.; Gómez, A.L.; Scheett, T.P.; Volek, J.S. A ketogenic diet favorably affects serum biomarkers for cardiovascular disease in normal-weight men. *J. Nutr.* **2002**, *132*, 1879–1885. [PubMed]
81. Volek, J.S.; Sharman, M.J.; Forsythe, C.E. Modification of lipoproteins by very low-carbohydrate diets. *J. Nutr.* **2005**, *135*, 1339–1342. [PubMed]
82. Foster, G.D.; Wyatt, H.R.; Hill, J.O.; Makris, A.P.; Rosenbaum, D.L.; Brill, C.; Stein, R.I.; Mohammed, B.S.; Miller, B.; Rader, D.J.; et al. Weight and metabolic outcomes after 2 years on a low-carbohydrate versus low-fat diet: A randomized trial. *Ann. Intern. Med.* **2010**, *153*, 147–157. [CrossRef] [PubMed]
83. Brinkworth, G.D.; Noakes, M.; Buckley, J.D.; Keogh, J.B.; Clifton, P.M. Long-term effects of a very-low-carbohydrate weight loss diet compared with an isocaloric low-fat diet after 12 mo. *Am. J. Clin. Nutr.* **2009**, *90*, 23–32. [CrossRef] [PubMed]
84. Lima, P.A.; de Brito Sampaio, L.P.; Damasceno, N.R.T. Ketogenic diet in epileptic children: Impact on lipoproteins and oxidative stress. *Nutr. Neurosci.* **2015**, *18*, 337–344. [CrossRef] [PubMed]
85. Westman, E.C.; Yancy, W.S.; Mavropoulos, J.C.; Marquart, M.; McDuffie, J.R. The effect of a low-carbohydrate, ketogenic diet versus a low-glycemic index diet on glycemic control in type 2 diabetes mellitus. *Nutr. Metab.* **2008**, *5*, 36. [CrossRef] [PubMed]
86. Stern, L.; Iqbal, N.; Seshadri, P.; Chicano, K.L.; Daily, D.A.; McGrory, J.; Williams, M.; Gracely, E.J.; Samaha, F.F. The effects of low-carbohydrate versus conventional weight loss diets in severely obese adults: One-year follow-up of a randomized trial. *Ann. Intern. Med.* **2004**, *140*, 778–785. [CrossRef] [PubMed]
87. De Souza, R.J.; Mente, A.; Maroleanu, A.; Cozma, A.I.; Ha, V.; Kishibe, T.; Uleryk, E.; Budylowski, P.; Schünemann, H.; Beyene, J.; et al. Intake of saturated and trans unsaturated fatty acids and risk of all cause mortality, cardiovascular disease, and type 2 diabetes: Systematic review and meta-analysis of observational studies. *BMJ* **2015**, *351*, h3978. [CrossRef] [PubMed]
88. Fung, T.T.; van Dam, R.M.; Hankinson, S.E.; Stampfer, M.; Willett, W.C.; Hu, F.B. Low-carbohydrate diets and all-cause and cause-specific mortality: Two cohort studies. *Ann. Intern. Med.* **2010**, *153*, 289–298. [CrossRef] [PubMed]
89. Ye, F.; Li, X.-J.; Jiang, W.-L.; Sun, H.-B.; Liu, J. Efficacy of and Patient Compliance with a Ketogenic Diet in Adults with Intractable Epilepsy: A Meta-Analysis. *J. Clin. Neurol.* **2015**, *11*, 26. [CrossRef] [PubMed]

90. Santos, F.L.; Esteves, S.S.; da Costa Pereira, A.; Yancy, W.S., Jr.; Nunes, J.P. Systematic review and meta-analysis of clinical trials of the effects of low carbohydrate diets on cardiovascular risk factors: Low carbohydrate diets and cardiovascular risk factors. *Obes. Rev.* **2012**, *13*, 1048–1066. [CrossRef] [PubMed]
91. Bueno, N.B.; de Melo, I.S.; de Oliveira, S.L.; da Rocha Ataide, T. Very-low-carbohydrate ketogenic diet v. low-fat diet for long-term weight loss: A meta-analysis of randomised controlled trials. *Br. J. Nutr.* **2013**, *110*, 1178–1187. [CrossRef] [PubMed]
92. Naude, C.E.; Schoonees, A.; Senekal, M.; Young, T.; Garner, P.; Volmink, J. Low carbohydrate versus isoenergetic balanced diets for reducing weight and cardiovascular risk: A systematic review and meta-analysis. *PLoS ONE* **2014**, *9*, e100652. [CrossRef] [PubMed]
93. Bergqvist, A.G.C. Long-term monitoring of the ketogenic diet: Do's and Don'ts. *Epilepsy Res.* **2012**, *100*, 261–266. [CrossRef] [PubMed]
94. Kossoff, E.; Wang, H.-S. Dietary Therapies for Epilepsy. *Biomed. J.* **2013**, *36*, 2. [CrossRef] [PubMed]
95. Lagiou, P.; Sandin, S.; Weiderpass, E.; Lagiou, A.; Mucci, L.; Trichopoulos, D.; Adami, H.-O. Low carbohydrate-high protein diet and mortality in a cohort of Swedish women. *J. Intern. Med.* **2007**, *261*, 366–374. [CrossRef] [PubMed]
96. Trichopoulou, A.; Psaltopoulou, T.; Orfanos, P.; Hsieh, C.-C.; Trichopoulos, D. Low-carbohydrate-high-protein diet and long-term survival in a general population cohort. *Eur. J. Clin. Nutr.* **2007**, *61*, 575–581. [CrossRef] [PubMed]

5

Cross-Sectional and Longitudinal Association between Glycemic Status and Body Composition in Men: A Population-Based Study

Khaleal Almusaylim, Maggie Minett, Teresa L. Binkley, Tianna M. Beare and Bonny Specker *

EA Martin Program in Human Nutrition, South Dakota State University, SWC, Box 506, Brookings, SD 57007, USA; khalealabdulha.almusaylim@jacks.sdstate.edu (K.A.); maggie.minett@sdstate.edu (M.M.); teresa.binkley@sdstate.edu (T.L.B.); tianna.beare@sdstate.edu (T.M.B.)

* Correspondence: Bonny.Specker@sdstate.edu

Abstract: This study sought to evaluate the associations between changes in glycemic status and changes in total body (TB), trunk, and appendicular fat (FM) and lean mass (LM) in men. A population-based study of men aged 20–66 years at baseline were included in cross-sectional ($n = 430$) and three-year longitudinal ($n = 411$) analyses. Prediabetes was defined as fasting glucose 100–125 mg/dL. Type 2 diabetes (T2D) was determined by: self-reported diabetes, current anti-diabetic drug use (insulin/oral hypoglycemic agents), fasting glucose ($\geq$126 mg/dL), or non-fasting glucose ($\geq$200 mg/dL). Body composition was evaluated by dual-energy X-ray absorptiometry. Longitudinal analyses showed that changes in TB FM and LM, and appendicular LM differed among glycemic groups. Normoglycemic men who converted to prediabetes lost more TB and appendicular LM than men who remained normoglycemic (all, $p < 0.05$). Normoglycemic or prediabetic men who developed T2D had a greater loss of TB and appendicular LM than men who remained normoglycemic (both, $p < 0.05$). T2D men had greater gains in TB FM and greater losses in TB and appendicular LM than men who remained normoglycemic (all, $p < 0.05$). Dysglycemia is associated with adverse changes in TB and appendicular LM.

Keywords: prediabetes; type 2 diabetes; total body fat; total body lean; appendicular fat; appendicular lean; body composition; cohort study

1. Introduction

Prediabetes and type 2 diabetes (T2D) are major public health issues in the United States. The national prevalence of prediabetes and T2D among adults aged $\geq$20 years has increased over time, with the prevalence of prediabetes rising from 26% in 1988–1994 [1] to 37% in 2009–2012 [2]. Recent estimates from the Centers for Disease Control and Prevention indicate that 15–30% of prediabetic cases progress from impaired fasting glucose or impaired glucose tolerance to T2D within five years. There are currently 25.8 million adults in the United States with prediabetes that will develop T2D by 2020, which will double the number of individuals affected by T2D [3]. The prevalence of T2D rose from 7% in 2005 to 12% in 2011 [4], and is projected to increase 165% by 2050 [5].

Case-control and cross-sectional studies have reported inconsistent associations of total body (TB), trunk, and appendicular fat mass (FM) and lean mass (LM) with prediabetes and T2D diabetes in middle-aged and older adults, including a positive association [6], an inverse association [7–10], and no association [6,8,9]. Prospective studies aimed at investigating the relationship between baseline glycemic status and subsequent changes in TB and regional distribution of FM and LM are sparse and inconclusive. Some studies reported differences in body composition measurements among glycemic groups [11–14], but others did not find differences [15,16]. The possible explanation for inconsistent findings includes different durations of follow-up period, sample size, and other covariates that were not adjusted for when investigating the association between various measures of body composition and glycemic status. We found no epidemiological studies that investigated the association between glycemic status (men with prediabetes who revert to normoglycemia, or men who are normoglycemic or prediabetic at baseline and convert to T2D) and changes in the TB and regional distribution of FM and LM.

The objective of the present analysis was to examine the associations between baseline and changes in glycemic status with baseline and changes over three years in TB, trunk, and appendicular FM and LM. The following *a priori* hypotheses were tested: (1) men with prediabetes or T2D at baseline would have higher TB and trunk fat measurements but lower appendicular fat than normoglycemic men; (2) men who were normoglycemic at baseline and developed either prediabetes or T2D would have increases in TB and trunk FM, and decreases in TB and appendicular LM over the three-year study compared with men who remained normoglycemic; (3) among men with prediabetes at baseline, the changes in TB and trunk FM and LM would differ over the three-year study depending on whether they remained prediabetic or developed T2D versus reverting to a normoglycemic state. Those who develop T2D would gain TB FM and lose LM, while those reverting to normoglycemia would lose FM and maintain or gain LM; and (4) men with T2D at baseline would have decreases in TB and trunk LM over the three-year study compared to normoglycemic men.

2. Materials and Methods

2.1. Study Population

The South Dakota Rural Bone Health Study is a population-based longitudinal study designed to investigate the impact of lifestyle factors on bone and body composition. The design and rationale of the study have been described elsewhere [17]. Briefly, adults aged 20 to 66 years, from eight counties in eastern South Dakota, were eligible for enrollment. A total of 1271 participants were recruited between 2001–2004 (baseline), and followed for an average of 3.0 years (range of 2.8 to 3.8 years), and the current analysis was limited to men (n = 544). Among those participants, 410 men farmed at least 75% of their lives (rural) and 134 men never lived on an active farm (non-rural). The rural population was divided into Hutterites and non-Hutterites. A Hutterite was defined as a participant of Hutterite descent who resided on a Hutterite colony. Hutterites are an Anabaptist religious group who believe in isolated communal living and self-sufficiency through an agriculturally advanced lifestyle. Non-Hutterites were randomly selected from the eight-county region as described elsewhere [17].

Men with chronic use (> six months) of immunosuppressants, anticonvulsants, or steroids or a diagnosis of type 1 diabetes mellitus at baseline were not eligible for inclusion in the original cohort. For baseline analyses, we excluded men with missing glucose measures at either baseline (n = 12) or follow-up (n = 34), baseline body composition measurements (n = 23), or men who withdrew from the study (n = 45) (Figure 1). For follow-up analyses, we further excluded men who did not have body composition measurements at follow-up (n = 19). These exclusions led to 430 men in the baseline analyses and 411 in the follow-up analyses. The study was approved by the South Dakota State University Institutional Review Board (IRB#1406004), and informed consent was obtained from all of the participants.

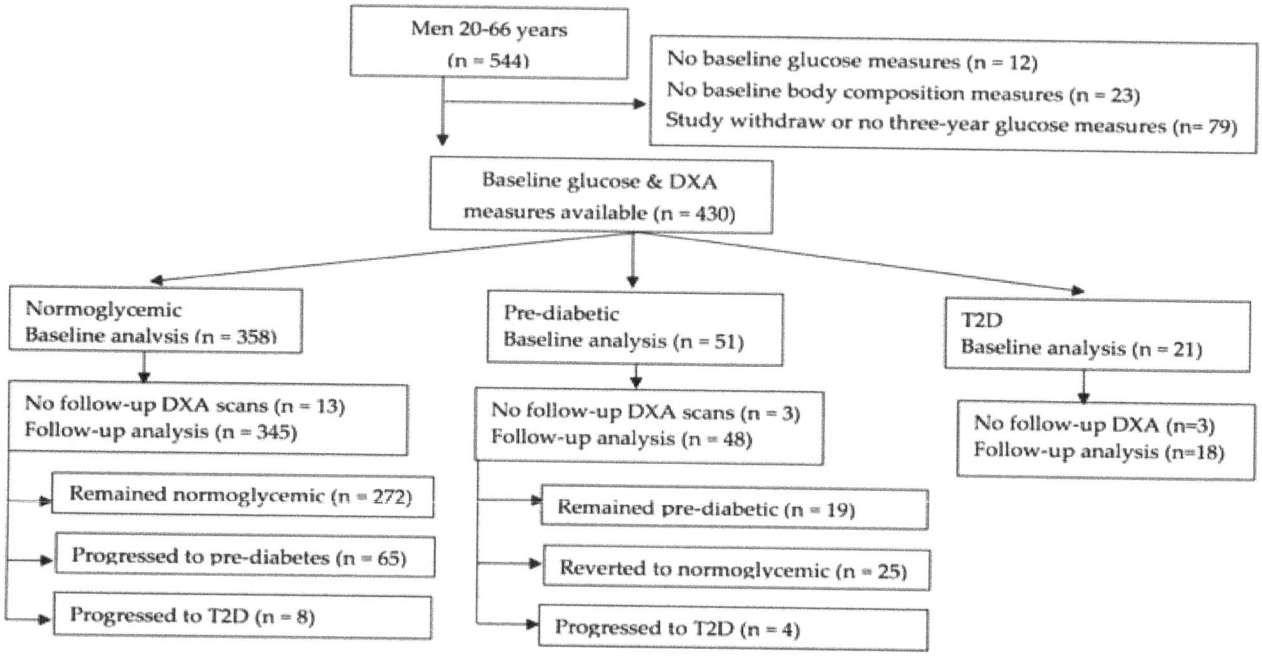

Figure 1. Flowchart of participants. Abbreviations: DXA, dual-energy X-ray absorptiometry; T2D, type 2 diabetic. Individuals who were unable to be categorized into glycemic groups were excluded.

2.2. *Assessment of Covariates*

Questionnaires were administered at study enrollment and at three years to obtain information on demographic and lifestyle characteristics as well as quarterly physical activity and dietary intake recalls. Information on smoking status and specific details regarding the use of prescription drugs was not collected at baseline; however, an 18-month survey was used to obtain this information. Participants were asked to provide information on types of smoking, such as cigarettes, cigars, and pipes, and were classified as smokers or non-smokers. The presence or absence of hypertension at 18 months was based on self-reported information on the use of antihypertensive medication.

2.2.1. Anthropometric Measures

Body height and weight were measured in lightweight clothes without shoes using a calibrated stadiometer and scale. Standing height was measured to the nearest 0.5 cm in duplicate with a stadiometer (Seca, Chino, CA, USA). A third measurement was taken if the discrepancy between the duplicate height measurements was more than 0.5 cm. Weight was measured to the nearest 0.1 kg with a digital scale (Seca Model 770, Chino, CA, USA).

2.2.2. Physical Activity Assessment

The Paffenbarger Physical Activity Questionnaire (PPAQ) was used to measure the average amount of time spent in sedentary behaviors and different intensity levels of physical activity during the past week [18]. Participants were asked to recall how many hours on their usual weekday and weekend day they spent sleeping, sitting, and engaging in moderate or vigorous intensity activity. Since the time spent in sleeping, sitting, and participating in moderate plus vigorous activity was measured, the remaining time was considered light activity. The PPAQ was administered quarterly over the first three years of the study. To properly report participants' physical activity, trained personnel administered the PPAQ by interview. The average time spent in sitting and moderate-plus-vigorous activity, as well as the average sleeping time, was calculated. The validity and reliability of the PPAQ have been established to measure physical activity intensities in men [19] and rural populations [20].

2.2.3. Dietary Assessment

Dietary intake was assessed using 24-h dietary recalls that were conducted at similar times as the activity recall. Trained interviewers administered 24-h dietary recalls, and dietary recall data were analyzed using Nutritionist Pro software (version 2.3.1, 2004, First DataBank, Inc., San Bruno, CA, USA) to estimate macronutrient and micronutrient intakes. For foods not available in the Nutritionist Pro software, the nutrient composition of the foods was obtained from recipes and entered into the diet analysis software. Activity levels and nutrient intakes at baseline were the averages of the baseline, three-month and six-month recalls, and measures at the 36-month visit were the averages of the 30-month, 33-month, and 36-month recalls.

2.3. *Ascertainment of Glycemic Status*

According to American Diabetes Association classifications, individuals with a fasting blood glucose of 100 mg/dL to 125 mg/dL were classified as having prediabetes [21]. T2D was determined by one of the following criteria: self-reported T2D, current use of an anti-diabetic drug (insulin or oral hypoglycemic agents), or a fasting blood glucose concentration $\geq$126 mg/dL or a non-fasting blood glucose concentration $\geq$200 mg/dL [21]. The same criteria for the diagnosis of prediabetes and T2D were applied at both the baseline and three-year visits. Attempts were made to obtain fasting blood samples at each visit, and measurements were made in the field from a sample of venous whole blood (with added ethylenediaminetetraacetic acid) using an Accu-Check Advantage glucometer (Roche Diagnostics, Indianapolis, IN, USA).

2.4. *Body Composition Measurements*

Body composition was assessed using dual-energy x-ray absorptiometry (DXA) (Discovery, Software Version 12.01, Hologic, Waltham, MA, USA). A TB scan was completed with boundaries for the various anatomical regions set according to manufacturer's specifications. The step phantom scan for body composition calibration was completed weekly as suggested by the manufacturer. Prior to DXA measurements, the Hologic spine phantom was scanned for quality control. All of the scans were analyzed by the same technician who was certified by the International Society of Clinical Densitometry. Scan results were deleted for obese participants with an equivalent epoxy thickness greater than 12 inches, as determined by the Hologic software, per manufacturer recommendations (n = 16 men: n = seven Hutterite, n = four rural, n = five non-rural). DXA-derived measurements of TB, trunk and appendicular FM and LM were expressed in kilograms. Our coefficients of variation for TB FM and LM assessed in 15 adults (one male) using triplicate scans with repositioning between each scan are <1.5%.

2.5. *Statistical Analysis*

All of the continuous variables were tested for normality before performing the analyses. Analysis of variance adjusting for multiple comparisons for continuous variables and a Fisher's exact test for categorical variables were used to determine statistical significance in baseline characteristics among the glycemic categories. The annual absolute change in each body composition measure was calculated as the follow-up value minus baseline value divided by length of follow-up in years.

Multiple regression models were used to estimate marginal means $\pm$ standard error of the mean (sem) for baseline body composition parameters and changes in outcome measures by different categories of glycemic status. Differences in marginal means among glycemic groups were evaluated using post hoc contrast tests based on the hypotheses. A priori determined covariates (age at baseline, height, population group, percent time in moderate-plus-vigorous activity, and total daily caloric intake) were included in all of the models, since they were found to be associated with at least one body composition measure. The multiple regression models that were used for baseline analyses included these covariates, and the FM model included the LM of the same compartment (TB, trunk, or appendicular), and the LM model included covariates plus the FM of the same compartment. Multiple regression models for the longitudinal analyses were adjusted for the same covariates, as well as changes in percent time in moderate-plus-vigorous activity and total daily caloric intake between baseline and three-year follow-up, baseline measure of the specific body compartment (TB, trunk, or appendicular), and baseline and annual changes in the FM or LM of same compartment. Due to issues with multicollinearity and the problem of body composition measures being components of both body mass index (BMI) and weight, neither BMI nor weight was included as covariates. The assumptions of linearity, normality, and homoscedasticity were evaluated visually to ensure no violation of assumptions. All of the analyses were performed using JMP software (version 13, SAS Institute, Cary, NC, USA), and the statistical significance level was set at $p < 0.05$ (two-tailed).

3. Results

3.1. Subject Characteristics

At the baseline visit, 358 (83.2%) of the men were normoglycemic, 51 (11.9%) were prediabetic based on fasting glucose concentrations, and 21 (4.9%) had T2D (14 self-reported a medical diagnosis, six based on fasting glucose, and one based on non-fasting glucose). Of the 345 men who were normoglycemic at baseline and for whom glucose and body composition measurements were available at three years, 272 (78.9%) remained normoglycemic, 65 (18.8%) progressed to prediabetes, and eight (2.3%) progressed to T2D (five based on fasting glucose, one based on non-fasting glucose, one self-reported a medical diagnosis, and one taking anti-diabetic medication). Among the 48 prediabetic men, 19 (39.6%) remained prediabetic, 25 (52.1%) reverted to normoglycemic, and four (8.3%) progressed to T2D based on fasting glucose concentrations. Of the 18 T2D men who were diabetic throughout the study, four (22.2%) self-reported a medical diagnosis, 11 (61.1%) were taking anti-diabetic medication, and three (16.7%) had T2D based on fasting glucose concentrations.

Participant characteristics by glycemic categories at baseline and follow-up are summarized in Tables 1 and 2. The mean age (+ sem) was 42.7 ± 0.6 years (range: 20 to 66 years), and men with T2D at baseline were older than those who were normoglycemic. The study population was 37.4% Hutterite, 37.2% rural non-Hutterite, and 25.4% non-rural. Hutterites and married men had a higher prevalence of prediabetes and T2D than non-Hutterites and single men. Men with prediabetes weighed more than normoglycemic men. A higher percentage of prediabetic and T2D men were taking antihypertensive medication than normoglycemic men, and carbohydrate intake was greater in normoglycemic men than in prediabetic and T2D men. At follow-up, men with T2D had lower caloric and carbohydrate intake than men who remained normoglycemic throughout the study or men who were normoglycemic and developed prediabetes (Table 2). Prediabetic men who remained prediabetic at three years increased their carbohydrate intake, and men who remained normoglycemic throughout the study increased their weight, time spent in moderate-plus-vigorous activity, and average daily fat intake. The overall mean changes over the three-year study in percent time in moderate-plus-vigorous activity and average dietary intake of calories, carbohydrates, fat, and protein were not significant (mean changes were 0.6 ± 0.4%, 10 ± 28 kcal, 1.0 ± 3.8 g, 3.0 ± 1.6 g, and 0.0 ± 1.5 g, respectively), and changes in caloric and macronutrient intakes did not differ by glycemic categories (data not shown).

Table 1. Baseline characteristics of the 430 men from the South Dakota Rural Bone Health Study cohort. NH: non-Hutterite.

	Normoglycemic	Prediabetic	T2D	*p*-Value [1]
Participants (*n*)	358	51	21	
Demographics				
Age (years)	41.6 ± 0.6 [a]	45.8 ± 1.7	53.0 ± 2.6 [a]	<0.001
Population Group (%)				0.001
Hutterite ($n = 161$)	73.3	18.0	8.7	
NH Rural ($n = 160$)	89.3	8.8	1.9	
NH Non-rural ($n = 109$)	89.0	7.3	3.7	
Ever Married (%)	81.3	92.2	95.2	0.06
Anthropometrics				
Height (cm)	177.9 ± 0.4	177.9 ± 0.9	174.3 ± 1.5	0.06
Weight (kg)	91.1 ± 0.8 [a]	98.5 ± 2.1 [a]	95.9 ± 3.3	0.003
Lifestyle Variables				
Smokers (%)	33.2	24.0	38.1	0.43
BP Meds (%)	8.7	23.5	47.6	<0.001
% Time in MVPA [2]	21.8 ± 0.5	23.1 ± 1.4	19.3 ± 2.1	0.32
Daily Macronutrient Intake [2]				
Total energy (kcal)	2373 ± 33	2218 ± 87	2060 ± 135	0.03 [3]
Carbohydrate (g)	265 ± 5 [ab]	224 ± 12 [b]	202 ± 19 [a]	<0.001
Fat (g)	97 ± 2	98 ± 4	90 ± 7	0.55
Protein (g)	105 ± 2	102 ± 4	102 ± 7	0.80

Values are means ± sem or *n* (percentages). [1] Significance based on ANOVA for continuous variables and Fisher's exact test for categorical variables; means with similar superscripts are different using a *post hoc* Tukey test. [2] Physical activity levels and nutrient intakes at baseline were the average of the baseline, 3-and 6-month recalls. [3] No means differed by post-hoc Tukey test for multiple comparisons. Abbreviations: T2D, type 2 diabetic; NH, non-Hutterite; BP Meds, hypertensive medications; MVPA, moderate-plus-vigorous physical activity.

Table 2. Anthropometrics, activity levels, and diet intake of the 411 men from the South Dakota Rural Bone Health Study cohort, according to glycemic categories after three years of follow-up.

Baseline:	**Normoglycemic**		**Prediabetic**		**Normoglycemic or Prediabetic**	**T2D**	
Follow-Up:	**Normoglycemic**	**Prediabetic**	**Normoglycemic**	**Prediabetic**	**T2D**	**T2D**	***p*-Value** [1]
Participants (*n*)	272	65	25	19	12	18	
Baseline Age (years)	41.0 ± 0.7 [ab]	42.6 ± 1.5 [c]	43.9 ± 2.6	47.1 ± 2.3	51.9 ± 2.3 [b]	53.0 ± 2.2 [ac]	<0.001
Baseline Height (cm)	177.9 ± 0.4	177.0 ± 0.8	179.4 ± 1.0	176.9 ± 2.0	175.3 ± 1.7	175.1 ± 1.7	0.17
Weight (kg)							
Baseline	90.3 ± 0.9 ‡	92.5 ± 2.0	96.1 ± 3.3	98.8 ± 3.9	100.4 ± 4.1	96.0 ± 3.1	0.01 [3]
Follow-Up	91.5 ± 0.9	93.3 ± 2.0	95.2 ± 3.4	100.1 ± 4.3	98.3 ± 4.0	96.0 ± 3.3	0.08
% Time MVPA [2]							
Baseline	21.0 ± 0.6 ‡	23.7 ± 1.2	22.6 ± 1.7	24.4 ± 2.3	26.2 ± 3.0	19.8 ± 2.1	0.11
Follow-Up	22.5 ± 0.6	22.1 ± 1.1	19.9 ± 1.6	21.9 ± 2.1	24.5 ± 2.5	22.8 ± 2.4	0.77
Daily Intake [2]							
Total Energy (kcal)							
Baseline	2344 ± 38	2435 ± 75	2284 ± 130	2140 ± 106	2248 ± 183	2067 ± 108	0.18
Follow-Up	2382 ± 38 [a]	2386 ± 81 [b]	2268 ± 102	2211 ± 95	2176 ± 189	1898 ± 132 [ab]	0.02
Carbohydrate (g)							
Baseline	263 ± 5 [a]	268 ± 11	239 ± 17	208 ± 14 ‡	233 ± 21	204 ± 15 [a]	0.003
Follow-Up	265 ± 5 [a]	267 ± 13 [b]	248 ± 16	232 ± 14	208 ± 19	186 ± 16 [ab]	0.001
Fat (g)							
Baseline	95 ± 2	102 ± 4	101 ± 7	94 ± 6	94 ± 10	91 ± 8	0.57
Follow-Up	101 ± 2 ‡	100 ± 3	95 ± 5	98 ± 6	99 ± 11	90 ± 8	0.75
Protein (g)							
Baseline	103 ± 2	107 ± 4	105 ± 7	96 ± 5	101 ± 11	101 ± 6	0.79
Follow-Up	104 ± 2	106 ± 3	105 ± 5	98 ± 5	107 ± 11	93 ± 8	0.50

Values are unadjusted means ± sem or *n* (percentages). ‡ Significant change from baseline to follow-up based on paired *t*-test. [1] Significance among glycemic categories based on ANOVA for continuous variables and Fisher's exact test for categorical variables; means with similar superscripts are different using a post hoc Tukey test. [2] Physical activity (PA) levels and nutrient intakes at baseline were the averages of the baseline, three-month, and six-month recalls, and at follow-up were the averages of 30-month, 33-month, and 36-month recalls. [3] No means differed by post hoc Tukey test for multiple comparisons. Abbreviations: T2D, type 2 diabetic; MVPA, moderate-plus-vigorous physical activity.

3.2. Cross-Sectional Assessment of Baseline Body Composition in Men with Prediabetes or Type 2 Diabetes

There were no differences in TB, trunk, or appendicular FM or LM among the three glycemic groups at baseline when covariates were included in the analyses (Table 3). Prediabetic men weighed more than normoglycemic men.

Table 3. Total body and regional body composition in the 430 men from the South Dakota Rural Bone Health Study cohort, according to glycemic status at baseline.

	Normoglycemic	Prediabetic	T2D	p-Value [1]
Participants (n)	358	51	21	
Body Weight (kg)				
Unadjusted Model	91.1 ± 0.8 [a]	98.5 ± 2.1 [a]	95.9 ± 3.3	0.003
Basic Model [2]	91.0 ± 0.8 [a]	97.0 ± 3.2 [a]	95.9 ± 3.2	0.01
Fat Mass (kg)				
Total Body				
Unadjusted Model	22.1 ± 0.5 [ab]	26.4 ± 1.2 [b]	26.7 ± 1.9 [a]	0.001
Full Model [3]	22.6 ± 0.3	24.0 ± 0.9	23.3 ± 1.5	0.38
Trunk				
Unadjusted Model	11.4 ± 0.3 [ab]	14.2 ± 0.8 [b]	15.1 ± 1.2 [a]	<0.001
Full Model [3]	11.8 ± 0.2	12.6 ± 0.5	11.8 ± 0.9	0.38
Appendicular				
Unadjusted Model	9.6 ± 0.2 [a]	11.1 ± 0.5 [a]	10.4 ± 0.8	0.01
Full Model [3]	9.7 ± 0.2	10.3 ± 0.4	10.1 ± 0.7	0.66
Lean Mass (kg)				
Total Body				
Unadjusted Model	67.0 ± 0.4	69.9 ± 1.2	66.8 ± 1.8	0.07
Full Model [4]	67.1 ± 0.3	67.9 ± 0.8	67.9 ± 1.2	0.56
Trunk				
Unadjusted Model	32.7 ± 0.2 [a]	34.5 ± 0.6 [a]	34.1 ± 0.9	0.01
Full Model [4]	32.7 ± 0.1	33.1 ± 0.4	33.8 ± 0.6	0.24
Appendicular				
Unadjusted Model	30.5 ± 0.2	31.6 ± 0.6 [a]	28.9 ± 0.9 [a]	0.04
Full Model [4]	30.5 ± 0.2	31.0 ± 0.4	30.3 ± 0.7	0.44

Data are means and marginal means ± sem. [1] p-values are from multiple regression models. Means with similar superscripts are different using a post hoc contrast test. [2] Basic model adjusted for age, height, population group, percent time in moderate-plus-vigorous activity, and average daily calories. [3] Fat mass models included covariates in basic model plus lean mass of same compartment (total body, trunk, or appendicular). [4] Lean mass models included covariates in basic model plus fat mass of same compartment. Abbreviations: T2D, type 2 diabetic.

3.3. Association between Development of Prediabetes and Type 2 Diabetes and Changes in Body Composition

Changes in body composition for the six glycemic groups are shown in Figures 2 and 3. There were differences among men who developed prediabetes or T2D and men who remained normoglycemic regarding the annual change in TB and appendicular LM. Among men who were normoglycemic at baseline, those who progressed to prediabetic lost more TB and appendicular LM than those who remained normoglycemic (Figure 3). Normoglycemic or prediabetic men who developed T2D also had greater losses in TB and appendicular LM than men who remained normoglycemic (Figure 3).

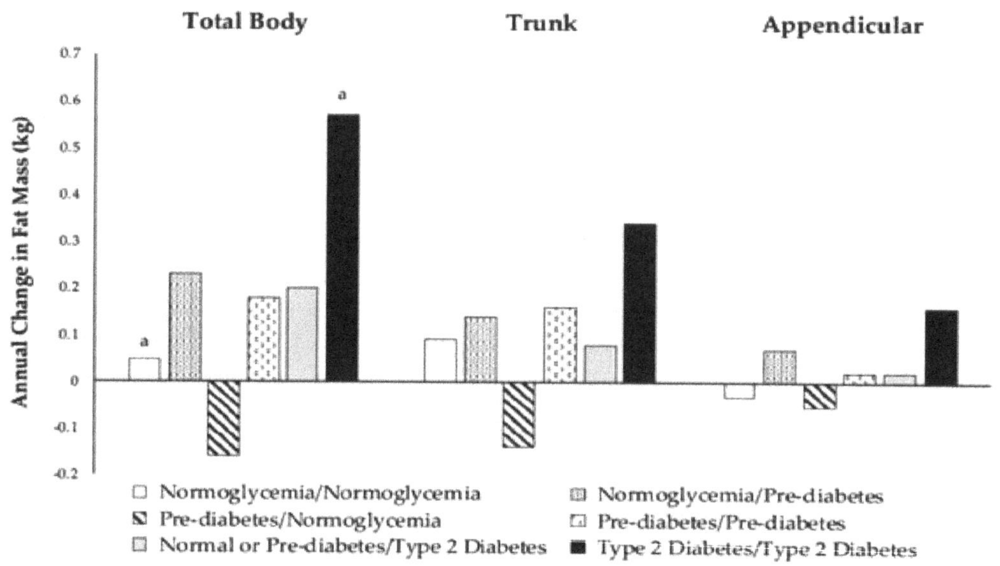

Figure 2. Adjusted marginal means of annual change from baseline in total body (p = 0.02), trunk (p = 0.06), and appendicular (p = 0.06) fat mass according to categories of glycemic status during the three-year follow-up. Model included baseline age, height, population group, percent time in moderate-plus-vigorous activity, average caloric intake, baseline measures of fat and lean mass in the specific body compartment (total body, trunk, or appendicular), changes in percent time in moderate-plus-vigorous activity and average caloric intake, and annual change in lean mass of the same compartment. Means with similar superscripts are different using post hoc contrast tests based on hypotheses.

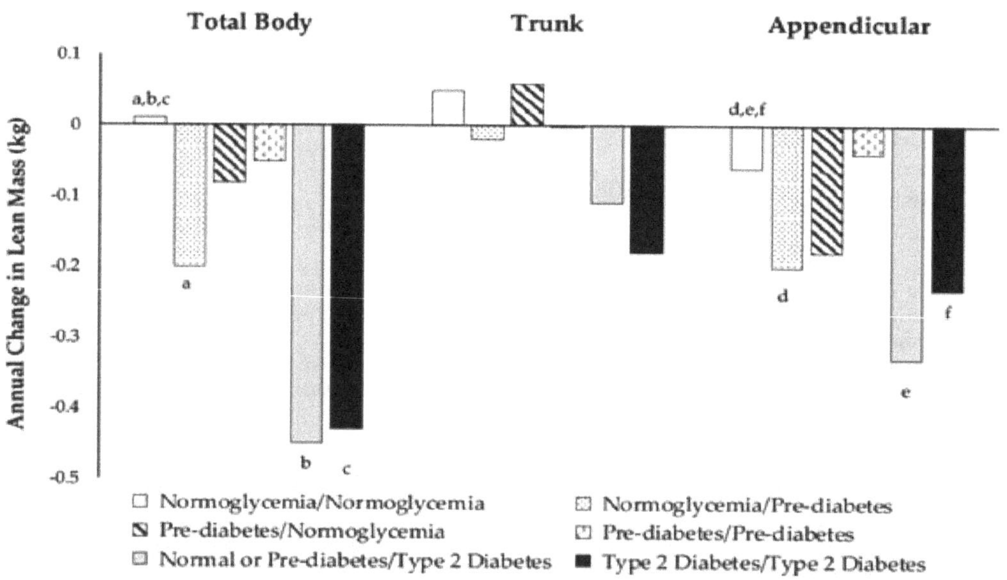

Figure 3. Adjusted marginal means of annual change from baseline in total body (p = 0.004), trunk (p = 0.24), and appendicular (p < 0.001) lean mass according to categories of glycemic status during the three-year follow-up. Model included baseline age, height, population group, percent time in moderate-plus-vigorous activity, average caloric intake, baseline measures of fat and lean mass in the specific body compartment (total body, trunk, or appendicular), changes in percent time in moderate-plus-vigorous activity and average caloric intake, and annual change in the fat mass of the same compartment. Means with similar superscripts are different using post hoc contrast tests based on hypotheses.

3.4. Changes in Body Composition among Prediabetic Men Depending on Reversion to Normoglycemia

There were no differences in the FM or LM between prediabetic men who remained prediabetic and those that reverted to normoglycemia (Figures 2 and 3). In general, prediabetic men who reverted to normoglycemia had negative changes in FM, whereas men who remained prediabetic had positive changes.

3.5. Changes in Body Composition among Type 2 Diabetic Men

Men who were T2D at baseline had greater gains in TB FM (Figure 2) and greater losses in TB and appendicular LM (Figure 3) than men who remained normoglycemic over the three-year follow-up.

4. Discussion

This is the first prospective population-based cohort study investigating the association of baseline glycemic status and changes in glycemic status over time with changes in TB, trunk, and appendicular FM and LM. Consequently, the findings of prior observational longitudinal studies cannot be compared to our findings. The findings of the current study indicate that there were no baseline differences among glycemic groups in TB, trunk, or appendicular FM and LM. Normoglycemic men who developed prediabetes or T2D had greater losses in TB and appendicular LM than men who remained normoglycemic. Men who had T2D throughout the study period had greater gains in TB FM, and greater losses in TB and appendicular LM, than men who were normoglycemic throughout the study. No differences were observed in changes in weight or body composition measures among prediabetic men who reverted to normoglycemia compared to those who remained prediabetic.

Contrary to our first hypothesis, we did not find differences in TB and regional FM and LM at baseline among the glycemic groups. The present study differs from other studies [6–8,10,22,23] due to the adjustment for covariates and inclusion of other body composition compartments (e.g., when determining whether TB FM was associated with glycemic status, TB LM was included in the statistical model). The inclusion of these covariates resulted in the relationships becoming non-significant.

Consistent with our hypothesis, normoglycemic men who developed prediabetes or T2D had greater losses in TB and appendicular LM than men who remained normoglycemic, but we found no association with changes in FM. A positive association between glucose concentrations and intermuscular adipose tissue has been reported [24], and it has been suggested that hyperglycemia stimulates the differentiation of mesenchymal stem cells derived from adipose and muscle tissues into adipocytes by activating the protein kinase C β pathway [25]. Other studies also have reported an association between hyperglycemia and reduced TB and appendicular LM in men [10]. The underlying mechanisms of the decline in LM may include elevated circulating concentrations of inflammatory markers and oxidative stress. Biomarkers of inflammation, tumor necrosis factor alpha, and C-reactive protein stimulate the loss of skeletal muscle through the activation of nuclear factor kappa B [26] and the inhibition of protein synthesis [27]. Oxidative stress contributes to a catabolic and anabolic imbalance in skeletal muscle, mitochondrial damage, and muscle atrophy and apoptosis [28]. These findings indicate that elevated inflammation markers in the presence of oxidative stress in prediabetic and T2D men can induce the loss of TB and appendicular LM. The present findings from the study support these reports.

The association of changes in prediabetes status over time with changes in body composition by compartments have not been previously investigated. A few prospective studies have examined changes in TB and appendicular FM and LM in prediabetic individuals compared to normoglycemic controls. Our findings are similar to other studies reporting no difference in longitudinal changes in TB and lower extremity LM between individuals with and without prediabetes [14,16,29]. On the contrary, others have reported a loss in TB FM and appendicular LM that was greater in prediabetics compared to their normoglycemic counterparts [14,29].

In addition to greater gains in TB FM among men with T2D than among normoglycemic men, we found a significant loss in TB and appendicular LM among men who either had T2D at baseline or developed T2D during the study compared to men who remained normoglycemic. By contrast, Park et al. [15] reported no differences in longitudinal changes in TB and appendicular FM and LM between older adults with normoglycemia and those diagnosed T2D. Our findings are consistent with longitudinal studies that have found T2D men gained TB FM and lost TB and appendicular LM [12–14]. The mechanism for fat gain and muscle loss may stem from insulin resistance in T2D. An excessive influx of free fatty acids into the systemic circulation resulting from the adipose tissue contributes to insulin resistance by increasing fat accumulation in the liver leading to decreased insulin clearance, and increasing fat accumulation in skeletal muscle by impairing glucose transport, decreasing muscle protein synthesis, and inducing muscle protein breakdown, leading to a reduced muscle surface area and insulin signaling [30,31].

The strengths of our study include the first prospective population-based study of the association between changes in glycemic status and changes in TB and regional body composition measured by DXA, our low dropout rate, and our statistical adjustment for the same body composition compartments. Our study has several limitations. The present study included predominantly white men, and our findings may not be generalizable to women or other races. The majority of the men were farmers who may have different activity patterns and dietary intake than non-farmers, which may influence the relationship between dysglycemia and body composition. However, a study conducted on a representative sample of the United States (U.S.) population reported a similar association between dysglycemia and reduced lean mass [10]. Another limitation is the sample size of some of the glycemic categories. We did not observe differences between those men who were prediabetic at baseline and remained prediabetic, or reverted to normoglycemia as we hypothesized. It is likely that our sample size ($n = 19$ and 25, respectively) was too small. Based on the observed means and standard deviations in changes in TB FM, we estimate that 72 men per group would be needed ($\alpha = 0.05$, $\beta = 0.20$). Despite the small sample size in some categories, we did observe other differences that we hypothesized, including differences in changes in TB and appendicular LM between normoglycemic men who developed prediabetes or T2D and those who remained normoglycemic throughout the study. We relied on participants' recall of diagnosis of T2D, antidiabetic medication usage, dietary intake, and physical activity. A self-reported diagnosis of T2D or the use of antidiabetic medication can lead to misclassification due to recall or reporting errors. Dietary and physical activity recalls may result in overestimation or underestimation. However, dietary intake and physical activity assessments were performed quarterly to consider seasonality. The 24-h diet recall [32] and PPAQ [19] are valid measures of dietary intake and physical activity in adults. Although this was a longitudinal study, given the period of time between measurements (three years), it is not possible to determine whether changes in glycemic status preceded changes in body composition or vice versa. Future studies should be over longer periods of time with more frequent measures of glycemic status and body composition in order to determine which factor comes first: dysglycemia or body composition changes. Only one fasting or non-fasting blood glucose measurement per visit was obtained for defining prediabetes and T2D. Although the American Diabetes Association recommends different criteria for screening for prediabetes and T2D using glycated hemoglobin, fasting blood glucose, and two-hour plasma glucose after an oral glucose tolerance test [21], numerous studies have reported that using two-hour plasma glucose test detects more cases of prediabetes and diabetes than using glycated hemoglobin or a fasting blood glucose test [33–38]; thus, we might have missed men with prediabetes and T2D using only one fasting blood glucose measurement, which would have made it more difficult to identify group differences in changes in body composition.

5. Conclusions

In conclusion, (1) there were no differences among glycemic groups in baseline TB and regional distribution of FM and LM; (2) men who were normoglycemic at baseline and developed prediabetes or

T2D had greater losses in TB and appendicular LM than men who remained normoglycemic; (3) there were no differences in changes in body weight or composition among men who were prediabetic at baseline and remained prediabetic compared to those who reverted back to normoglycemia; and (4) men who had T2D at baseline had greater gains in TB FM and greater losses in TB and appendicular LM than normoglycemic men. These findings add to a growing body of literature on the associations between changes in glycemic status and body composition.

Author Contributions: Conceptualization, K.A. and B.S.; Data curation, M.M., T.L.B., T.M.B. and B.S.; Formal analysis, K.A. and B.S.; Funding acquisition, B.S.; Investigation, M.M., T.L.B., T.M.B. and B.S.; Methodology, T.L.B. and B.S.; Project administration, M.M., T.L.B., T.M.B. and B.S.; Resources, B.S.; Software, T.L.B., T.M.B. and B.S.; Supervision, M.M., T.L.B., T.M.B. and B.S.; Validation, M.M. and T.L.B.; Visualization, K.A. and B.S.; Writing—original draft, K.A. and B.S.; Writing—review & editing, M.M., T.L.B., T.M.B. and B.S. All authors read and approved the final manuscript.

Acknowledgments: We would like to acknowledge the willingness and time the participants contributed to this research.

References

1. Cowie, C.C.; Rust, K.F.; Ford, E.S.; Eberhardt, M.S.; Byrd-Holt, D.D.; Li, C.; Williams, D.E.; Gregg, E.W.; Bainbridge, K.E.; Saydah, S.H. Full accounting of diabetes and pre-diabetes in the US population in 1988–1994 and 2005–2006. *Diabetes Care* **2009**, *32*, 287–294. [CrossRef] [PubMed]
2. Centers for Disease Control and Prevention. *National Diabetes Statistics Report: Estimates of Diabetes and its Burden in the United States, 2014*; US Department of Health and Human Services: Atlanta, GA, USA, 2014.
3. Centers for Disease Control and Prevention. Prediabetes: Could It Be You? Available online: http://www.cdc.gov/diabetes/pubs/images/prediabetes-inforgraphic.jpg (accessed on 12 July 2017).
4. O'Brien, M.J.; Whitaker, R.C.; Yu, D.; Ackermann, R.T. The comparative efficacy of lifestyle intervention and metformin by educational attainment in the Diabetes Prevention Program. *Prev. Med.* **2015**, *77*, 125–130. [CrossRef] [PubMed]
5. Steeves, J.A.; Murphy, R.A.; Crainiceanu, C.M.; Zipunnikov, V.; Van Domelen, D.R.; Harris, T.B. Daily patterns of physical activity by type 2 diabetes definition: Comparing diabetes, prediabetes, and participants with normal glucose levels in nhanes 2003–2006. *Prev. Med. Rep.* **2015**, *2*, 152–157. [CrossRef] [PubMed]
6. Rabijewski, M.; Papierska, L.; Piątkiewicz, P. The relationships between anabolic hormones and body composition in middle-aged and elderly men with prediabetes: A cross-sectional study. *J. Diabetes Res.* **2016**, *2016*. [CrossRef] [PubMed]
7. Heshka, S.; Ruggiero, A.; Bray, G.A.; Foreyt, J.; Kahn, S.E.; Lewis, C.E.; Saad, M.; Schwartz, A.V. Altered body composition in type 2 diabetes mellitus. *Int. J. Obes. (Lond.)* **2008**, *32*, 780–787. [CrossRef] [PubMed]
8. Azuma, K.; Heilbronn, L.K.; Albu, J.B.; Smith, S.R.; Ravussin, E.; Kelley, D.E. Adipose tissue distribution in relation to insulin resistance in type 2 diabetes mellitus. *Am. J. Physiol. Endocrinol. Metab.* **2007**, *293*, E435–E442. [CrossRef] [PubMed]
9. Leenders, M.; Verdijk, L.B.; van der Hoeven, L.; Adam, J.J.; van Kranenburg, J.; Nilwik, R.; van Loon, L.J. Patients with type 2 diabetes show a greater decline in muscle mass, muscle strength, and functional capacity with aging. *J. Am. Med. Dir. Assoc.* **2013**, *14*, 585–592. [CrossRef] [PubMed]
10. Kalyani, R.R.; Tra, Y.; Egan, J.; Ferrucci, L.; Brancati, F. Hyperglycemia is associated with relatively lower lean body mass in older adults. *J. Nutr. Health Aging* **2014**, *18*, 737–743. [CrossRef] [PubMed]
11. Lee, C.G.; Boyko, E.J.; Strotmeyer, E.S.; Lewis, C.E.; Cawthon, P.M.; Hoffman, A.R.; Everson-Rose, S.A.; Barrett-Connor, E.; Orwoll, E.S. Association between insulin resistance and lean mass loss and fat mass gain in older men without diabetes mellitus. *J. Am. Geriatr. Soc.* **2011**, *59*, 1217–1224. [CrossRef] [PubMed]
12. Pownall, H.J.; Bray, G.A.; Wagenknecht, L.E.; Walkup, M.P.; Heshka, S.; Hubbard, V.S.; Hill, J.; Kahn, S.E.; Nathan, D.M.; Schwartz, A.V. Changes in body composition over 8 years in a randomized trial of a lifestyle intervention: The Look Ahead Study. *Obesity* **2015**, *23*, 565–572. [CrossRef] [PubMed]
13. Pownall, H.J.; Schwartz, A.V.; Bray, G.A.; Berkowitz, R.I.; Lewis, C.E.; Boyko, E.J.; Jakicic, J.M.; Chen, H.; Heshka, S.; Gregg, E.W. Changes in regional body composition over 8 years in a randomized lifestyle trial: The Look Ahead Study. *Obesity* **2016**, *24*, 1899–1905. [CrossRef] [PubMed]

14. Lee, C.G.; Boyko, E.J.; Barrett-Connor, E.; Miljkovic, I.; Hoffman, A.R.; Everson-Rose, S.A.; Lewis, C.E.; Cawthon, P.M.; Strotmeyer, E.S.; Orwoll, E.S. Insulin sensitizers may attenuate lean mass loss in older men with diabetes. *Diabetes Care* **2011**, *34*, 2381–2386. [CrossRef] [PubMed]
15. Park, S.W.; Goodpaster, B.H.; Lee, J.S.; Kuller, L.H.; Boudreau, R.; De Rekeneire, N.; Harris, T.B.; Kritchevsky, S.; Tylavsky, F.A.; Nevitt, M. Excessive loss of skeletal muscle mass in older adults with type 2 diabetes. *Diabetes Care* **2009**, *32*, 1993–1997. [CrossRef] [PubMed]
16. Kalyani, R.R.; Metter, E.J.; Egan, J.; Golden, S.H.; Ferrucci, L. Hyperglycemia predicts persistently lower muscle strength with aging. *Diabetes Care* **2015**, *38*, 82–90. [CrossRef] [PubMed]
17. Specker, B.; Binkley, T.; Fahrenwald, N. Rural versus nonrural differences in BMC, volumetric BMD, and bone size: A population-based cross-sectional study. *Bone* **2004**, *35*, 1389–1398. [CrossRef] [PubMed]
18. Paffenbarger, R.S.; Wing, A.L.; Hyde, R.T. Physical activity as an index of heart attack risk in college alumni. *Am. J. Epidemiol.* **1978**, *108*, 161–175. [CrossRef] [PubMed]
19. Simpson, K.; Parker, B.; Capizzi, J.; Thompson, P.; Clarkson, P.; Freedson, P.; Pescatello, L.S. Validity and reliability question 8 of the Paffenbarger physical activity questionnaire among healthy adults. *J. Phys. Act. Health* **2015**, *12*, 116–123. [CrossRef] [PubMed]
20. Samra, H.A.; Beare, T.; Specker, B. Pedometer readings and self-reported walking distances in a rural Hutterite population. *J. Rural Health* **2008**, *24*, 99–100. [CrossRef] [PubMed]
21. American Diabetes Association. Classification and diagnosis of diabetes. Sec. 2. In standards of medical care in diabetes—2015. *Diabetes Care* **2015**, *38*, S8–S16.
22. Kim, T.N.; Park, M.S.; Yang, S.J.; Yoo, H.J.; Kang, H.J.; Song, W.; Seo, J.A.; Kim, S.G.; Kim, N.H.; Baik, S.H. Prevalence and determinant factors of sarcopenia in patients with type 2 diabetes: The Korean Sarcopenic Obesity Study (KSOS). *Diabetes Care* **2010**, *33*, 1497–1499. [CrossRef] [PubMed]
23. Julian, V.; Blondel, R.; Pereira, B.; Thivel, D.; Boirie, Y.; Duclos, M. Body composition is altered in pre-diabetic patients with impaired fasting glucose tolerance: Results from the NHANES survey. *J. Clin. Med. Res.* **2017**, *9*, 917–925. [CrossRef] [PubMed]
24. Yim, J.; Heshka, S.; Albu, J.; Heymsfield, S.; Kuznia, P.; Harris, T.; Gallagher, D. Intermuscular adipose tissue rivals visceral adipose tissue in independent associations with cardiovascular risk. *Int. J. Obes. (Lond.)* **2007**, *31*, 1400–1405. [CrossRef] [PubMed]
25. Aguiari, P.; Leo, S.; Zavan, B.; Vindigni, V.; Rimessi, A.; Bianchi, K.; Franzin, C.; Cortivo, R.; Rossato, M.; Vettor, R. High glucose induces adipogenic differentiation of muscle-derived stem cells. *Proc. Natl. Acad. Sci. USA* **2008**, *105*, 1226–1231. [CrossRef] [PubMed]
26. Li, Y.-P.; Reid, M.B. Nf-κb mediates the protein loss induced by TNF-α in differentiated skeletal muscle myotubes. *Am. J. Physiol. Regul. Integr. Comp. Physiol.* **2000**, *279*, R1165–R1170. [CrossRef] [PubMed]
27. Wåhlin-Larsson, B.; Wilkinson, D.J.; Strandberg, E.; Hosford-Donovan, A.; Atherton, P.J.; Kadi, F. Mechanistic links underlying the impact of c-reactive protein on muscle mass in elderly. *Cell Physiol. Biochem.* **2017**, *44*, 267–278. [CrossRef] [PubMed]
28. Bianchi, L.; Volpato, S. Muscle dysfunction in type 2 diabetes: A major threat to patient's mobility and independence. *Acta Diabetol.* **2016**, *53*, 879–889. [CrossRef] [PubMed]
29. Piaggi, P.; Thearle, M.S.; Bogardus, C.; Krakoff, J. Fasting hyperglycemia predicts lower rates of weight gain by increased energy expenditure and fat oxidation rate. *J. Clin. Endocrinol. Metab.* **2015**, *100*, 1078–1087. [CrossRef] [PubMed]
30. Frayn, K.N. Visceral fat and insulin resistance—causative or correlative? *Br. J. Nutr.* **2000**, *83*, S71–S77. [CrossRef] [PubMed]
31. Brøns, C.; Grunnet, L.G. Mechanisms in endocrinology: Skeletal muscle lipotoxicity in insulin resistance and type 2 diabetes: A causal mechanism or an innocent bystander? *Eur. J. Endocrinol.* **2017**, *176*, R67–R78. [CrossRef] [PubMed]
32. Conway, J.M.; Ingwersen, L.A.; Moshfegh, A.J. Accuracy of dietary recall using the USDA five-step multiple-pass method in men: An observational validation study. *J. Am. Diet. Assoc.* **2004**, *104*, 595–603. [CrossRef] [PubMed]
33. Menke, A.; Casagrande, S.; Geiss, L.; Cowie, C.C. Prevalence of and trends in diabetes among adults in the United States, 1988–2012. *JAMA* **2015**, *314*, 1021–1029. [CrossRef] [PubMed]

34. Menke, A.; Rust, K.F.; Cowie, C.C. Diabetes based on 2-h plasma glucose among those classified as having prediabetes based on fasting plasma glucose or A1c. *Diab. Vasc. Dis. Res.* **2018**, *15*, 46–54. [CrossRef] [PubMed]
35. Cowie, C.C.; Rust, K.F.; Byrd-Holt, D.D.; Eberhardt, M.S.; Flegal, K.M.; Engelgau, M.M.; Saydah, S.H.; Williams, D.E.; Geiss, L.S.; Gregg, E.W. Prevalence of diabetes and impaired fasting glucose in adults in the US population. *Diabetes Care* **2006**, *29*, 1263–1268. [CrossRef] [PubMed]
36. Cowie, C.C.; Rust, K.F.; Byrd-Holt, D.D.; Gregg, E.W.; Ford, E.S.; Geiss, L.S.; Bainbridge, K.E.; Fradkin, J.E. Prevalence of diabetes and high risk for diabetes using A1c criteria in the US population in 1988–2006. *Diabetes Care* **2010**, *33*, 562–568. [CrossRef] [PubMed]
37. DECODE Study Group. Age-and sex-specific prevalences of diabetes and impaired glucose regulation in 13 European cohorts1. *Diabetes Care* **2003**, *26*, 61–69. [CrossRef]
38. NCD Risk Factor Collaboration. Effects of diabetes definition on global surveillance of diabetes prevalence and diagnosis: A pooled analysis of 96 population-based studies with 331 288 participants. *Lancet Diabetes Endocrinol.* **2015**, *3*, 624–637. [CrossRef]

6

Nutrient Patterns Associated with Fasting Glucose and Glycated Haemoglobin Levels in a Black South African Population

Tinashe Chikowore [1,*], Pedro T. Pisa [2], Tertia van Zyl [1], Edith J. M. Feskens [3], Edelweiss Wentzel-Viljoen [1,4] and Karin R. Conradie [1]

1 Centre for Excellence in Nutrition, North-West University, Potchefstroom 2520, North West Province, South Africa; tertia.vanzyl@nwu.ac.za (T.v.Z.); edelweiss-wentzel-viljoen@nwu.ac.za (E.W.-V.); karin.conradie@nwu.ac.za (K.R.C.)
2 Wits Reproductive Health and HIV Institute, University of the Witwatersrand, Johannesburg 2000, South Africa; ppisa@wrhi.ac.za
3 Division of Human Nutrition, Wageningen University, P.O. Box 17, 6700 AA Wageningen, The Netherlands; edith.feskens@wur.nl
4 Medical Research Council Research Unit for Hypertension and Cardiovascular Disease, Faculty of Health Sciences, North-West University, Potchefstroom 2520, South Africa
* Correspondence: tinashedoc@gmail.com

Abstract: Type 2 diabetes (T2D) burden is increasing globally. However, evidence regarding nutrient patterns associated with the biomarkers of T2D is limited. This study set out to determine the nutrient patterns associated with fasting glucose and glycated haemoglobin the biomarkers of T2D. Factor analysis was used to derive nutrient patterns of 2010 participants stratified by urban/rural status and gender. Principal Component Analysis (PCA) was applied to 25 nutrients, computed from the quantified food frequency questionnaires (QFFQ). Three nutrient patterns per stratum, which accounted for 73% of the variation of the selected nutrients, were identified. Multivariate linear regression models adjusted for age, BMI, smoking, physical activity, education attained, alcohol intake, seasonality and total energy intake were computed. Starch, dietary fibre and B vitamins driven nutrient pattern was significantly associated with fasting glucose ($\beta = -0.236$ (-0.458; -0.014); $p = 0.037$) and glycated haemoglobin levels ($\beta = -0.175$ (-0.303; -0.047); $p = 0.007$) in rural women. Thiamine, zinc and plant protein driven nutrient pattern was associated with significant reductions in glycated haemoglobin and fasting glucose (($\beta = -0.288$ (-0.543; -0.033); $p = 0.027$) and ($\beta = -0.382$ (-0.752; -0.012); $p = 0.043$), respectively) in rural men. Our results indicate that plant driven nutrient patterns are associated with low fasting glucose and glycated haemoglobin levels.

Keywords: plant based; fasting glucose and glycated haemoglobin; T2D; dietary patterns

---

1. Introduction

Type 2 diabetes (T2D) prevalence and the burden it places on populations is increasing globally, thereby making it a public health challenge which requires urgent attention [1]. For instance, the global prevalence of T2D among women increased from 5% to 7.9% from 1980 to 2014 [2]. The diabetes prevalence in Africa is projected to have the largest increase of 109% compared to other regions in the world by 2035 [3]. Urban black South Africans have not been spared from the T2D burden. The highest prevalence of T2D in Sub Saharan Africa was reported among urban black South Africans, with 60% of these cases being reported amongst women [4]. Black South African women also have the highest prevalence of obesity, which has been reported to be rising together with T2D in this population [5].

The adoption of Westernised lifestyles by urban dwellers is suggested to be among the leading factors resulting in the increase in non-communicable diseases (NCDs) such as T2D in developing countries [6]. The migration of populations from rural to urban areas has been accompanied by an increase in meat consumption as well as an increase in the consumption of sugary foods in South Africa [7]. Both of these foods are recognised as dietary risk factors for T2D [6]. However, improvements in micronutrient intake among black South African women in urban areas is suggested to be a result of the increased consumption of fruits and vegetables which are protective of T2D risk [8–10]. Thus, the role of diet as a risk factor for T2D is complex among the black South African women. In addition, people eat meals with a variety of nutrients which have interactive and synergistic effects on health [11]. Therefore, it is difficult to determine the separate effect of a food or nutrient on disease development as it is highly interrelated with other nutrients [11]. There is need of dietary pattern analysis methods which are able to evaluate the diet as a whole and clarify the effects of the consumption of sugary foods and meat products, together with improved intakes of fruits and vegetables, related to T2D risk amongst this population group.

Dietary pattern (or food pattern) approaches comprise data driven methods such as factor analysis, which allow the dietary information (or food intake) at hand to determine the unique dietary pattern for the population group being evaluated [10]. Although dietary patterns have been associated with disease risk, their effect is considered to be through nutrient intake; therefore, it is pivotal to determine nutrient patterns that are associated with T2D risk [12]. This information will aid in the understanding of the aetiology of T2D. The foods that people eat are governed by their cultural norms and beliefs, which vary amongst ethnic groups, making dietary patterns limited and not applicable across divergent population groups [12]. Evidence exists that the Western dietary pattern association with fasting glucose varies among different ethnic groups [13]. However, nutrients are universal, thereby making nutrient patterns associations with disease risk applicable for multiple population groups [14]. To the best of our knowledge, no study has reported on the association of the nutrient patterns with fasting glucose and glycated haemoglobin levels among apparently healthy individuals. T2D is a complex and multifactorial diseases, however glycated haemoglobin and fasting glucose levels are proxies for the development of this disease which are affected by diet [15]. Fasting glucose levels are indicative of the short term changes in glucose metabolism, while glycated haemoglobin depicts the long term changes [15]. This study seeks to evaluate the association of nutrient patterns derived by factor analysis with fasting glucose and glycated haemoglobin levels among apparently healthy black South Africans.

2. Materials and Methods

2.1. Study Population

The study participants (n = 2010) were recruited from two urban and rural areas of the North West Province into the South African arm of the Prospective urban and rural epidemiological (PURE) study using a population based sampling strategy. Apparently healthy male and female volunteers between the ages of 35 and 60 years were recruited by the fieldworkers. Individuals were considered to be apparently healthy if they were not using any medication for chronic disease and if they were not diagnosed with a chronic medical condition/disease. The international PURE study is a large-scale epidemiological study, which comprises research participants recruited from 17 low, middle, and high income countries [16]. The South African arm of the PURE study was initiated in 2005 with initial five-year follow-up intervals up to 2015. At baseline in 2005 and at the five-year intervals during the course of the study, medical history, lifestyle behaviour (physical activity and dietary intake), blood collection (for both genetic and biochemical analyses), an electrocardiogram, and anthropometric assessments were performed to determine the role of risk factors in the development of cardiovascular diseases [16]. Our study was nested in the 2005 PURE study baseline data. Stratified nutrient pattern analysis was conducted according to gender and urban/rural status among the 2010 participants of the PURE study. However, significant associations of the nutrient patterns with fasting glucose and glycated haemoglobin were noted only among the rural women and rural men. Therefore, the detailed nutrient pattern and association results of the rural participants are elaborated in the main text while results of the urban men and women are illustrated in the Supplementary Materials.

2.2. Ethical Approval

The participants gave written informed consent before participating in the study and the study was conducted according to the Declaration of Helsinki principles [17]. Ethical approval was granted by the Ethics Committee of the North-West University, Potchefstroom Campus, with ethics number NWU-00016-10-A1.

2.3. Dietary, Anthropometric and Physical Activity Assessments

The trained fieldworkers captured the dietary intake of the participants using a standardised quantitative food frequency questionnaire (QFFQ) which had been validated for the same ethnic population group of the study participants [18,19]. The reproducibility of the QFFQ was also assessed and found to be good in this specific study population [20]. The dietary intake data were coded, analysed and nutrient intakes were computed using the South African Food Composition Database [21]. Body weight measurements were performed in duplicate by the PURE research team members using a portable electronic scale (Precision Health Scale, A & D Company, Tokyo, Japan), after which the mean was recorded. The heights of the subjects were determined by the PURE study research team members using a stadiometer (IP 1465, Invicta, and London, UK). The BMI of the participants was computed using the formula: BMI = weight (kg/height (m^2)). The Baecke physical activity questionnaire (BPAQ) which was validated for South Africa was used to collect the physical activity information of the participants [22]. The questionnaire was used to compute a physical activity index score as described elsewhere [22,23]. This physical activity index scores were used in the multivariate regression analysis to adjust for physical activity.

2.4. Biochemical Measurements

The research participants were required to fast (at least 8 h with no food or beverages, including water before measurements) and their blood glucose levels were measured by the PURE research team. These fasting glucose levels were measured using the SYNCHRON® System from fluoride plasma. The Bio-Rad D-10™, HbA1c kit (Bio-Rad Laboratories, Inc., Hercules, France), which operates via cation exchange high performance liquid chromatography was used to assess HbA1c levels from whole blood ethylenediaminetetraacetic acid (EDTA) treated samples. The coefficient of variation of the glycated haemoglobin and fasting glucose tests were 1.16% and 2.1%, respectively.

2.5. Statistical Analysis

The statistical analysis was performed using the statistical package for social scientists (SPSS) version 23. Normality tests for the continuous variables were performed using the Q-Q plots. Twenty-five nutrients were used to determine the nutrient patterns as has been reported previously by Pisa et al. [24]. Among these 25 nutrients, total protein was split into animal protein and plant protein; total carbohydrates were divided into total sugar, starch, and total dietary fibre; and total fat was categorised into saturated fat, monounsaturated fat and polyunsaturated fat. The total dietary fibre comprised soluble and insoluble dietary fibre. Alcohol was not regarded as a nutrient and not included in deriving the nutrient pattern analysis. However, in view of the reported association of alcohol intake with glycated haemoglobin, it was adjusted for in the multivariate linear models for the association of the derived nutrient patterns with glycated haemoglobin and fasting glucose [25]. The nutrient intake variables from the quantitative food frequency questionnaire (QFFQ) were log transformed to remove bias due to variance as a result of the different measures of scale used to quantify the nutrients. These nutrients were adjusted for log alcohol free energy using the multivariate (standard) method [11]. The multivariate method was selected as it yielded more cumulative variance and interpretable nutrient patterns compared to the standard nutrient density method of adjusting for total energy intake [11]. Principal component analysis (PCA) was the factor reduction tool used to determine the nutrient patterns from the 25 selected nutrients. The PCA was performed with the variance based on the covariance matrix and Varimax rotation. The retained principal components (PC) were used to identify the nutrient patterns. The scree plot (Figure 1) was used to determine the number of PCs to retain. The nutrient patterns were named using the nutrients with loadings greater than ±0.47 on the PCs. The total variances explained by the retained PCs were also evaluated to determine the relevance of the extracted PCs. The PCA was a suitable data reduction approach for the nutrient data in this study as was indicated by a Kaiser–Meyer–Olkin measure of sampling adequacy of 0.911, and a Bartlett's test of sphericity which was significant at $p < 0.001$. The PCs were categorised into tertiles and analysis of variance ANOVA (for continuous variables) and Chi-square (for categorical variables) tests were used to determine the descriptive characteristics of the study participants across the tertiles of the extracted PCs.

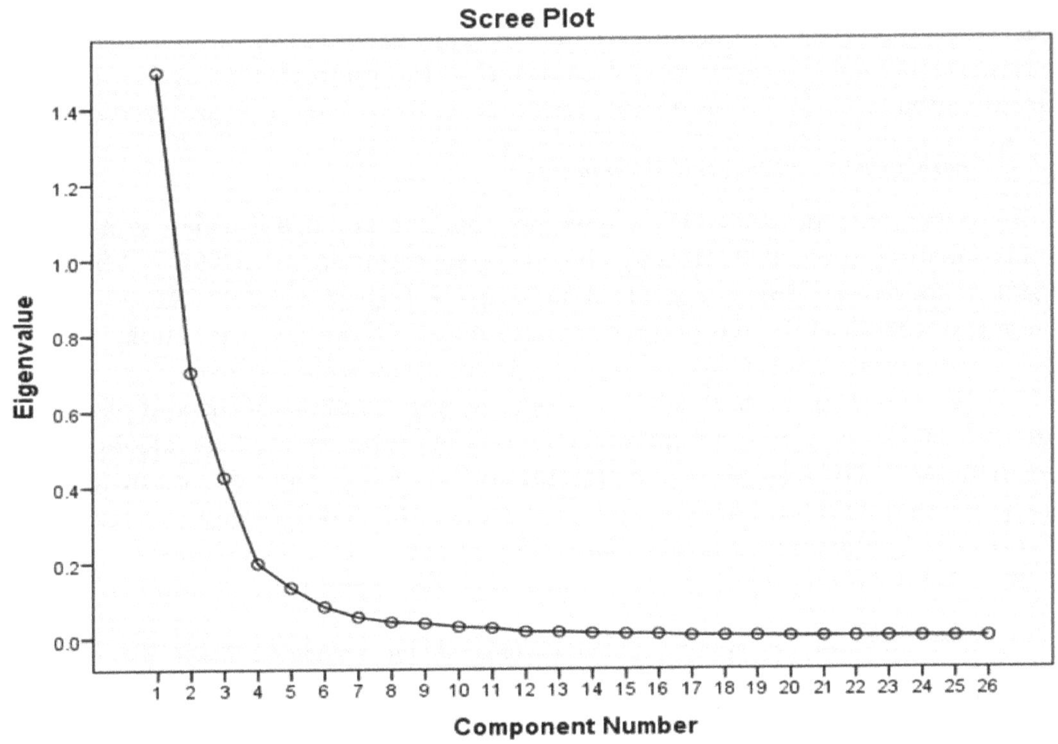

Figure 1. Scree plot of the nutrients and the extracted principal components among rural women.

Crude and adjusted multiple linear regression models were computed to assess the association between the extracted PCs with glycated haemoglobin and fasting glucose as dependent variables separately through varied models. In these models, regression coefficients for 1 standard deviation (SD) increase in the PC scores (and their 95% confidence intervals) were computed for four models: M1: (crude); M2: (adjusted for M1 plus Log Total Energy); M3: (adjusted for M2 plus Body Mass Index); and M4: (adjusted for M3 plus age, smoking, physical activity, education level, seasonality, alcohol intake and other PCs). Seasonality was adjusted based on the months in which the dietary assessments were conducted. Thus, for the rural participants, seasonality was adjusted basing on August and September; and the months of October and November were used to adjust for seasonality in the urban participants. Partial R^2 values were computed to express the variance explained by each model. Statistical significance was regarded at p value less than 0.05.

3. Results

3.1. Nutrient Patterns

Three nutrient patterns (Table S1) were extracted from the PCA, which explained 73% of the total variation of the selected nutrient factors among the rural women. The first nutrient pattern was depicted as "Magnesium, phosphorus and plant protein driven nutrients". This pattern consisted of higher loadings for magnesium, phosphorus and plant protein. The second nutrient pattern was termed "Fat and animal protein driven nutrients" as it had higher loadings of cholesterol, monounsaturated fat, animal protein, polyunsaturated fat and saturated fat. The "Starch, dietary fibre and B vitamins driven" based nutrient pattern was the third extracted nutrient pattern. This nutrient pattern had high loadings of starch, folate, vitamin B6, dietary fibre and thiamine as illustrated in Table S1.

Three nutrient patterns were extracted among rural men and named according to the nutrients with the highest loadings as indicated in Table S1. These were the "Thiamine, zinc and plant protein driven nutrients", "Fat and animal protein driven nutrients", and "Retinol and vitamin B12 driven nutrients". Three similar nutrients patterns were extracted among the rural men, urban men and urban women, which explained 76%, 77% and 76% (Tables S1 and S2) variance of the nutrients, respectively. However, some considerable differences were noted in the plant driven nutrient patterns, which accounted for the greater variation of the nutrients among the urban and rural participants (Table S3).

3.2. Descriptive Characteristics of the Study Population

The study participants included 659 rural women, 347 rural men, 605 urban women and 399 urban men. The mean fasting glucose levels and glycated haemoglobin were 4.96 $\pm$ 1.57 mmol·L^{-1} and 5.64% $\pm$ 0.88%, respectively [26]. The women had a mean BMI of 26.73 $\pm$ 7.21, which signified that a considerable proportion of the women were overweight. Overall, in the whole study population, 39.4% of the participants were overweight and 87.3% of these were women. The mean total energy intake was 7707.13 $\pm$ 3692.36 KJ. The high scores of magnesium, phosphorus and plant protein driven nutrient pattern were associated with high total energy intake and energy from alcohol in rural women, as indicated in Table 1. The high scores for the fat and animal protein driven nutrient pattern was significantly associated with tertiary education status, as indicated inTable 1.

High scores for the thiamine, zinc and plant protein nutrient pattern were associated with higher energy and alcohol intake compared to other nutrient patterns among the rural men (Table 2).

3.3. Nutrient Patterns Associations with Fasting and Glycated Haemoglobin Levels

The association results of glycated haemoglobin and fasting glucose levels with 1 SD increases in the extracted nutrient patterns are shown in Tables 3–6 for the rural women and rural men. The magnesium, phosphorus and plant protein driven nutrient pattern was associated with a consistent trend of increases in fasting glucose and glycated haemoglobin among rural women, as illustrated in Table 3.

Conversely, the starch, dietary fibre and B vitamins nutrient pattern was consistently associated with reduced glycated haemoglobin and fasting glucose levels in all evaluated linear models, for instance the M4 model: -0.175% (-0.303; -0.047); $p = 0.007$) and -0.236 mmol·L^{-1} (-0.458; -0.014); $p = 0.037$), respectively, as indicated in Tables 3 and 4 among rural women.

The thiamine, zinc and plant protein nutrient pattern was associated with reduced glycated haemoglobin and fasting glucose levels in rural men as illustrated in Tables 5 and 6. For instance, the M4 models, which explained the highest variances of the fasting glucose and glycated haemoglobin, indicated reductions of these outcome variables to be -0.382 mmol·L^{-1} (-0.752; -0.012; $p = 0.043$) and -0.288% (-0.543; -0.033; $p = 0.027$), respectively, as illustrated in Tables 5 and 6.

Table 1. Descriptive characteristics for the rural women of the study population according to the lowest and highest tertiles of the three nutrient patterns (PC).

	Magnesium, Phosphorus and Plant Protein Driven Nutrients			Fat and Animal Protein Driven Nutrients			Starch, Dietary Fibre and B Vitamin Driven Nutrients		
	T1	T3	*p*	T1	T3	*p*	T1	T3	*p*
Age	48.72 ± 10.23	47.51 ± 9.57	0.247	47.94 ± 8.89	47.73 ± 10.16	0.837	49.15 ± 10.40	46.94 ± 8.99	0.036
Body Mass Index	25.28 ± 6.63	25.27 ± 6.58	0.988	25.31 ± 6.75	26.13 ± 6.85	0.262	25.26 ± 6.41	25.65 ± 7.11	0.605
Total energy	4322.96 ± 1217.30	8365.01 ± 2476.92	<0.001	5631.33 ± 2816.62	6883.88 ± 2189.38	<0.001	5893.08 ± 2645.21	6567.51 ± 2425.60	0.013
Alcohol (%TE)	0.76 ± 2.56	7.42 ± 12.56	<0.001	5.54 ± 11.70	1.47 ± 4.40	<0.001	5.36 ± 11.91	1.69 ± 5.01	<0.001
Protein (%TE)	11.26 ± 1.96	10.77 ± 1.64	0.008	10.27 ± 1.33	11.67 ± 1.81	<0.001	11.23 ± 2.05	10.91 ± 1.31	0.092
Current Smokers (%)	33.5	36.8	0.168	38.0	34.7	0.005	30.6	36.4	0.595
Physical Activity Index	8.19 ± 1.42	8.28 ± 1.42	0.593	8.29 ± 1.29	8.32 ± 1.55	0.854	8.23 ± 1.37	8.44 ± 1.45	0.205
Tertiary education (%)	33.7	24.5	0.058	26.5	42.9	0.028	28.6	38.8	0.854
Fasting glucose (mmol·L^{-1})	4.73 ± 0.78	4.93 ± 1.47	0.219	4.91 ± 1.18	4.87 ± 1.02	0.784	5.12 ± 2.41	4.88 ± 0.83	0.160
HbA1C (%)	5.64 ± 0.53	5.67 ± 0.93	0.785	5.68 ± 0.91	5.69 ± 0.58	0.843	5.84 ± 1.23	5.62 ± 0.55	0.027

p = *p* value based on ANOVA or Chi-square test where appropriate; Alcohol (%TE) = percentage of total energy due to alcohol intake; Protein (%TE) = percentage of total energy due to protein intake; T1 = lowest tertile; T3 = highest tertile, TE = total energy; HbA1C = glycated haemoglobin.

Table 2. Descriptive characteristics for the rural men of the study population according to the lowest and highest tertiles of the three nutrient patterns (PC).

	Thiamine, Zinc and Plant Protein Driven Nutrients			Fat and Animal Protein Driven Nutrients			Retinol and Vitamin B12 Driven Nutrients		
	T1	T3	*p*	T1	T3	*p*	T1	T3	*p*
Age	47.95 ± 9.99	50.19 ± 10.69	0.156	48.43 ± 9.97	51.42 ± 11.45	0.057	49.66 ± 10.01	49.57 ± 9.95	0.954
Body Mass Index	20.86 ± 4.15	20.54 ± 4.31	0.606	20.86 ± 3.99	20.94 ± 4.65	0.894	20.30 ± 3.57	20.95 ± 4.19	0.297
Total energy	4693.60 ± 1584.26	10,637.00 ± 2887.76	<0.001	6319.63 ± 3228.51	8220.85 ± 3228.51	<0.001	7164.14 ± 2975.31	7855.83 ± 3672.65	0.159
Alcohol (%TE)	5.98 ± 9.40	13.82 ± 13.70	<0.001	11.19 ± 13.41	5.70 ± 9.16	0.002	6.65 ± 11.23	9.19 ± 11.79	0.159
Protein (%TE)	11.51 ± 2.69	10.76 ± 1.53	0.014	10.09 ± 1.43	12.19 ± 2.33	<0.001	10.64 ± 1.69	11.50 ± 2.48	0.005
Current Smokers (%)	32.4	35.9	0.636	40.0	26.2	0.003	31.7	31.7	0.577
Physical Activity Index	8.25 ± 1.64	8.02 ± 1.44	0.380	8.03 ± 1.65	7.99 ± 1.79	0.861	7.92 ± 1.61	7.97 ± 1.63	0.847
Tertiary education (%)	44.2	20.9	0.141	23.3	37.2	0.514	27.9	37.2	0.451
Fasting glucose (mmol·L^{-1})	4.90 ± 0.93	4.68 ± 0.90	0.113	4.75 ± 0.79	4.96 ± 1.24	0.138	4.94 ± 2.41	4.75 ± 0.78	0.190
HbA1C (%)	5.59 ± 0.52	5.51 ± 0.81	0.386	5.49 ± 0.34	5.62 ± 0.97	0.169	5.57 ± 0.83	5.53 ± 0.49	0.678

p = *p* value based on ANOVA or Chi-square test where appropriate; Alcohol (%TE) = percentage of total energy due to alcohol intake; Protein (%TE) = percentage of total energy due to protein intake; T1 = lowest tertile; T3 = highest tertile; TE = total energy; HbA1C = glycated haemoglobin.

Table 3. Regression coefficients for fasting glucose for 1 SD increase in the derived nutrient pattern scores among rural black South African women.

	Magnesium, Phosphorus and Plant Protein Driven Nutrients			Fat and Animal Protein Driven Nutrients			Starch, Dietary Fibre and B Vitamin Driven Nutrients		
	B (95% CI)	*p* Value	R^2	B (95% CI)	*p* Value	R^2	B (95% CI)	*p* Value	R^2
M1	0.129 (−0.014; 0.271)	0.077	0.007	0.009 (−0.141; 0.160)	0.902	0.000	−0.164 (−0.311; −0.018)	0.027	0.008
M2	0.196 (−0.063; 0.455)	0.138	0.007	−0.020 (−0.183; 0.143)	0.813	0.003	−0.197 (−0.349; −0.049)	0.011	0.016
M3	0.278 (−0.001; 0.280)	0.034	0.045	−0.038 (−0.198; 0.123)	0.645	0.037	−0.203 (−0.351; −0.054)	0.008	0.051
M4	0.147 (−0.360; 0.655)	0.569	0.086	−0.004 (−0.290; 0.281)	0.976	0.086	−0.236 (−0.458; −0.014)	0.037	0.086

M1: (crude); M2: (adjusted for M1 plus Log Total Energy); M3: (adjusted for M2 plus Body Mass Index); M4: (adjusted for M3 plus age, smoking, physical activity, alcohol intake, seasonality, education level, PC1, PC2 and PC3); M1 = model 1; M2 = model 2; M3 = model 3; M4 = model 4; PC1 = Magnesium, phosphorus and plant protein driven nutrients; PC2 = Fat and animal protein driven nutrients; PC3 = Starch, dietary fibre and B vitamin driven nutrients Fasting glucose units $mmol{\cdot}L^{-1}$ = millimoles per litre; SD = standard deviation; CI = confidence interval.

Table 4. Regression coefficients for glycated haemoglobin for 1 SD increase in the derived nutrient pattern scores among rural black South African women.

	Magnesium, Phosphorus and Plant Protein Driven Nutrients			Fat and Animal Protein Driven Nutrients			Starch, Dietary Fibre and B Vitamin Driven Nutrients		
	B (95% CI)	*p* Value	R^2	B (95% CI)	*p* Value	R^2	B (95% CI)	*p* Value	R^2
M1	0.029 (−0.055; 0.112)	0.502	0.001	0.032 (−0.056; 0.120)	0.477	0.001	−0.138 (−0.224; −0.053)	0.002	0.020
M2	0.048 (−0.104; 0.199)	0.538	0.001	0.028 (−0.067; 0.123)	0.563	0.001	−0.145 (−0.234; −0.056)	0.001	0.021
M3	0.112 (−0.036; 0.260)	0.139	0.069	0.014 (−0.078; 0.106)	0.766	0.065	−0.151 (−0.237; −0.065)	0.001	0.087
M4	0.107 (−0.188; 0.401)	0.478	0.150	−0.011 (−0.175; 0.154)	0.478	0.150	−0.175 (−0.303; −0.047)	0.007	0.150

M1: (crude); M2: (adjusted for M1 plus Log Total Energy); M3: (adjusted for M2 plus Body Mass Index); M4: (adjusted for M3 plus age, smoking, physical activity, alcohol intake, seasonality, education level, PC1, PC2 and PC3); M1 = model 1; M2 = model 2; M3 = model 3; M4 = model 4; PC1 = Magnesium, phosphorus and plant protein driven nutrients; PC2 = Fat and animal protein driven nutrients; PC3 = Starch, dietary fibre and B vitamin driven nutrients. Glycated haemoglobin unit = per cent; SD = standard deviation; CI = confidence interval.

Table 5. Regression coefficients for fasting glucose for 1 SD increase in the derived nutrient pattern scores among rural black South African men.

	Thiamine, Zinc and Plant Protein Driven Nutrients			Fat and Animal Protein Driven Nutrients			Retinol and Vitamin B12 Driven Nutrients		
	B (95% CI)	p Value	R^2	B (95% CI)	p Value	R^2	B (95% CI)	p Value	R^2
M1	−0.057 (−0.172; 0.057)	0.326	0.004	0.054 (−0.061; 0.169)	0.355	0.003	−0.039 (−0.156; 0.077)	0.504	0.002
M2	−0.237 (−0.492; 0.019)	0.069	0.013	0.061 (−0.064; 0.186)	0.335	0.004	−0.055 (−0.173; 0.064)	0.363	0.003
M3	−0.255 (−0.496; 0.014)	0.038	0.117	0.055 (−0.063; 0.172)	0.363	0.115	−0.082 (−0.194; 0.030)	0.153	0.120
M4	−0.382 (−0.752; −0.012)	0.043	0.182	−0.051 (−0.241; 0.139)	0.596	0.182	−0.109 (−0.229; 0.032)	0.074	0.182

M1: (crude); M2: (adjusted for M1 plus Log Total Energy); M3: (adjusted for M2 plus Body Mass Index); M4: (adjusted for M3 plus age, smoking, physical activity, alcohol intake, seasonality, education level, PC1, PC2 and PC3); M1 = model 1; M2 = model 2; M3 = model 3; M4 = model 4; PC1 = Magnesium, phosphorus and plant protein driven nutrients; PC2 = Fat and animal protein driven nutrients; PC3 = Starch, dietary fibre and B vitamin driven nutrients Fasting glucose units mmol·L^{-1} = millimoles per litre; SD = standard deviation; CI = confidence interval.

Table 6. Regression coefficients for glycated haemoglobin for 1 SD increase in the derived nutrient pattern scores among rural black South African women.

	Thiamine, Zinc and Plant Protein Driven Nutrients			Fat and Animal Protein Driven Nutrients			Retinol and Vitamin B12 Driven Nutrients		
	B (95% CI)	p Value	R^2	B (95% CI)	p Value	R^2	B (95% CI)	p Value	R^2
M1	−0.039 (−0.117; 0.038)	0.320	0.000	0.046 (−0.031; 0.123)	0.241	0.005	0.012 (−0.065; 0.090)	0.754	0.000
M2	−0.214 (−0.384; 0.044)	0.014	0.024	0.053 (−0.031; 0.138)	0.213	0.006	0.015 (−0.065; 0.094)	0.713	0.001
M3	−0.230 (−0.392; −0.067)	0.006	0.113	0.050 (−0.030; 0.131)	0.219	0.092	0.001 (−0.075; 0.077)	0.975	0.086
M4	−0.288 (−0.543; −0.033)	0.027	0.174	−0.057 (−0.189; 0.075)	0.396	0.174	−0.018 (−0.100; 0.064)	0.662	0.174

M1: (crude); M2: (adjusted for M1 plus Log Total Energy); M3: (adjusted for M2 plus Body Mass Index); M4: (adjusted for M3 plus age, smoking, physical activity, alcohol intake, seasonality, education level, PC1, PC2 and PC3); M1 = model 1; M2 = model 2; M3 = model 3; M4 = model 4; PC1 = Magnesium, phosphorus and plant protein driven nutrients; PC2 = Fat and animal protein driven nutrients; PC3 = Starch, dietary fibre and B vitamin driven nutrients. Glycated haemoglobin unit = per cent; SD = standard deviation; CI = confidence interval.

The plant driven nutrient patterns had significant results as has been shown above among the urban and rural participants. However, some notable differences were depicted in the plant driven nutrient patterns illustrated in Table S3. The following nutrient patterns, "thiamine, zinc and plant protein driven nutrients", "thiamine, starch and folate driven nutrients", and "magnesium, phosphorus and plant protein driven nutrients" extracted from the urban men, urban women and rural women, respectively, had higher loadings for animal protein, saturated fat, mono-saturated fat and sugar compared to the "thiamine, zinc and plant protein driven nutrients" and "the starch, dietary fibre and B vitamin driven nutrients patterns", which were associated with significant reductions in fasting and glycated haemoglobin among the rural men and women respectively (see factor loadings in bold in Table S3). These two nutrient patterns that had significant associations with fasting glucose and glycated haemoglobin had very low cholesterol and saturated fat as illustrated in Table S3.

4. Discussion

We set out to determine the nutrient patterns associated with fasting glucose and glycated haemoglobin levels among apparently healthy volunteers. The principal component analysis method enabled the extraction of three nutrient patterns among a black South African population which explained about 73% of the variation of the nutrient factors in the urban/rural and gender stratifications. The magnesium, phosphorus and plant protein driven nutrient pattern was associated with a trend of increasing fasting glucose and glycated haemoglobin levels per 1 SD increase in the pattern in the rural women while the thiamine, zinc and plant protein nutrient pattern was associated with a positive trend of increasing glycated haemoglobin among urban men. Notably, the starch, dietary fibre and B vitamin nutrient pattern was associated with decreases in glycated haemoglobin and fasting glucose levels, −0.175% ((−0.303; −0.047); $p = 0.007$) and −0.236 mmol·L^{-1} ((−0.458; −0.014); $p = 0.037$), respectively, among rural women. The thiamine, zinc and plant protein driven nutrient pattern was associated with significant reductions in fasting glucose and glycated haemoglobin of −0.382 mmol·L^{-1} (−0.752; −0.012; $p = 0.043$) and −0.288% (−0.543; −0.033; $p = 0.027$) in rural men. These associations were significantly maintained after adjusting for age, BMI, log total energy intake, smoking, physical activity, alcohol intake, seasonality and education level attained thus indicating an independent association of the starch, dietary fibre and B vitamin nutrient pattern and the thiamine, zinc and plant protein driven nutrient pattern with fasting glucose and glycated haemoglobin in the rural women and rural men strata's, respectively.

Comparable studies evaluating the associations of nutrients patterns with fasting glucose and glycated haemoglobin are scarce. However, evidence exists of dietary patterns which have evaluated this phenomenon [10]. The Health/Prudent dietary pattern has been associated with decreases in fasting glucose and glycated haemoglobin levels while the Western dietary pattern has been associated with increases in these biomarkers of T2D [27,28]. However, the association of the Western dietary pattern, which is characterised with high intakes of animal proteins and snacks, with fasting glucose levels was noted to vary among ethnic groups [13]. The Western dietary pattern was reported in one study to be only significantly associated with high fasting glucose levels and glycated haemoglobin levels among Dutch and not among the Moroccans and Turkish groups [13]. Dietary patterns are known to vary among different ethnic groups, therefore nutrient patterns that were considered in our study are considered helpful in indicating a non-ethnic insight into this phenomenon.

In our study, we noted that fat and animal protein driven nutrients were also not associated with fasting glucose and glycated levels, as had been depicted in dietary pattern analysis studies among different ethnic groups [13]. This disparity from the Western populations where the animal based/Western dietary patterns are associated with increasing fasting glucose levels has been explained by the realisation that ethnic groups such as Asians may adopt the Western diets but their intake of animal products will remain lower as they also continue to consume traditional cereals and vegetables [29]. Similarly, in this study population, the intake of fat and animal protein nutrients were lower in the plant driven nutrients patterns that accounted for the greatest variance among the three nutrients patterns extracted per stratum as illustrated in Table S3. In other local studies, the protein and fat intakes as percentage of total energy intake for urban women from 1975 to 2005 did not change drastically though evidences of the adoption of Western dietary patterns were being noted and the greater proportion of the energy intake was still being contributed by the carbohydrate intake as had been noted in the Asians [6]. From 1975 to 2005, the percentage of energy of protein intake changed from 14% to 13%, while fat intake as percentage of energy changed from 21% to 30% and carbohydrate intake changed from 67% to 57% of total energy intake [6]. Thus, the intake of fat and animal protein driven nutrients in this population group might have been lower and thus not associated with increases in fasting glucose and glycated haemoglobin as was expected.

The magnesium, phosphorus and plant protein driven nutrient pattern indicated a positive trend association with increases in fasting glucose and glycated haemoglobin levels among rural women, while the thiamine, zinc and plant protein driven nutrient pattern was associated with a trend of increasing glycated haemoglobin levels in the urban men (Table S7). However, plant protein and zinc, which were high in these nutrient patterns, have been reported to independently lower fasting glucose levels [30–33]. In addition, the thiamine, zinc and plant protein driven nutrient pattern was associated with a trend of decreasing glycated haemoglobin and fasting glucose levels in the rural men. In view that the study population comprised people who consumed diets with both animal and plant based nutrients and not purely vegetarians, the discrepancies in the associations of the plant driven nutrients can be explained by the varied proportions of animal protein, saturated fat, mono-saturated fat, cholesterol and sugar among these plant driven nutrient patterns, as illustrated in Table S3. The magnesium, phosphorus and plant protein driven nutrient pattern in rural women and the thiamine, zinc and plant protein driven nutrient pattern in urban men had higher loadings of animal protein, saturated fat, mono-saturated fat, cholesterol and sugar compared to the other nutrient patterns discussed below such as the starch, dietary fibre and B vitamins driven nutrient pattern among rural women and the thiamine, zinc and plant protein nutrient pattern among rural men which associated with low fasting glucose and glycated haemoglobin levels. Animal protein, saturated fat, cholesterol and sugar are high in Western dietary patterns which have been previously associated with increased risk of T2D and this helps clarify the positive trend of association of the magnesium, phosphorus and plant protein driven nutrient pattern in rural women and the thiamine, zinc and plant protein driven nutrient pattern in urban men with the study outcome variables [34]. The comparisons of the varied constituents of the plant driven nutrients as discussed above and illustrated in Table S3 indicates the attractiveness of the PCA approach of nutrient pattern determination as it allows a whole based approach of the effect of nutrients to particular outcomes to be evaluated.

The starch, dietary fibre and B vitamins driven nutrient pattern was consistently associated with reduced fasting glucose and glycated haemoglobin levels in all the multivariate linear models which were considered in this study among rural women. The thiamine, zinc and plant protein nutrient pattern was also associated with significant reductions in glycated haemoglobin and fasting glucose among rural men. These findings are similar to the results of other studies on plant based dietary patterns and T2D risk [10,34]. It has been consistently reported that plant based diets are protective against T2D risk [10,34,35]. A number of mechanisms have been proposed to explain this phenomenon [10]. Plant based diets which are rich in dietary fibre are suggested to reduce T2D risk by reducing postprandial insulin demand, improving insulin sensitivity and the antioxidants found in these diets may help enhance β-cell function [36,37]. Dietary fibre from cereal foods which are also high in starch has been consistently shown across eight European countries to be associated with reduced T2D risk [38]. Maize meal fortified with iron, zinc and B vitamins which is largely consumed among the black South African population group is known to contain resistant starches that are partially digested and have been associated with improved insulin sensitivity which may then lead to reductions in fasting glucose levels [39,40]. Thiamine was also high in this nutrient pattern. Evidence exists that dietary fibre beneficial effects might also be due to its concomitant intake together with thiamine [41]. The results of this study suggest that starch, dietary fibre and B vitamins nutrients, zinc and plant protein consumed together may lead to the lowering of fasting and glycated haemoglobin levels as has been postulated elsewhere [35].

The strengths of the current study include the use of a validated QFFQ and recruitment criteria of selecting apparently healthy individuals who were not taking chronic medications or suffering from chronic diseases. This might have helped to prevent the confounding of drugs and T2D to the nutrient pattern association results with glycated haemoglobin and fasting glucose levels. The factor analysis approach used to derive the nutrient patterns is known for depicting real-world dietary behaviours [42]. However, this approach is based on a number of subjective decisions such as naming nutrient patterns, method of rotation and selection of food groups which can lead to an overall measurement error [10,42]. Since this approach is a posteriori analysis tool, it derives nutrient patterns based on data at hand and this makes comparisons with other studies difficult [10,42]. However, regardless of the differences in the constituents of the nutrient patterns due to the data driven approaches used to derive them, consistent similarities of the dietary factors associated with T2D risk as reported in this study, has been depicted in multiple populations [10,34,37]. It might be probable that the residual confounding effect of total energy intake might have led to distortions in the association of the nutrient patterns with fasting glucose and glycated haemoglobin levels. Residual confounding is a result of measurement error in a confounder included in the model [43]. Although the nutrient and total energy intake based on the QFFQs are not precisely measured, adjustment for total energy intake should control for total energy intake confounding [44]. However, evidence exists that the control of total energy intake is not complete in epidemiological studies involving QFFQs thereby leading to residual confounding [44,45]. Therefore, there is need to further explore the association of the nutrient patterns in isocaloric clinical trials which are better designed to control for confounding for total energy intake [45].

5. Conclusions

In summary, our results indicate the beneficial associations of plant driven nutrient patterns with reductions in fasting glucose and glycated haemoglobin levels. However, the small variances that were explained by the models explored in this study are suggestive of the presence of other factors that affect the variation of fasting glucose and glycated haemoglobin which were not accounted for in this study. Thus, more studies are required to further explore the association of nutrient patterns with fasting glucose and glycated haemoglobin.

Table S1. Extracted nutrient patterns and factor loadings of rural women and rural men, Table S2. Nutrient patterns and factor loadings for urban participants, Table S3. Comparison of the factors loadings in the plant driven nutrient patterns among the urban and rural participants, Table S4. Regression coefficients for fasting glucose for 1 SD increase in the derived nutrient pattern scores among urban black South African women, Table S5. Regression coefficients for glycated haemoglobin for 1 SD increase in the derived nutrient pattern scores among urban black South African women, Table S6. Regression coefficients for fasting glucose for 1 SD increase in the derived nutrient pattern scores among urban black South African men, Table S7. Regression coefficients for glycated haemoglobin for 1 SD increase in the derived nutrient pattern scores among urban black South African men.

Acknowledgments: This research was supported by a grant National Research Foundation of South Africa (87970). Tinashe Chikowore is supported by the National Research Foundation of South Africa (89117). We would like to acknowledge A. Kruger and the PURE research team, funders and participants.

Author Contributions: T.C. conceptualized the paper, analysed the data and wrote the draft article. P.T.P. designed the data analysis plan and contributed to the writing of the paper. E.W.-V. designed the dietary data collection tools, coded and analysed the data for nutrients and contributed to the writing of the paper. T.v.Z., E.J.M.F. and K.R.C. supervised and contributed to the writing of the paper.

References

1. Chen, L.; Magliano, D.J.; Zimmet, P.Z. The worldwide epidemiology of type 2 diabetes mellitus—Present and future perspectives. *Nat. Rev. Endocrinol.* **2012**, *8*, 228–236. [CrossRef] [PubMed]

2. Collaboration, N.C.D.R.F. Worldwide trends in diabetes since 1980: A pooled analysis of 751 population-based studies with 4.4 million participants. *Lancet* **2016**, *387*, 1513–1530.
3. Guariguata, L.; Whiting, D.R.; Hambleton, I.; Beagley, J.; Linnenkamp, U.; Shaw, J.E. Global estimates of diabetes prevalence for 2013 and projections for 2035. *Diabetes Res. Clin. Pract.* **2014**, *103*, 137–149. [CrossRef] [PubMed]
4. Peer, N.; Steyn, K.; Lombard, C.; Lambert, E.V.; Vythilingum, B.; Levitt, N.S. Rising diabetes prevalence among urban-dwelling black South Africans. *PLoS ONE* **2012**, *7*, e43336. [CrossRef] [PubMed]
5. Sartorius, B.; Veerman, L.J.; Manyema, M.; Chola, L.; Hofman, K. Determinants of obesity and associated population attributability, South Africa: Empirical evidence from a national panel survey, 2008–2012. *PLoS ONE* **2015**, *10*, e0130218. [CrossRef] [PubMed]
6. Vorster, H.H.; Kruger, A.; Margetts, B.M. The nutrition transition in Africa: Can it be steered into a more positive direction? *Nutrients* **2011**, *3*, 429–441. [CrossRef] [PubMed]
7. Vorster, H.H.; Kruger, A.; Wentzel-Viljoen, E.; Kruger, H.S.; Margetts, B.M. Added sugar intake in South Africa: Findings from the adult prospective urban and rural epidemiology cohort study. *Am. J. Clin. Nutr.* **2014**, *99*, 1479–1486. [CrossRef] [PubMed]
8. Vorster, H.H.; Margetts, B.M.; Venter, C.S.; Wissing, M.P. Integrated nutrition science: From theory to practice in South Africa. *Public Health Nutr.* **2005**, *8*, 760–765. [CrossRef] [PubMed]
9. Hattingh, Z.; Walsh, C.M.; Bester, C.J.; Oguntibeju, O.O. Evaluation of energy and macronutrient intake of black women in Bloemfontein: A cross-sectional study. *Afr. J. Biotechnol.* **2008**, *7*, 4019–4024.
10. McEvoy, C.T.; Cardwell, C.R.; Woodside, J.V.; Young, I.S.; Hunter, S.J.; McKinley, M.C. A posteriori dietary patterns are related to risk of type 2 diabetes: Findings from a systematic review and meta-analysis. *J. Acad. Nutr. Diet.* **2014**, *114*, 1759–1775. [CrossRef] [PubMed]
11. Hu, F.B. Dietary pattern analysis: A new direction in nutritional epidemiology. *Curr. Opin. Lipidol.* **2002**, *13*, 3–9. [CrossRef] [PubMed]
12. Salehi-Abargouei, A.; Esmaillzadeh, A.; Azadbakht, L.; Keshteli, A.H.; Feizi, A.; Feinle-Bisset, C.; Adibi, P. Nutrient patterns and their relation to general and abdominal obesity in Iranian adults: Findings from the Sepahan study. *Eur. J. Nutr.* **2016**, *55*, 505–518. [CrossRef] [PubMed]
13. Dekker, L.H.; van Dam, R.M.; Snijder, M.B.; Peters, R.J.; Dekker, J.M.; de Vries, J.H.; de Boer, E.J.; Schulze, M.B.; Stronks, K.; Nicolaou, M. Comparable dietary patterns describe dietary behavior across ethnic groups in The Netherlands, but different elements in the diet are associated with glycated hemoglobin and fasting glucose concentrations. *J. Nutr.* **2015**, *145*, 1884–1891. [CrossRef] [PubMed]
14. Freisling, H.; Fahey, M.T.; Moskal, A.; Ocke, M.C.; Ferrari, P.; Jenab, M.; Norat, T.; Naska, A.; Welch, A.A.; Navarro, C.; et al. Region-specific nutrient intake patterns exhibit a geographical gradient within and between European countries. *J. Nutr.* **2010**, *140*, 1280–1286. [CrossRef] [PubMed]
15. Koenig, R.J.; Peterson, C.M.; Jones, R.L.; Saudek, C.; Lehrman, M.; Cerami, A. Correlation of glucose regulation and hemoglobin A_{Ic} in diabetes mellitus. *N. Engl. J. Med.* **1976**, *295*, 417–420. [CrossRef] [PubMed]
16. Teo, K.; Chow, C.K.; Vaz, M.; Rangarajan, S.; Yusuf, S. The Prospective Urban Rural Epidemiology (PURE) study: Examining the impact of societal influences on chronic noncommunicable diseases in low-, middle-, and high-income countries. *Am. Heart J.* **2009**, *158*, 1–7. [CrossRef] [PubMed]
17. Arie, S. Revision of Helsinki declaration aims to prevent exploitation of study participants. *BMJ* **2013**, *347*, f6401. [CrossRef] [PubMed]
18. MacIntyre, U.E.; Venter, C.S.; Vorster, H.H.; Steyn, H.S. A combination of statistical methods for the analysis of the relative validation data of the quantitative food frequency questionnaire used in the THUSA study. *Public Health Nutr.* **2001**, *4*, 45–51. [CrossRef] [PubMed]
19. Wolmarans, P.; Danster, N.; Dalton, A.; Rossouw, K.; Schönfeldt, H. *Condensed Food Composition Tables for South Africa*; Medical Research Council: Cape Town, South Africa, 2010.
20. Wentzel-Viljoen, E.; Laubscher, R.; Kruger, A. Using different approaches to assess the reproducibility of a culturally sensitive quantified food frequency questionnaire. *S. Afr. J. Clin. Nutr.* **2011**, *24*, 143–148. [CrossRef]
21. Wolmarans, P.; Chetty, J.; Danster-Christians, N. Food composition activities in South Africa. *Food Chem.* **2013**, *140*, 447–450. [CrossRef] [PubMed]

22. Kruger, H.; Venter, C.; Steyn, H. A standardised physical activity questionnaire for a population in transition: The THUSA study. *Afr. J. Phys. Health Educ. Recreat. Dance* **2000**, *6*, 54–64.
23. Oyeyemi, A.L.; Moss, S.J.; Monyeki, M.A.; Kruger, H.S. Measurement of physical activity in urban and rural South African adults: A comparison of two self-report methods. *BMC Public Health* **2016**, *16*, 1004. [CrossRef] [PubMed]
24. Pisa, P.T.; Pedro, T.M.; Kahn, K.; Tollman, S.M.; Pettifor, J.M.; Norris, S.A. Nutrient patterns and their association with socio-demographic, lifestyle factors and obesity risk in rural South African adolescents. *Nutrients* **2015**, *7*, 3464–3482. [CrossRef] [PubMed]
25. Boeing, H.; Weisgerber, U.M.; Jeckel, A.; Rose, H.J.; Kroke, A. Association between glycated hemoglobin and diet and other lifestyle factors in a nondiabetic population: Cross-sectional evaluation of data from the Potsdam cohort of the European Prospective Investigation into Cancer and Nutrition Study. *Am. J. Clin. Nutr.* **2000**, *71*, 1115–1122. [PubMed]
26. Alberti, K.G.; Zimmet, P.Z. Definition, diagnosis and classification of diabetes mellitus and its complications. Part 1: Diagnosis and classification of diabetes mellitus provisional report of a who consultation. *Diabet. Med.* **1998**, *15*, 539–553. [CrossRef]
27. Kim, H.S.; Park, S.Y.; Grandinetti, A.; Holck, P.S.; Waslien, C. Major dietary patterns, ethnicity, and prevalence of type 2 diabetes in rural Hawaii. *Nutrition* **2008**, *24*, 1065–1072. [CrossRef] [PubMed]
28. Liese, A.D.; Weis, K.E.; Schulz, M.; Tooze, J.A. Food intake patterns associated with incident type 2 diabetes: The insulin resistance atherosclerosis study. *Diabetes Care* **2009**, *32*, 263–268. [CrossRef] [PubMed]
29. Gilbert, P.A.; Khokhar, S. Changing dietary habits of ethnic groups in Europe and implications for health. *Nutr. Rev.* **2008**, *66*, 203–215. [CrossRef] [PubMed]
30. Roberts-Toler, C.; O'Neill, B.T.; Cypess, A.M. Diet-induced obesity causes insulin resistance in mouse brown adipose tissue. *Obesity (Silver Spring)* **2015**, *23*, 1765–1770. [CrossRef] [PubMed]
31. Capdor, J.; Foster, M.; Petocz, P.; Samman, S. Zinc and glycemic control: A meta-analysis of randomised placebo controlled supplementation trials in humans. *J. Trace Elem. Med. Biol.* **2013**, *27*, 137–142. [CrossRef] [PubMed]
32. Hruby, A.; Ngwa, J.S.; Renstrom, F.; Wojczynski, M.K.; Ganna, A.; Hallmans, G.; Houston, D.K.; Jacques, P.F.; Kanoni, S.; Lehtimaki, T.; et al. Higher magnesium intake is associated with lower fasting glucose and insulin, with no evidence of interaction with select genetic loci, in a meta-analysis of 15 CHARGE Consortium Studies. *J. Nutr.* **2013**, *143*, 345–353. [CrossRef] [PubMed]
33. Khattab, M.; Abi-Rashed, C.; Ghattas, H.; Hlais, S.; Obeid, O. Phosphorus ingestion improves oral glucose tolerance of healthy male subjects: A crossover experiment. *Nutr. J.* **2015**, *14*, 112. [CrossRef] [PubMed]
34. Alhazmi, A.; Stojanovski, E.; McEvoy, M.; Garg, M.L. The association between dietary patterns and type 2 diabetes: A systematic review and meta-analysis of cohort studies. *J. Hum. Nutr. Diet.* **2014**, *27*, 251–260. [CrossRef] [PubMed]
35. Sabate, J.; Wien, M. A perspective on vegetarian dietary patterns and risk of metabolic syndrome. *Br. J. Nutr* **2015**, *113* (Suppl. 2), S136–143. [CrossRef] [PubMed]
36. Barclay, A.W.; Petocz, P.; McMillan-Price, J.; Flood, V.M.; Prvan, T.; Mitchell, P.; Brand-Miller, J.C. Glycemic index, glycemic load, and chronic disease risk—A meta-analysis of observational studies. *Am. J. Clin. Nutr.* **2008**, *87*, 627–637. [PubMed]
37. Montonen, J.; Knekt, P.; Harkanen, T.; Jarvinen, R.; Heliovaara, M.; Aromaa, A.; Reunanen, A. Dietary patterns and the incidence of type 2 diabetes. *Am. J. Epidemiol.* **2005**, *161*, 219–227. [CrossRef] [PubMed]
38. InterAct Consortium. Dietary fibre and incidence of type 2 diabetes in eight European countries: The epic-interact study and a meta-analysis of prospective studies. *Diabetologia*, 2015; 58, 1394–1408.
39. Brites, C.M.; Trigo, M.J.; Carrapico, B.; Alvina, M.; Bessa, R.J. Maize and resistant starch enriched breads reduce postprandial glycemic responses in rats. *Nutr. Res.* **2011**, *31*, 302–308. [CrossRef] [PubMed]
40. Gower, B.A.; Bergman, R.; Stefanovski, D.; Darnell, B.; Ovalle, F.; Fisher, G.; Sweatt, S.K.; Resuehr, H.S.; Pelkman, C. Baseline insulin sensitivity affects response to high-amylose maize resistant starch in women: A randomized, controlled trial. *Nutr. Metab. (Lond.)* **2016**, *13*, 2. [CrossRef] [PubMed]
41. Bakker, S.J.; Hoogeveen, E.K.; Nijpels, G.; Kostense, P.J.; Dekker, J.M.; Gans, R.O.; Heine, R.J. The association of dietary fibres with glucose tolerance is partly explained by concomitant intake of thiamine: The hoorn study. *Diabetologia* **1998**, *41*, 1168–1175. [CrossRef] [PubMed]

42. Moeller, S.M.; Reedy, J.; Millen, A.E.; Dixon, L.B.; Newby, P.K.; Tucker, K.L.; Krebs-Smith, S.M.; Guenther, P.M. Dietary patterns: Challenges and opportunities in dietary patterns research an experimental biology workshop, April 1, 2006. *J. Am. Diet. Assoc.* **2007**, *107*, 1233–1239. [CrossRef] [PubMed]
43. Fewell, Z.; Davey Smith, G.; Sterne, J.A. The impact of residual and unmeasured confounding in epidemiologic studies: A simulation study. *Am. J. Epidemiol.* **2007**, *166*, 646–655. [CrossRef] [PubMed]
44. Willett, W. *Nutritional Epidemiology*; Oxford University Press: New York, NY, USA, 1998.
45. Jakes, R.W.; Day, N.E.; Luben, R.; Welch, A.; Bingham, S.; Mitchell, J.; Hennings, S.; Rennie, K.; Wareham, N.J. Adjusting for energy intake—What measure to use in nutritional epidemiological studies? *Int. J. Epidemiol.* **2004**, *33*, 1382–1386. [CrossRef] [PubMed]

7

A Randomized Controlled Trial to Compare the Effect of Peanuts and Almonds on the Cardio-Metabolic and Inflammatory Parameters in Patients with Type 2 Diabetes Mellitus

Yun-Ying Hou [1,†], Omorogieva Ojo [2,†], Li-Li Wang [1], Qi Wang [1], Qing Jiang [3], Xin-Yu Shao [3] and Xiao-Hua Wang [1,*]

1 School of Nursing, Medical College, Soochow University, Suzhou 215006, China; houyunying@suda.edu.cn (Y.-Y.H.); wanglili83476@suda.edu.cn (L.-L.W.); xuweipan@whu.edu.cn (Q.W.)
2 Faculty of Education and Health, University of Greenwich, London SE9 2UG, UK; o.ojo@greenwich.ac.uk
3 Medical College, Soochow University, Suzhou 215006, China; jiangqing2015@suda.edu.cn (Q.J.); wudan@suda.edu.cn (X.-Y.S.)
* Correspondence: wangxiaohua@suda.edu.cn
† Yun-Ying Hou and Omorogieva Ojo are co-first authors.

Abstract: A low carbohydrate diet (LCD), with some staple food being replaced with nuts, has been shown to reduce weight, improve blood glucose, and regulate blood lipid in patients with type 2 diabetes mellitus (T2DM). These nuts include tree nuts and ground nuts. Tree nut consumption is associated with improved cardio-vascular and inflammatory parameters. However, the consumption of tree nuts is difficult to promote in patients with diabetes because of their high cost. As the main ground nut, peanuts contain a large number of beneficial nutrients, are widely planted, and are affordable for most patients. However, whether peanuts and tree nuts in combination with LCD have similar benefits in patients with T2DM remains unknown; although almonds are the most consumed and studied tree nut. This study sought to compare the effect of peanuts and almonds, incorporated into a LCD, on cardio-metabolic and inflammatory measures in patients with T2DM. Of the 32 T2DM patients that were recruited, 17 were randomly allocated to the Peanut group ($n = 17$) and 15 to the Almond group ($n = 15$) in a parallel design. The patients consumed a LCD with part of the starchy staple food being replaced with peanuts (Peanut group) or almonds (Almond group). The follow-up duration was three months. The indicators for glycemic control, other cardio-metabolic, and inflammatory parameters were collected and compared between the two groups. Twenty-five patients completed the study. There were no significant differences in the self-reported dietary compliance between the two groups. Compared with the baseline, the fasting blood glucose (FBG) and postprandial 2-h blood glucose (PPG) decreased in both the Peanut and Almond groups ($p < 0.05$). After the intervention, no statistically significant differences were found between the Peanut group and the Almond group with respect to the FBG and PPG levels. A decrease in the glycated hemoglobin A1c (HbA1c) level from the baseline in the Almond group was found ($p < 0.05$). However, no significant difference was found between the two groups with respect to the HbA1c level at the third month. The peanut and almond consumption did not increase the body mass index (BMI) and had no effect on the blood lipid profile or interleukin-6 (IL-6).In conclusion, incorporated into a LCD, almonds and peanuts have a similar effect on improving fasting and postprandial blood glucose among patients with T2DM. However, more studies are required to fully establish the effect of almond on the improvement of HbA1c.

Keywords: type 2 diabetes mellitus; peanut; almond; glycemic control; body mass index; lipids; interleukin-6

1. Introduction

Type 2 diabetes mellitus (T2DM) is a chronic disease that involves a heterogeneous group of disorders of the intermediary metabolism, characterized by glucose intolerance [1]. The incidence and prevalence of T2DM have increased markedly worldwide, and its complications are the leading causes of morbidity and premature mortality [2]. The use of diet in the prevention, treatment, and control of T2DM has been recommended, and is one of the strategies for managing the condition. According to the American Diabetes Association (ADA), the nutritional goals for patients with T2DM are to achieve normoglycemia and a cardio protective lipid profile that reduces the risk for cardiovascular disease (CVD) [3].

In recent years, a low carbohydrate diet (LCD) has gained popularity [4],and its effectiveness in reducing weight, improving blood glucose, and regulating blood lipid in patients with T2DM has been confirmed by the American Diabetes Association and Diabetes UK [5,6]. ALCD combined with a low saturated fat intake may be best for patients [7].

Nuts are high in unsaturated fat and are a rich source of bioactive nutrients that have the potential to provide metabolic and cardiovascular benefits [8]. Bodies concerned with diabetes and CVD (e.g., the Canadian Cardiovascular Society and the European Atherosclerosis Society) are now advocating for an increase in nut consumption as part of their dietary recommendations [9–12].

Nuts include tree nuts (almond, walnut, hazelnut, pistachio, pine nut, cashew, pecan, macadamia, and Brazil nut) and ground nuts (mainly peanut). Almonds are the most studied tree nut. Clinical trials have shown that the consumption of almonds as well as other tree nuts is associated with improved glycemic control, insulin sensitivity, decreased inflammation, and reduced/sustained body weight [13–16]. However, tree nuts are difficult to promote in patients with diabetes because of their high cost, especially in developing and under-developed countries.

As the main ground nut, peanuts have a similar nutrient composition to tree nuts, thus being nutrient-dense and rich in monounsaturated fatty acid (MUFA) (40% of energy).They are also a good source of arginine, fiber, phytosterols, polyphenols, niacin, folic acid, and vitamin E [17]. In addition, peanuts are widely planted and are much cheaper than tree nuts, and they are affordable for most T2DM patients. Randomized controlled and cross-over trials have shown that peanut consumption helps to moderate glucose concentrations [18], improve the postprandial lipid response, and preserve endothelial function [19]. However, whether peanuts and tree nuts have similar benefits forT2DM patients remains unknown.

Almonds are the most consumed tree nut [20]. We aim to compare the effect of peanuts and almonds incorporated into LCD on cardio-metabolic and inflammatory measures in T2DM patients.

2. Materials and Methods

2.1. Subjects

The participants were recruited from a diabetes club and from the Endocrine Division of the First Affiliated Hospital of Soochow University. The inclusion criteria were as follows: The patients were diagnosed with T2DM, had glycated hemoglobin A1c (HbA1c) of less than 10%, had no change in oral antidiabetic drugs or in insulin half a month before the intervention, were between 40 to 80 years old [15,21], were able to communicate, had volunteered to participate in this study, and were willing to provide informed consent. Those that were excluded were the patients who ate nuts regularly ($\geq$four per day/week) [22]; were allergic to nuts or other food; had difficulty in chewing nuts as a result of fewer teeth or for other reasons; could not adhere to a LCD strategy; received other dietary interventions; had severe conditions including indigestion, hepatic failure, renal failure, severe gallbladder and pancreatic diseases, stroke, malignant tumors, or unstable cardiovascular diseases (such as myocardial infarction, ketosis, or hyperthyroidism); those who were taking glucocorticoid; and those whose fasting blood glucose (FBG) was more than 16.7 mmol/L [23] during the intervention.

2.2. Study Design

This study is a prospective, randomized controlled trial (RCT) that was performed between December 2015 and April 2016. The recruited patients were randomly allocated to the Peanut and Almond groups using a table of random numbers. The random numbers were generated by one researcher, and were concealed to the researcher who was responsible for the allocation, and the participants were blinded prior to assignment. Before the intervention, all of the subjects underwent a one-week washout period [23] to diminish the effect of background diets on the study. This study followed the Declaration of Helsinki and the Guidelines for Good Clinical Practice, and was approved by the ethics committee of the First Affiliated Hospital of Soochow University (no. 2015106). All of the enrolled participants signed a consent form.

2.3. Sample Size Calculation

Evidence from the literature showed that the mean difference of the changes in the HbA1c levels were 1.6% between the Peanut group and the Almond group [21,24]. Therefore, we calculated 13 participants for each group, with $\alpha = 0.05$ and power = 0.80. In light of the sample loss of 10%, the number for each group was calculated to be 16. Finally, we recruited 15 participants for the Peanut group and 17 participants for the Almond group in this study.

2.4. Intervention

We incorporated peanuts or almonds into a low-carbohydrate diet (LCD), which is a dietary strategy that refers to a carbohydrate intake of between 30–200 g/day or calories from carbohydrates/total calories <45%, being supplemented instead with fat or protein [24]. Our team developed a LCD education handbook [24] for patients with T2DM based on evidence from the literature, guidelines regarding T2DM dietary management, consultation with diabetes experts and nutritionists, and reviews by patients. The researcher and patients reviewed the LCD handbook, and the researcher trained the patients to restrict their intake of starchy staple food (such as potatoes and broad beans) to 50 g/meal per day during the one-on-one education session. The reduced staple food/meal was substituted by consuming 60 g/day peanuts for men and 50 g/day for women in the Peanut group [25], and 55 g/day almonds for men and 45 g/day for women in the Almond group [25,26]. The peanuts and almonds (without salt and with the skin intact, and free of charge) were prepared in vacuum packing, according to a daily amount. The patients were instructed to consume nuts between meals or with breakfast, or when hungry. For those whose fasting plasma glucose were higher than normal (>6.1 mmol/L), the nuts were required to be consumed before 10:00 a.m. in the morning [27]. The patients were instructed to consume 50% of the nuts before bedtime if there was a risk of a nocturnal hypoglycemic event. The intervention duration was three months for the two groups.

The follow-ups were conducted once a week in the first month of the intervention, and once every two weeks in the second and third months. The duration of each follow-up session was about 10 min. The patients' compliance to the dietary plan was reviewed and those with a poor compliance were supported in order to adhere to the plan. The data relating to modification of hypoglycemic agents and the occurrence of hypoglycemia were also collected. Those whose diets did not meet the requirements of the dietary program in the intervention period were excluded from the study.

2.5. Diet Record

The patients maintained a diet record, including details of the diet of any day over the weekend and two working days, as well as the time of nut consumption. The types and quantities of the food consumed were assessed to determine the patients' adherence to a LCD strategy. Among the patients who met the dietary requirements for a LCD, the number of bags of nuts consumed per week was assessed to determine the patients' dietary adherence.

2.6. *Cardio-Metabolic and Anthropometric Parameters*

The cardio-metabolic and anthropometric parameters included the FBG, postprandial 2-h blood glucose (PPG) levels, HbA1c, total cholesterol, low density lipoprotein cholesterol (LDL-C), high density lipoprotein cholesterol (HDL-C), triglycerides, and body mass index (BMI). The HbA1c, blood lipids, and BMI were measured at the baseline and at the end of the third month. Venous blood samples were collected at the School of Nursing of Soochow University after a 12 h overnight fast. The HbA1c was measured by high-performance liquid chromatography using Afinion AS100 Analyzer (Alere, Inc., Shanghai, China), and the total cholesterol, LDL-C, HDL-C, and triglycerides were measured using the spectrophotometry method in the molecular laboratory of the School of Nursing of Soochow University. The height and weight were measured using a calibrated stadiometer, and the patients were weighed wearing light clothing and without shoes. The BMI was calculated as the weight (in kilograms) divided by the square of the height (in meters). The FBG and PPG levels were measured by collecting the peripheral blood from the fingers using a rapid glycemic apparatus by patients once a week at home. The glycemic meters were checked by the research staff and the patients were educated to measure the FBG and PPG correctly so as to reduce the subject bias.

2.7. *Hypoglycemic Episodes and Antidiabetic Medication Modification*

Hypoglycemic episodes in this study were determined by the patients' self-reported hypoglycemic symptoms, with or without a measured plasma glucose concentration of ≤70 mg/dL (≤3.9 mmol/L), according to the definition of hypoglycemia in diabetes, given by the American Diabetes Association [28]. To assess the modification of the hypoglycemic agents, the use and changes of the doses of oral antidiabetic drugs and insulin were recorded at the baseline and in the third month.

2.8. *Interleukin-6*

Interleukin-6 (IL-6) was measured to assess the impact of peanuts and almonds on inflammation. The fasting venous blood was collected and the serum was separated in the molecular laboratory of the School of Nursing of Soochow University. Human IL-6 ELISA kit (R&D Systems™, Emeryville, CA, USA) was used to determine the IL-6 levels in the Hematology Center of the Cyrus Tang Medical Institute at Soochow University.

2.9. *Ratio of Urinary Albumin/Creatinine*

In order to determine the safety of peanuts and almonds in patients with diabetes, a mid-stream specimen of random urine was collected, and the ratio of urinary albumin/creatinine (ACR) was measured using a dry immune marker scattering quantitative method [29].

2.10. *Statistical Analysis*

A statistical analysis was performed using SPSS 18.0 software (SPSS, Inc., Dhicago, IL, USA). For continuous variables, the results were presented as mean ± standard deviation (SD). Comparisons were performed using a *t*-test for the independent samples for general baseline demographic, and clinical characteristics, and one-way analysis of variance (ANOVA) for the outcomes of interest. To eliminate the problem of imbalance in the baseline characteristics, the comparisons of anthropometric and metabolic variables between the groups after the intervention were performed using a covariance analysis with the baseline measurements adjusted. The trends in the dietary adherence, FBG, and PPG in the two groups, which were assessed once a week during the intervention, were analyzed using repeated ANOVA, and have been presented as a fold line diagram. The intention-to-treat (ITT) of HbA1c was performed so as to ensure the reliability of the research results. For the categorical variables, the results were presented as numbers and percentages, and comparisons between the groups were performed using the Chi-squared test or the Fisher's exact test. A p value of <0.05 was considered statistically significant.

3. Results

3.1. Study Participants

On the basis of inclusion and exclusion criteria, 32 T2DM participants were recruited and randomly allocated to the Peanut group (n = 15) and the Almond group (n = 17). Four participants in the Peanut group and three participants in the Almond group withdrew from the study. In the Peanut group, one participant did not like peanuts, one showed abnormally elevated FPG after the first week, one's uric acid increased during the second week (with a history of increased uric acid), and one showed a poor adherence (<four per day/week). In the Almond group, one did not like almonds, one was lost to follow-up, and one could not adhere to the diet program because of toothache. Finally, the data of 11 patients in the Peanut group and 14 in the Almond group were analyzed (Figure 1). The mean age of the participants was 69.60 ± 7.25 years, and 15 (60.0%) were men. The general characteristics of the enrolled participants in each group are shown in Table 1. There were no statistically significant differences in any of the parameters between the two groups ($p > 0.05$, Table 1). The time of exercise per week in the two groups did not change significantly from the baseline, and there was no statistically significant difference found at the third month.

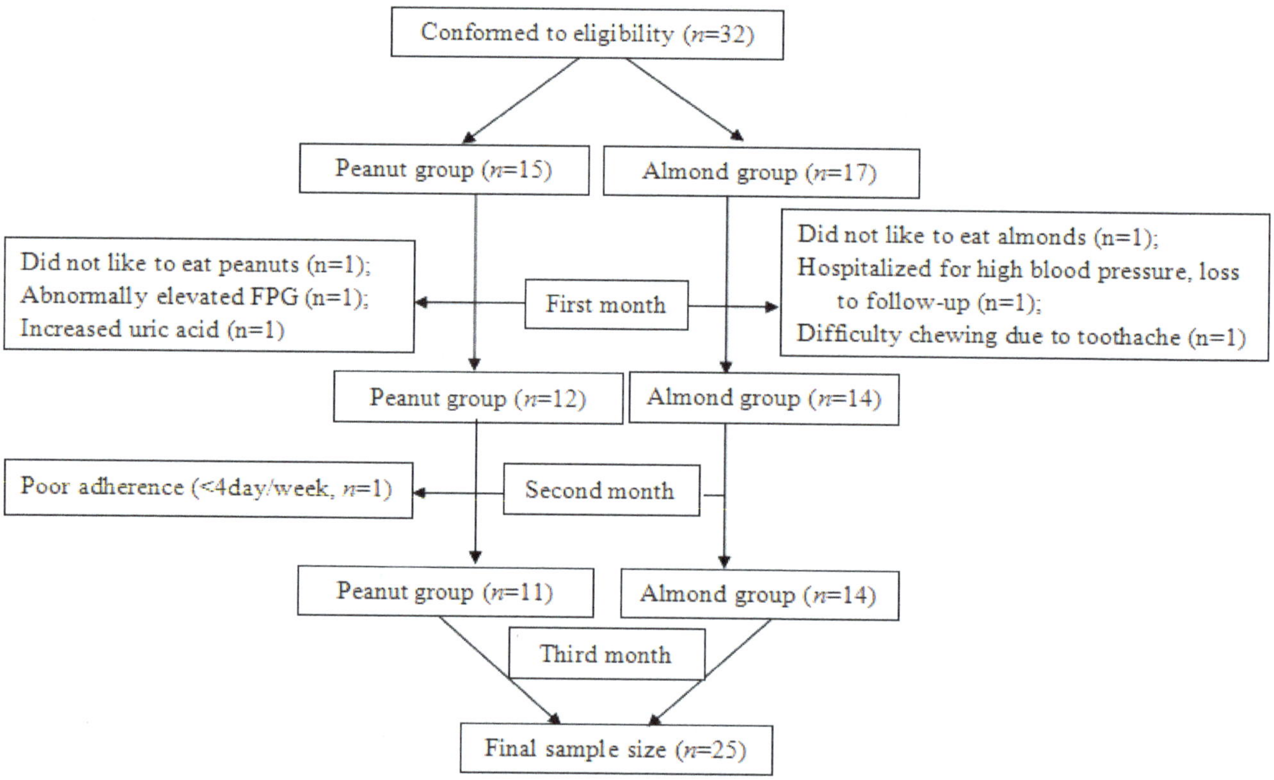

Figure 1. Flow diagram of the patients included in the study.

Table 1. Baseline characteristics.

Variables		Peanut (n = 11) $\bar{x} \pm$ SD/n (%)	Almond (n = 14) $\bar{x} \pm$ SD/n (%)	t/χ^2	p
Demographic data					
Age (years)		68.00 ± 5.80	70.86 ± 8.21	−0.977 [a]	NS
Gender—male		5 (45.5)	10 (71.4)	- [b]	NS
Exercise (min/week)		430.9 ± 222.2	421.4 ± 318.5	0.084 [a]	NS
Exercise habits	Never regular exercise	4 (36.4)	10 (71.4)	- [b]	NS
	Regular exercise	7 (63.6)	4 (28.6)		
Like sweets or rice or noodles—no		1 (9.1)	1 (7.1)	- [b]	NS
The amount of staple food, liang/day (1 liang = 50 g)		3.77 ± 1.75	3.61 ± 2.02	0.215 [a]	NS
Consuming nuts—yes		9 (81.8)	13 (92.9)	- [b]	NS
Clinical data					
Smoking—yes		2 (18.2)	0 (0)	- [b]	NS
SBP (mmHg)		130.73 ± 7.56	128.00 ± 13.77	0.589 [a]	NS
DBP (mmHg)		79.55 ± 10.25	75.71 ± 8.89	1.000 [a]	NS
Family history of diabetes—yes		5 (45.5)	6 (42.9)	- [b]	NS
Diabetes duration, years		11.27 ± 6.36	15.21 ± 8.82	−1.247 [a]	NS
Complications—yes		4 (36.4)	6 (42.9)	- [b]	NS
Accompanying diseases—yes		9 (81.8)	7 (50.0)	- [b]	NS

p-value for comparisons between the treatment diets by an independent samples t-test or Chi-square test. [a] t-test; [b] Fisher's exact test. SBP—systolic blood pressure; DBP—diastolic blood pressure; NS: Differences were not significant. SD—standard deviation. Complications included diabetic retinopathy, nephropathy, neuropathy, cardiopathy, foot ulcers, and cognitive impairment.

3.2. Dietary Adherence

The dietary adherence was assessed through the bags of nuts consumed by the participants per week. A fold line diagram was performed to compare the dietary compliance between the two groups (Peanut versus Almond). The results showed that there were no significant differences in the self-reported dietary compliance per week between the two groups ($p > 0.05$, Figure 2).

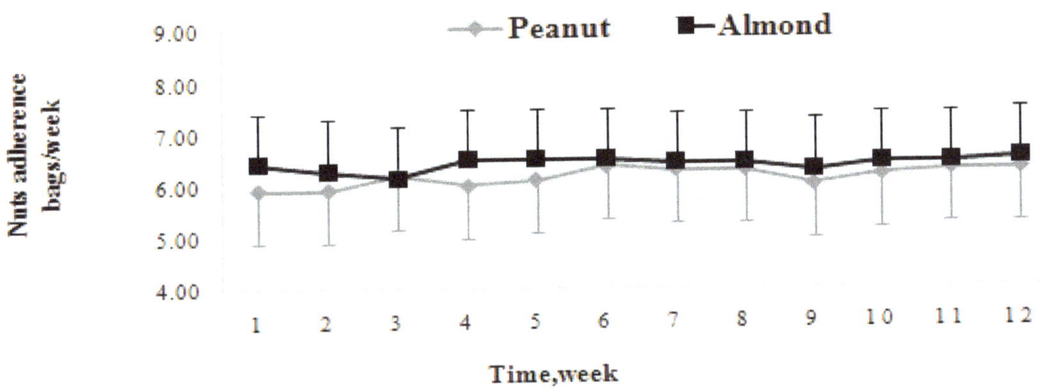

Figure 2. The changing trends of dietary adherence in the Peanut and Almond groups. Values are means, with their standard deviations represented by vertical bars.

3.3. Effect of Peanuts and Almonds on Glycemic Control

3.3.1. Fasting Blood Glucose

Changing Trends of Fasting Blood Glucose

The changing trends of FBG in the two groups during the intervention are described by the fold line diagram (Figure 3). The results show that, for the Peanut group, the levels of FBG were stable with a slight decline, down to the tenth week to the lowest level. For the Almond group, the levels of FBG decreased significantly for the first three weeks, and then fluctuated around the level of the third month.

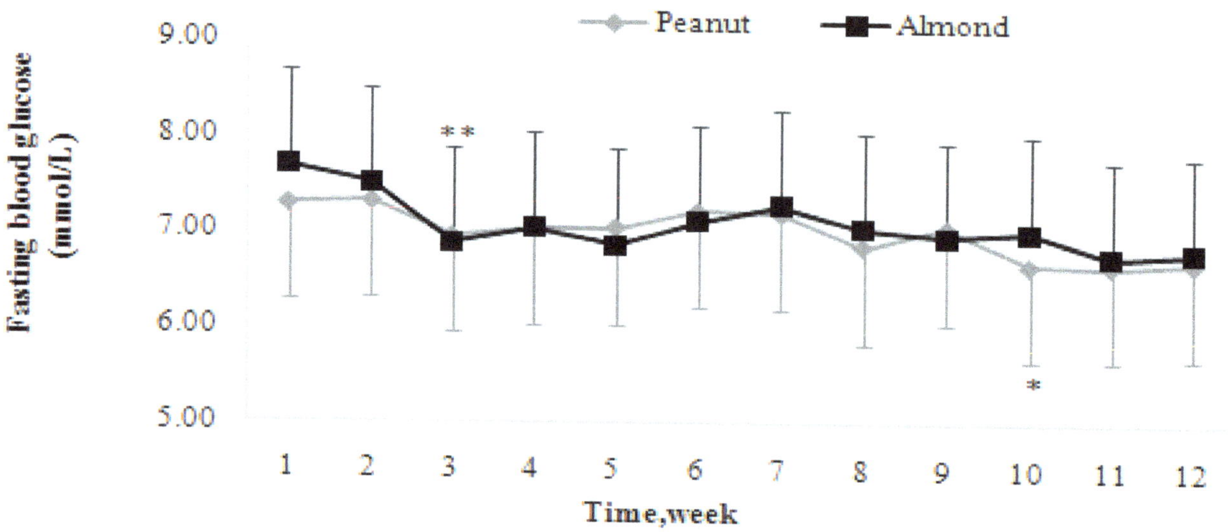

Figure 3. The changing trends of fasting blood glucose (FBG) in the Peanut and Almond groups. Values are means, with their standard deviations represented by vertical bars. For the Peanut group, * FBG was significantly lower at the tenth week than that at the sixth week ($p = 0.035$). For the Almond group, ** FBG was significantly lower at the third week than that at the first week ($p = 0.001$).

Comparison of Fasting Blood Glucose Levels

Compared to the baseline, the FBG levels of the two groups decreased significantly ($p < 0.05$). However, the differences between the two groups, with respect to FBG, were not statistically significant ($p > 0.05$) (Table 2).

Table 2. Comparison of fasting blood glucose (mmol/L) between the two groups.

Study Period	**Peanut ($n = 11$)**	**Almond ($n = 14$)**	F	p
Baseline	7.73 ± 1.19	8.28 ± 2.05	0.537	NS
Third month	6.69 ± 0.54 (adjusted: 6.77 ± 0.20)	6.79 ± 0.92 (adjusted: 6.73 ± 0.17)	0.016	NS
F	6.945	5.785	-	-
p	0.016 *	0.024 *	-	-

F-value and p-value for comparisons by one-way analysis of variance or covariance analysis for between-group differences at the third month, with adjusted data presented as mean ± standard error. * $p < 0.05$; NS: differences were not significant.

3.3.2. Postprandial Two-Hour Blood Glucose

Trends in Postprandial Two-Hour Blood Glucose

The changing trends of PPG in the two groups during the intervention are described by the fold line diagram (Figure 4). Both of the groups showed fluctuation, and the amplitude of the fluctuation of the Peanut group was significantly larger than that of the Almond group.

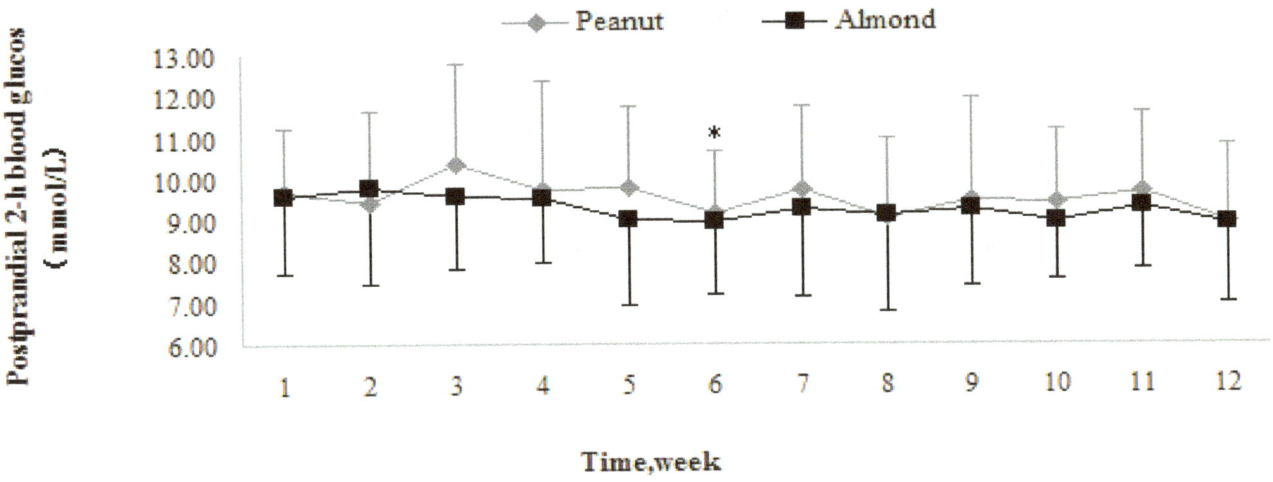

Figure 4. The changing trends of postprandial 2-h blood glucose in the Peanut and Almond groups. Values are means, with their standard deviations represented by vertical bars. For the Peanut group, * PPG was significantly lower at the sixth week than that at the third week ($p = 0.027$).

Comparison of Postprandial Two-Hour Blood Glucose

Compared to the baseline, the PPG in the two groups improved significantly ($p < 0.05$). However, there were no significant differences between the two groups at the third month ($p > 0.05$) (Table 3).

Table 3. Comparison of postprandial 2-h blood glucose (mmol/L) in the two groups.

Study Period	Peanut (n = 11)	Almond (n = 14)	F	p
Baseline	10.36 ± 1.40	10.61 ± 2.83	0.072	NS
Third month	8.94 ± 1.55 (adjusted: 9.03 ± 0.38)	8.91 ± 1.89 (adjusted: 8.85 ± 0.34)	0.115	NS
F	5.011	4.487	-	-
p	0.037 *	0.044 *	-	-

F-value and p-value for comparisons by one-way analysis of variance or covariance analysis for between-group differences at the third month, with adjusted data presented as mean ± standard error. * $p < 0.05$; NS: differences were not significant.

3.3.3. Glycated Hemoglobin

At the baseline, the HbA1c levels were not significantly different between the Peanut and Almond groups. Compared with the baseline, the HbA1c decreased significantly in the Almond group ($p< 0.05$, Table 4). However, there were no significant differences between the two groups by the third month. The intention-to-treat (ITT) in relation to the HbA1c levels were performed so as to ensure the stability of the above results. The ITT results were found to be in agreement with the earlier findings (Table 5).

Table 4. Comparison of glycated hemoglobin (%) between the two groups.

Study Period	Peanut (n = 11)	Almond (n = 14)	F	p
Baseline	6.81 ± 0.82	7.39 ± 1.16	0.072	NS
Third month	6.76± 0.91 (adjusted: 6.97 ± 0.15)	6.81 ± 0.73 (adjusted: 6.65 ± 0.13)	2.453	NS
F	0.015	4.541	-	-
p	NS	0.043 *	-	-

F-value and p-value for comparisons by one-way analysis of variance or covariance analysis for between-group differences at the third month, with adjusted data presented as mean ± standard error. * $p < 0.05$; NS: differences were not significant.

Table 5. Glycated hemoglobin (%) between the two groups in intention-to-treat (ITT).

Study Period	Peanut (n = 15)	Almond (n = 17)	F	p
Baseline	6.96 ± 0.89	7.36 ± 1.07	2.119	NS
Third month	6.93 ± 0.96 (adjusted: 6.90 ± 0.18)	6.88 ± 0.71 (adjusted: 6.65 ± 0.11)	2.361	NS
F	0.015	4.210	-	-
p	NS	0.048 *	-	-

F-value and p-value for comparisons by one-way analysis of variance or covariance analysis for between-group difference at the third month, with adjusted data presented as mean ± standard error. * $p < 0.05$; ITT—intention-to-treat; NS: differences were not significant.

3.4. *Effect of Peanuts and Almonds on Other Cardio-Metabolic and Anthropometric Indicators*

Compared with the baseline, the BMI, total cholesterol, LDL-C, HDL-C, and triglycerides in the two groups did not improve significantly by the third month. After the intervention, the cardio-metabolic and anthropometric indicators were not significantly different between the two groups (Table 6).

Table 6. Comparison of other cardio-metabolic indicators between the two groups.

Variables	Study Period	Peanut (n = 11)	Almond (n = 14)	F	p
BMI (Kg/m^2)	Baseline	22.84 ± 2.48	24.08 ± 3.15	1.141	NS
	Third month	22.67 ± 2.44 (adjusted: 23.30 ± 0.22)	23.43 ± 2.90 (adjusted: 22.94 ± 0.20)	1.482	NS
	F	0.025	1.141	-	-
	p	NS	NS	-	-
Total cholesterol (mmol/L)	Baseline	4.48 ± 0.77	4.90 ± 1.00	1.362	NS
	Third month	4.25 ± 0.93 (adjusted: 4.40 ± 0.21)	4.51 ± 0.86 (adjusted:4.39 ± 0.19)	0.002	NS
	F	0.398	1.260	-	-
	p	NS	NS	-	-
LDL-C (mmol/L)	Baseline	2.48 ± 0.72	2.97 ± 0.84	2.290	NS
	Third month	2.51 ± 0.84 (adjusted: 2.69 ± 0.15)	2.74 ± 0.63 (adjusted: 2.59 ± 0.14)	0.234	NS
	F	0.006	0.653	-	-
	p	NS	NS	-	-
HDL-C (mmol/L)	Baseline	1.49 ± 0.28	1.36 ± 0.30	1.219	NS
	Third month	1.53 ± 0.22 (adjusted: 1.49 ± 0.05)	1.34 ± 0.26 (adjusted: 1.38 ± 0.04)	3.123	NS
	F	0.197	0.029	-	-
	p	NS	NS	-	-
Triglycerides (mmol/L)	Baseline	1.05 ± 0.46	1.87 ± 1.19	2.184	NS
	Third month	0.96 ± 0.46 (adjusted: 0.98 ± 0.23)	1.26 ± 0.87 (adjusted: 1.25 ± 0.20)	0.777	NS
	F	0.207	1.317	-	-
	p	NS	NS	-	-

F-value and p-value for comparisons by one-way analysis of variance or covariance analysis for between-group differences at the third month, with adjusted data presented as mean ± standard error.BMI—body mass index; LDL-C—low density lipoprotein cholesterol; HDL-C—high density lipoprotein cholesterol; NS: differences were not significant.

3.5. *Hypoglycemia and Medication Changes*

3.5.1. Incidence of Hypoglycemia

The incidence of hypoglycemia in the two groups showed no significant differences during the three months before the intervention (baseline) and during the intervention period. One patient in the Almond group and none in the Peanut group sustained a hypoglycemic episode during the trial.

3.5.2. Antidiabetic Drugs Used

During the study, one subject in the Peanut group and two subjects in the Almond group had a decrease in the dose of oral hypoglycemic drugs, and one subject in the Almond group had an increase in the dose of oral hypoglycemic drugs, according to the recommendations of physicians. There were no significant differences in the antidiabetic drugs used between the two groups at baseline and by the third month (Table 7).

Table 7. Comparison of antidiabetic drugs between the two groups.

Study Period		Peanut (n = 11)	Almond (n = 14)	F/χ^2	p
		$\bar{x} \pm$ SD/n (%)	$\bar{x} \pm$ SD/n (%)		
Baseline	No Oral antidiabetic drugs Insulin Both	1 (9.1%) 7 (63.6%) 0 (0%) 3 (27.3)	2 (14.3%) 9 (64.3%) 0 (0%) 3 (21.4%)	0.423 [a]	NS
Third month	No Oral antidiabetic drugs Insulin Both	1 (9.1%) 7 (63.6%) 0 (0%) 3 (27.3)	1 (7.1%) 10 (71.4%) 0 (0%) 3 (21.4%)	0.581 [a]	NS
Insulin dose (IU)	Baseline	28.33 ± 11.59	36.00 ± 24.58	0.239 [b]	NS
	Third month	27.00 ± 10.82 (adjusted: 30.19 ± 1.18 [d])	33.33 ± 20.03 (adjusted: 30.14 ± 1.18 [d])	0.001 [c]	NS

[a] Fisher's exact test; [b] one-way analysis of variance; [c] covariance analysis; [d] standard error; NS: differences were not significant.

3.6. *Effect of Peanuts and Almonds onInterleukins-6*

Compared with the baseline, theIL-6 in the two groups did not improve significantly by the third month. After the intervention, the IL-6 was not significantly different between the two groups (Table 8).

Table 8. Comparison of interleukin-6 (IL-6) ($\bar{x} \pm$ s, pg/mL) in the two groups.

Study Period	Peanut (n = 11)	Almond (n = 14)	F	p
Baseline	12.78 ± 30.62	2.18 ± 1.10	1.696	NS
Third month	10.65 ± 26.91 (adjusted: 5.44 ± 0.52)	2.70 ± 1.83 (adjusted: 6.79 ± 0.45)	3.761	NS
F	0.030	0.832	-	-
p	NS	NS	-	-

p-value for comparisons by one-way analysis of variance or covariance analysis for between-group differences at the third month, with adjusted data presented as mean ± standard error. NS: differences were not significant.

3.7. *Effect of Peanuts and Almonds on Ratio of Urinary Albumin/Creatinine*

There were no significant differences between the two groups at baseline and by the third month (Table 9).

Table 9. Comparison of albumin/creatinine (ACR) ($\bar{x} \pm$ s, mg/g) in the two groups.

Study Period	Peanut (n = 11)	Almond (n = 14)	F	p
Baseline	25.58 ± 26.40	18.53 ± 16.19	0.679	NS
Third month	31.47 ± 48.70 (adjusted: 25.55 ± 5.26)	17.88 ± 21.87 (adjusted: 22.54 ± 4.65)	0.182	NS
F	0.124	0.008	-	-
p	NS	NS	-	-

p-value for comparisons by one-way analysis of variance or covariance analysis for between-group difference at the third month, with adjusted data presented as mean ± standard error. ACR—ratio of urinary albumin/creatinine; NS: differences were not significant.

4. Discussion

This is the first study that compared the effect of peanuts and almonds in patients with T2DM, when incorporated into a LCD diet in order to replace some staple food. The diet diaries revealed that the participants had a good adherence to the dietary intervention, and no significant difference with respect to nut adherence was found between the two groups. This RCT showed that, in combination with a LCD diet, peanuts yielded similar reductions in FBG and PPG compared to almonds.

4.1. Effect of Peanuts and Almonds on Glycemic Control

High levels of FBG, PPG, and HbA1c are some of the most difficult challenges faced by patients with T2DM, and these parameters could be used as the main indicators in order to establish a glycemic control [30]. This study showed that both peanuts and almonds incorporated into a LCD diet resulted in reductions in FBG and PPG after the intervention, which is consistent with previous research results [18,21,31]. The reason might lie in the fact that there is a decrease in the total amount of carbohydrate rich foods in a LCD. In addition, peanuts and almonds are rich in fat, they possess a low-glycemic index, and could alter the glycemic index of co-consumed foods [32]. What is more, the greater fat availability may reduce the gastric emptying rate, and may decrease the carbohydrate absorption rate [33].

However, the content of unsaturated fatty acids (UFAs) and soluble fiber in almonds is higher than that in peanuts [17]. UFAs could facilitate the movement of the glucose receptor to the cell surface, thus increasing the insulin sensitivity [34]. UFAs also act through the stimulation of GLP-1 secretion, which improves the efficacy of the β-cell function [35]. Soluble fiber increases the gastric distention, viscosity in the gastrointestinal tract, and the slower absorption of macronutrients [36]. In this way, it lowers the speed of carbohydrate absorption and the concentration of PPG [37]. Based on the above reasons, the glycemic effect of almonds may be more stable than that of peanuts. In our study, although peanuts and almonds yielded similar reductions in FBG and PPG by the end of the three-months intervention, the amplitude of the fluctuation of the PPG in the Peanut group was significantly larger than that of the Almond group.

The HbA1c level can reflect the mean blood glucose level over the last 8–12 weeks, and can be used to evaluate the long-term glycemic control of patients [30]. HbA1c has a closer association with PPG than FPG [38]. In the present study, the effect of peanuts on the HbA1c reduction was not significant. This might be due to the fluctuation of PPG in the Peanut group. The result of our study is in line with the RCT by Wien et al. [39], which did not find that incorporating peanuts into an American Diabetes Association meal plan had a significant effect in decreasing HbA1c in adults with T2DM. Although there was a 0.48% decrease in HbA1c from the baseline caused by almond consumption, the greater effect of almonds on the improvement of HbA1c was not found by the third month, compared to peanuts. The short-term duration of the follow-up may be one of the reasons for this. After a 24-week almond intervention, Gulati et al. [40] found a statistically significant improvement in the levels of HbA1c compared with the control diet.

4.2. Other Cardio-Metabolic Indicators

The consumption of peanuts and almonds has not been associated with increased body weight, despite their high lipid content. Human feeding trials have shown that nut ingestion moderates appetite postprandially [41]. The inclusion of peanuts and almonds increases a feeling of satiety and leads to a strong dietary compensation effect. In addition, because of the inefficiency in energy absorption, nut consumption does not promote a greater energy intake than other foods [41]. In a randomized cross-over study, after 12 weeks of incorporating high oleic peanuts into the diet, a less than predicted increase in the body weight was found, despite a large additional amount of energy being consumed from the peanuts [25]. Similarly, Li et al. [26] and Gulati et al. [40] also reported no changes in the body weight and BMI with the almond diet, however, a statistically significant improvement was seen in the body fat [26], waist circumference, and waist-to-height ratio [40]. Sato et al. [42] reported a significant improvement of BMI on a LCD diet on in T2DM patients with higher baseline levels of BMI (26.5 Kg/m^2). Among the subjects with a relative normal baseline BMI, this study did not find that peanuts or almonds incorporated into a LCD diet had a significant reduction on the BMI.

The total cholesterol, LDL-C, HDL-C, and triglyceride levels were not altered significantly with an almond or peanut diet in this study, contrary to many other studies [14]. However, the cholesterol lowering effects of nuts are shown to be the greatest in individuals with higher baseline lipids [43]. The subjects in this study had an average healthy baseline lipid level. Barbour et al. [25] and Wien et al. [39] also reported no differences in lipids with peanut consumption in subjects with healthy baseline lipid levels.

4.3. Hypoglycemia and Medication Changes

The antidiabetic drugs and insulin doses used in the Peanut and Almond groups were identical. There was no interference caused by the agents when comparing the glycemic control effects between peanuts and almonds in this study.

We used hypoglycemia as a safety indicator. Although there was no significant difference in the between-group comparison, the percentage of hypoglycemia was reduced from 18.2% to zero in the Peanut group. Nocturnal hypoglycemia occurred in two participants in the Peanut group before the intervention, and it was recommended that they consume 50% of their prescribed peanuts before bedtime. The occurrence of hypoglycemia in the morning causes the body to produce a large amount of glucocorticoids, namely the Somogyi effect, leading to increased blood glucose in the morning [44]. Peanuts and almonds, which are rich in healthy fat, can delay the speed of gastric emptying, and can continuously supply energy [27] to the body so as to prevent the occurrence of the Somogyi effect. During the intervention in the Almond group, daytime hypoglycemia occurred in one case because of strenuous exercise, and there was no nocturnal hypoglycemia found.

4.4. Effect of Peanuts and Almonds on Interleukin-6

IL-6 was chosen as an indicator of inflammation. Chronic low-level inflammation plays an important role in the occurrence and development of DM [17,45]. IL-6 is the source of the metabolic syndrome induced by inflammation, and plays a core regulatory role in the inflammatory response [46,47]. IL-6 can inhibit insulin signaling transduction and could therefore impede the action of insulin [47].

Peanuts are rich in folic acid, which can inhibit the cascade of a reaction in the process of inflammation in vessel wall, and this may reduce the release of vascular inflammatory factors [48]. Although the administration of folic acid can cause a decrease in the concentration of homocysteine, and, as a consequence, could influence the decrease in the concentration of the indicators of inflammation [49], a decrease of IL-6 caused by peanut consumption was not found in this study. As an indicator of inflammation, the C reactive protein (CRP) did not improve after 12-week of peanut consumption in the study by Barbour et al. [25]. Contrary to our study, in the study by Gulati et al. [40], a significant improvement in the CRP was found after 24-weeks of almond consumption. Whether the inconsistency in the improvement of inflammation between studies is correlated to the different intervention duration needs to be further verified.

4.5. Effect of Peanuts and Almonds on Kidney Burden

ACR is a sensitive indicator of early renal damage [50], which is used to assess the impact of peanuts and almonds incorporated into a LCD on renal function in this study. Our study found that peanut and almond consumption with a LCD did not increase the burden on the kidney. Díaz-López et al. also reported no change in ACR after a one-year Mediterranean diet supplemented with nuts [51].

There are some limitations to this study. Firstly, the sample size was small. There was also an imbalance in the gender, diabetes duration, and baseline HbA1c level between groups, although there were no significant differences found. The prolonged effect of peanuts and almonds on the prognosis of T2DM was not observed because of the short follow-up duration. Finally, measurement differences might exist in the FBG and PPG levels, which were measured by the patients themselves, using different blood glucose meters at home.

6. Conclusions

Incorporated into a low-carbohydrate diet, both peanuts and almonds can improve the fasting blood glucose and postprandial 2-h blood glucose in patients with T2DM. The effect of almonds in promoting long-term glycemic control needs to be confirmed by more studies.

Author Contributions: Y.-Y.H., O.O., and X.-H.W. analyzed the data. Y.-Y.H. wrote the initial draft, which was revised by O.O., X.-H.W., and X.-Y.S. L.-L.W., Q.W., and Q.J. collected the data. X.-H.W. contributed most to the design of this research, and all of the other authors participated in the study design and quality control. Y.-Y.H. and O.O. contributed equally to this study. X.-H.W. was the corresponding author.

Acknowledgments: We thank the patients with DM who volunteered to participate in this study. We also thank all of the staff in the Endocrine Division of the First Affiliated Hospital of Soochow University—Huijuan Zhou, Xiaoyan Zhang, and Li Wang—who provided us with assistance so as to ensure that the study was conducted.

References

1. Adeghate, E.; Schattner, P.; Dunn, E. An Update on the Etiology and Epidemiology of Diabetes Mellitus. *Ann. N. Y. Acad. Sci.* **2006**, *1084*, 1–29. [CrossRef] [PubMed]
2. World Health Organization. World Health Organization Global Report on Diabetes: Executive Summary. 2016. Available online: http://www.who.int/diabetes/global-report (accessed on 20 May 2018).
3. American Diabetes Association; Bantle, J.P.; Wylie-Rosett, J.; Albright, A.L.; Apovian, C.M.; Clark, N.G.; Franz, M.J.; Hoogwerf, B.J.; Lichtenstein, A.H.; Mayer-Davis, E.; et al. Nutrition recommendations and interventions for diabetes: A position statement of the American Diabetes Association. *Diabetes Care* **2010**, *33*, S61–S78.
4. Forouhi, N.G.; Misra, A.; Mohan, V.; Taylor, R.; Yancy, W. Dietary and nutritional approaches for prevention and management of type 2 diabetes. *BMJ* **2018**, *361*, k2234. [CrossRef] [PubMed]
5. Dyson, P.A.; Kelly, T.; Deakin, T.; Duncan, A.; Frost, G.; Harrison, Z.; Khatri, D.; Kunka, D.; McArdle, P.; Mellor, D. Diabetes UK evidence-based nutrition guidelines for the prevention and management of diabetes. *Diabet. Med.* **2011**, *28*, 1282–1288. [CrossRef] [PubMed]
6. Wheeler, M.L.; Dunbar, S.A.; Jaacks, L.M.; Wahida, K.; Mayer-Davis, E.J.; Judith, W.R., Jr.; William, S. Macronutrients, Food Groups, and Eating Patterns in the Management of Diabetes. *Diabetes Care* **2010**, *35*, 434–445. [CrossRef] [PubMed]
7. Tay, J.; Luscombe-Marsh, N.D.; Thompson, C.H.; Noakes, M.; Buckley, J.D.; Wittert, G.A.; Yancy, W.S., Jr.; Brinkworth, G.D. Comparison of low- and high-carbohydrate diets for type 2 diabetes management: A randomized trial. *Am. J. Clin. Nutr.* **2015**, *102*, 780–790. [CrossRef] [PubMed]
8. Souza, R.G.M.; Gomes, A.C.; Naves, M.M.V.; Mota, J.F. Nuts and legume seeds for cardiovascular risk reduction: Scientific evidence and mechanisms of action. *Nutr. Rev.* **2015**, *73*, 335–347. [CrossRef] [PubMed]
9. Cheng, A.Y.Y.; Barnes, T. Canadian Diabetes Association 2013 Clinical Practice Guidelines for the Prevention and Management of Diabetes in Canada. *Can. J. Diabetes* **2013**, *373*, S291–S360. [CrossRef]
10. Anderson, T.J.; Gregoire, J.; Hegele, R.A.; Couture, P.; Mancini, G.B.J.; McPherson, R.; Francis, G.A.; Poirier, P.; Lau, D.C.; Grover, S.; et al. 2012 Update of the Canadian Cardiovascular Society Guidelines for the Diagnosis and Treatment of Dyslipidemia for the Prevention of Cardiovascular Disease in the Adult. *Can. J. Cardiol.* **2013**, *29*, 151–167. [CrossRef] [PubMed]

11. Stroes, E.S.; Thompson, P.D.; Corsini, A.; Vladutiu, G.D.; Raal, F.J.; Ray, K.K.; Roden, M.; Stein, E.; Tokgozoglu, L.; Nordestgaard, B.G.; et al. Statin-associated muscle symptoms: Impact on statin therapy-European Atherosclerosis Society Consensus Panel Statement on Assessment, Aetiology and Management. *Eur. Heart J.* **2015**, *36*, 1012–1022. [CrossRef] [PubMed]
12. Mann, J.I.; De Leeuw, I.; Hermansen, K.; Karamanos, B.; Karlstrom, B.; Katsilambros, N.; Riccardi, G.; Rivellese, A.A.; Rizkalla, S.; Slama, G.; et al. Evidence-based nutritional approaches to the treatment and prevention of diabetes mellitus. *Nutr. Metab. Cardiovasc.* **2004**, *14*, 373–394. [CrossRef]
13. Viguiliouk, E.; Kendall, C.W.C.; Mejia, B.S.; Cozma, A.I.; Ha, V. Effect of Tree Nuts on Glycemic Control in Diabetes: A Systematic Review and Meta-Analysis of Randomized Controlled Dietary Trials. *PLoS ONE* **2014**, *9*, e103376. [CrossRef] [PubMed]
14. Musa-Veloso, K.; Paulionis, L.; Poon, T.; Lee, H.Y. The effects of almond consumption on fasting blood lipid levels: A systematic review and meta-analysis of randomised controlled trials. *J. Nutr. Sci.* **2016**, *5*, e34. [CrossRef] [PubMed]
15. Liu, J.; Liu, Y.; Chen, C.; Chang, W.; Chen, C.O. The effect of almonds on inflammation and oxidative stress in Chinese patients with type 2 diabetes mellitus: A randomized crossover controlled feeding trial. *Eur. J. Nutr.* **2013**, *52*, 927–935. [CrossRef] [PubMed]
16. Jenkins, D.J.A.; Hu, F.B.; Tapsell, L.C.; Josse, A.R.; Kendall, C.W.C. Possible benefit of nuts in type 2 diabetes. *J. Nutr.* **2008**, *138*, 1752S–1756S. [CrossRef] [PubMed]
17. Ros, E. Health Benefits of Nut Consumption. *Nutrients* **2010**, *2*, 652–682. [CrossRef] [PubMed]
18. Reis, C.E.G.; Ribeiro, D.N.; Costa, N.M.B.; Bressan, J.; Alfenas, R.C.G.; Mattes, R.D. Acute and second-meal effects of peanuts on glycaemic response and appetite in obese women with high type 2 diabetes risk: A randomised cross-over clinical trial. *Brit. J. Nutr.* **2013**, *109*, 2015–2023. [CrossRef] [PubMed]
19. Liu, X.; Hill, A.; West, S.; Gabauer, R.; McCrea, C.; Fleming, J.; Kris-Etherton, P. Acute Peanut Consumption Alters Postprandial Lipids and Vascular Responses in Healthy Overweight or Obese Men. *J. Nutr.* **2017**, *147*, 835–840. [CrossRef] [PubMed]
20. Buzby, J.; Pollack, S. Almonds lead increase in tree nut consumption. *Amber Waves* **2008**, *6*, 5.
21. Cohen, A.E.; Johnston, C.S. Almond ingestion at mealtime reduces postprandial glycemia and chronic ingestion reduces hemoglobin A(1c) in individuals with well-controlled type 2 diabetes mellitus. *Metabolism* **2011**, *60*, 1312–1317. [CrossRef] [PubMed]
22. Asghari, G.; Ghorbani, Z.; Mirmiran, P.; Azizi, F. Nut consumption is associated with lower incidence of type 2 diabetes: The Tehran Lipid and Glucose Study. *Diabetes Metab.* **2017**, *43*, 18–24. [CrossRef] [PubMed]
23. Chen, L. A brief discussion on the increase of fasting blood glucose. *Health Guide* **2014**, *20*, 34–35.
24. Wang, Q. Effect of Loose Low Carbohydrate Diet on Metabolism in Patients with Type 2 Diabetes Mellitus. Master's Thesis, Soochow University, Suzhou, China, 2015.
25. Barbour, J.A.; Howe, P.R.C.; Buckley, J.D.; Bryan, J.; Coates, A.M. Effect of 12 Weeks High Oleic Peanut Consumption on Cardio-Metabolic Risk Factors and Body Composition. *Nutrients* **2015**, *7*, 7381–7398. [CrossRef] [PubMed]
26. Li, S.; Liu, Y.; Liu, J.; Chang, W.; Chen, C.; Chen, C.O. Almond consumption improved glycemic control and lipid profiles in patients with type 2 diabetes mellitus. *Metabolism* **2011**, *60*, 474–479. [CrossRef] [PubMed]
27. Collier, G.; O'Dea, K. He effect of coingestion of fat on the glucose, insulin, and gastric inhibitory polypeptide responses to carbohydrate and protein. *Am. J. Clin. Nutr.* **1983**, *37*, 941–944. [CrossRef] [PubMed]
28. Childs, B.P.; Clark, N.G.; Cox, D.J.; Cryer, P.E.; Davis, S.N.; Dinardo, M.M.; Kahn, R.; Kovatchev, B.; Shamoon, H. Defining and reporting hypoglycemia in diabetes—A report from the American Diabetes Association Workgroup on Hypoglycemia. *Diabetes Care* **2005**, *28*, 1245–1249.
29. Shi, H. The Change of Urinary Albumin-to-Creatinine Ratio in Patients with Coronary Heart Disease and the Relationship between Urinary Albumin-to-Creatinine Ratio and the Severity of Coronary Stenosis. Master's Thesis, Fudan University, Shanghai, China, 2010.
30. Chinese Diabetes Society. Guidelines for the prevention and treatment of type 2 diabetes in China. *Chin. Med. J.* **2017**, 4–67.
31. Reis, C.E.G.; Bordalo, L.A.; Rocha, A.L.C.; Freitas, D.M.O.; Da Silva, M.V.L.; de Faria, V.C.; Martino, H.S.D.; Costa, N.M.B.; Alfenas, R.C. Ground roasted peanuts leads to a lower post-prandial glycemic response than raw peanuts. *Nutr. Hosp.* **2011**, *26*, 745–751. [PubMed]

32. Hernandez-Alonso, P.; Camacho-Barcia, L.; Bullo, M.; Salas-Salvado, J. Nuts and Dried Fruits: An Update of Their Beneficial Effects on Type 2 Diabetes. *Nutrients* **2017**, *9*, 673. [CrossRef] [PubMed]
33. Gentilcore, D.; Chaikomin, R.; Jones, K.L.; Russo, A.; Feinle-Bisset, C.; Wishart, J.M.; Rayner, C.K.; Horowitz, M. Effects of fat on gastric emptying of and the glycemic, insulin, and incretin responses to a carbohydrate meal in type 2 diabetes. *J. Clin. Endocrinol. Metab.* **2006**, *91*, 2062–2067. [CrossRef] [PubMed]
34. Kien, C.L. Dietary interventions for metabolic syndrome: Role of modifying dietary fats. *Curr. Diabetes Rep.* **2009**, *9*, 43–50. [CrossRef]
35. Riserus, U.; Willett, W.C.; Hu, F.B. Dietary fats and prevention of type 2 diabetes. *Prog. Lipid Res.* **2009**, *48*, 44–51. [CrossRef] [PubMed]
36. Chandalia, M.; Garg, A.; Lutjohann, D.; von Bergmann, K.; Grundy, S.M.; Brinkley, L.J. Beneficial effects of high dietary fiber intake in patients with type 2 diabetes mellitus. *N. Engl. J. Med.* **2000**, *342*, 1392–1398. [CrossRef] [PubMed]
37. Hopping, B.N.; Etber, E.; Grandinetti, A.; Verheus, M.; Kolonel, L.N.; Maskarinec, G. Dietary Fiber, Magnesium, and Glycemic Load Alter Risk of Type 2 Diabetes in a Multiethnic Cohort in Hawaii. *J. Nutr.* **2010**, *140*, 68–74. [CrossRef] [PubMed]
38. Ketema, E.B.; Kibret, K.T. Correlation of fasting and postprandial plasma glucose with HbA1c in assessing glycemic control; systematic review and meta-analysis. *Arch. Public Health* **2015**, *73*, 43. [CrossRef] [PubMed]
39. Wien, M.; Oda, K.; Sabate, J. A randomized controlled trial to evaluate the effect of incorporating peanuts into an American Diabetes Association meal plan on the nutrient profile of the total diet and cardiometabolic parameters of adults with type 2 diabetes. *Nutr. J.* **2014**, *13*, 10. [CrossRef] [PubMed]
40. Gulati, S.; Misra, A.; Pandey, R.M. Effect of Almond Supplementation on Glycemia and Cardiovascular Risk Factors in Asian Indians in North India with Type 2 Diabetes Mellitus: A 24-Week Study. *Metab. Syndr. Relat. Disord.* **2017**, *15*, 98–105. [CrossRef] [PubMed]
41. Tan, S.Y.; Dhillon, J.; Mattes, R.D. A review of the effects of nuts on appetite, food intake, metabolism, and body weight. *Am. J. Clin. Nutr.* **2014**, *100*, 412S–422S. [CrossRef] [PubMed]
42. Sato, J.; Kanazawa, A.; Hatae, C.; Makita, S.; Komiya, K.; Shimizu, T.; Ikeda, F.; Tamura, Y.; Ogihara, T.; Mita, T.; et al. One year follow-up after a randomized controlled trial of a 130 g/day low-carbohydrate diet in patients with type 2 diabetes mellitus and poor glycemic control. *PLoS ONE* **2017**, *12*, e0188892. [CrossRef] [PubMed]
43. Sabate, J.; Oda, K.; Ros, E. Nut Consumption and Blood Lipid Levels A Pooled Analysis of 25 Intervention Trials. *Arch. Intern. Med.* **2010**, *170*, 821–827. [CrossRef] [PubMed]
44. Rybicka, M.; Krysiak, R.; Okopien, B. The dawn phenomenon and the Somogyi effect-two phenomena of morning hyperglycaemia. *Endokrynol. Pol.* **2011**, *62*, 276–283. [PubMed]
45. Yu, Z.; Malik, V.S.; Keum, N.; Hu, F.B.; Giovannucci, E.L.; Stampfer, M.J.; Willett, W.C.; Fuchs, C.S.; Bao, Y. Associations between nut consumption and inflammatory biomarkers. *Am. J. Clin. Nutr.* **2016**, *104*, 722–728. [CrossRef] [PubMed]
46. Chen, Y.; Zheng, S.; Meng, C.; Hao, J. The role of IL-6 on liver insulin resistance in type 2 diabetes mellitus rats. *Chin. J. Lab. Diagn.* **2013**, *17*, 436–439.
47. When, H.J.; Yang, J.S.; Zhang, J.J. Effect of folic acid combined with pravastatin on inflammatory factors in patients with carotid artery stenosis. *Chin. J. Integr. Med. Cardio-Cerebrovasc. Dis.* **2013**, *11*, 111–112.
48. Scheurig, A.C.; Thorand, B.; Fischer, B.; Heier, M.; Koenig, W. Association between the intake of vitamins and trace elements from supplements and C-reactive protein: Results of the MONICA/KORA Augsburg study. *Eur. J. Clin. Nutr.* **2008**, *62*, 127–137. [CrossRef] [PubMed]
49. Baszczuk, A.; Kopczynski, Z.; Kopczynski, J.; Cymerys, M.; Thielemann, A.; Bielawska, L.; Banaszewska, A. Impact of administration of folic acid on selected indicators of inflammation in patients with primary arterial hypertension. *Postep. Hig. Med. Dosw.* **2015**, *69*, 429–435. [CrossRef]
50. Hasanato, R.M. Diagnostic efficacy of random albumin creatinine ratio for detection of micro and macro-albuminuria in type 2 diabetes mellitus. *Saudi Med. J.* **2016**, *37*, 268–273. [CrossRef] [PubMed]
51. Diaz-Lopez, A.; Bullo, M.; Angel Martinez-Gonzalez, M.; Guasch-Ferre, M.; Ros, E.; Basora, J.; Covas, M.; Del Carmen Lopez-Sabater, M.; Salas-Salvado, J. Effects of Mediterranean Diets on Kidney Function: A Report from the PREDIMED Trial. *Am. J. Kidney Dis.* **2012**, *60*, 380–389. [CrossRef] [PubMed]

8

Cardiovascular Risk Factors and their Association with Vitamin D Deficiency in Mexican Women of Reproductive Age

Alejandra Contreras-Manzano, Salvador Villalpando *, Claudia García-Díaz and Mario Flores-Aldana

Center for Nutrition and Health Research, National Institute of Public Health, Cuernavaca 62100, Mexico; alejandra.contreras@insp.mx (A.C.-M.); clauw.g.diaz@gmail.com (C.G.-D.); mario.flores@insp.mx (M.F.-A.)
* Correspondence: svillalp@insp.mx

Abstract: Based on a nationally representative sample of young Mexican women aged 20 to 49 years ($n = 3260$), we sought to explore whether cardiovascular risk factors and acute myocardial infarction (AMI) were associated with vitamin D deficiency (VDD, defined as 25-OH-D <50 nmol/L). To this end, we obtained sociodemographic, serum and anthropometric data from the 2012 National Health and Nutrition Survey (ENSANUT 2012). Analyses were developed through logistic regression models adjusted for potential confounders. The prevalence of VDD was significantly higher in obese women (42.5%, 95% CI; 37.3–47.9) compared to women with a normal body mass index (29.9%, 95% CI; 23.5–37.1, $p = 0.05$), in those with high total cholesterol (TC) (45.6% 95% CI; 39.4–51.9) compared to those with normal TC levels (33.9%, 95% CI 30–38.1, $p = 0.03$), and in those with insulin resistance (IR) (44%, 95% CI; 36.9–51.7) or type 2 diabetes mellitus (T2DM) (58.6%, 95% CI 46.9–69.4) compared to those with normal glycemia (no insulin resistance: 34.7%, 95% CI; 30.9–38.8, $p = 0.04$ and no T2DM: 34.9%, 95% CI 31.4–38.6, $p < 0.001$). Utilizing individual models to estimate cardiovascular risk according to VDD, we found that the odds of being obese (odds ratio, OR: 1.53, 95% CI 1.02–2.32, $p = 0.05$), or having high TC levels (OR: 1.43, 95% CI; 1.05–2.01, $p = 0.03$), T2DM (OR: 2.64, 95% CI; 1.65–4.03, $p < 0.001$), or IR (OR: 1.48, 95% CI 1.04–2.10, $p = 0.026$) were significantly higher in women with VDD ($p < 0.05$). Odds were not statistically significant for overweight, high blood pressure, sedentarism, AMI, high serum concentration of triglycerides, homocysteine, or C-reactive protein models. In conclusion, our results indicate that young Mexican women with VDD show a higher prevalence of cardiovascular risk factors.

Keywords: vitamin D deficiency; 25-OH-D; women; cardiovascular risk factors; T2DM; obesity

1. Introduction

Receptors for vitamin D (VD) and VD activity have been found in many body tissues, suggesting non-calcemic effects of VD related to the regulation of cell proliferation and differentiation, immune response, insulin production, and insulin sensitivity [1–3]. These recognized actions of VD suggest that VD plays a role in the prevention of many chronic diseases such as cancer and cardiovascular disease (CVD) [4], but observational studies have not consistently found any association between VD deficiency (VDD) and chronic conditions such as type 2 diabetes mellitus (T2DM), metabolic syndrome, high blood pressure (HBP), and other cardiovascular risk factors [5–9]. Moreover, several supplementation experiments aimed at preventing pathologies associated with VDD have been carried out, but they have yielded contradictory results as regards to the association of VDD with obesity, insulin sensitivity, and insulin secretion, casting doubt on the association of these conditions with VDD [10–12].

In 2013, the three leading causes of disability-adjusted life years (DALYs) in Mexico were diabetes, ischemic heart disease, and chronic kidney disease, with fasting plasma glucose, high body-mass index (BMI), and HBP being the main risk factors [13]. It is crucial to understand the role of VDD in the occurrence of cardiovascular disease, particularly among young women, in order to help prevent negative health consequences not only for these women in the form of osteoporosis, preeclampsia, or chronic diseases [14,15], but also for their infants, whose bone health and neurological development are influenced by the VD status of their mothers [16,17].

Although little research has been performed concerning VDD in women of reproductive age [18], it is well known that long lactation periods and the use of sunscreen constitute risk factors for middle-aged and elderly women [19,20]. Studies in Mexico have revealed high rates of VDD among children and women of reproductive age (≈36%), with an even higher prevalence observed in the presence of obesity, in urban areas and in subjects with low dietary intake of VD [21,22].

A recent cohort study in Mexico documented an inverse association between VD intake and cardiovascular risk factors among adults; however, the sample was not nationally representative and 25-OH-D levels were not measured [23]. In addition, most international reports on the relationship between VDD and cardiovascular risks have not addressed several cardiovascular risks together, and few research efforts have focused on young and/or non-pregnant women [6]. Therefore, the objective of this study, conducted among a probabilistic national sample of Mexican women of reproductive age (20 to 49 years old), was to explore whether VDD was associated with sedentarism, overweight, obesity, T2DM, insulin resistance (IR), HBP, high total cholesterol (TC), low high-density lipoprotein cholesterol (HDL-C), high triglycerides (TGs), high homocysteine (Hcy) or C-reactive protein (CRP), and acute myocardial infarction (AMI).

2. Materials and Methods

Study population: This analysis was performed among a sample of 3260 women participating in the 2012 National Health and Nutrition Survey (ENSANUT 2012). The ENSANUT 2012 was a probabilistic population-based survey stratified by cluster and representative at the national, regional and urban/rural levels [24]. A detailed description of its sampling method has been published previously [25]. We analyzed the VD data of 3260 women aged 20–49 years with complete information on T2DM, serum concentrations of TC, HDL-C, TG, CRP, IR, and high levels of Hcy.

2.1. *Sociodemographic Information*

Sociodemographic information was collected using validated questionnaires. A Well-Being Index (WBI) was constructed according to the characteristics of and the property owned by households in a principal component analysis. The first component, representing 40% of total variability with a lambda of 3.4, was divided into tertiles in order to classify the WBI as low, medium, and high [26]. Localities with fewer than 2500 inhabitants were defined as rural and otherwise as urban. As in previous ENSANUTs, the country was divided into three regions: north, center (including Mexico City), and south. An individual was defined as indigenous where one of the members of the household spoke an indigenous language as his/her mother tongue.

2.2. *Anthropometry*

Body weight was measured using an electronic scale with a precision of 100 g, (Tanita Co., Tokyo, Japan), and height using a stadiometer with a precision of 1 mm (Dynatop, Mexico City). These measurements were performed by specialized personnel utilizing the Lohman method [27], and were standardized according to the Habitch method [28].

2.3. *Blood Samples*

Eight-hour-fasting blood samples were drawn from the winter of 2011 to the spring of 2012, between the latitudes of 14° 54′ and 32° 31′ N. Blood samples were drawn from an antecubital vein and collected in evacuated tubes. Serum was separated by in situ spinning-down at 3000 g. Serum samples were immediately stored in codified cryovials and preserved in liquid nitrogen until delivery to the Central Nutrition Laboratory at the National Institute of Public Health (INSP), in Cuernavaca, Morelos, Mexico. Thereafter, the samples were preserved at −70°C in a deep freezer until chemical analysis.

A chemiluminescence microparticle immunoassay was used to measure serum 25-OH-D, with intra- and inter-assay coefficient-of-variation (CV) results of 1.34 and 3.69%, respectively. This method has proved acceptable compared to LC/MS/MS ($r = 0.73$) [29]. Quality control was performed according to the reference standard serum NIST 968E of the National Institute of Standards & Technology. The serum concentrations of TC were measured using an enzymatic and oxidation method, glucose by the glucose oxidase technique, HDL-C by direct enzymatic assay after eliminating chylomicrons from the sample, TG by lipase hydrolysis, and Hcy and CRP using ultrasensitive monoclonal antibodies in an Architect CI8200 automatic analyzer (Abbott Lab, Michigan, MI, USA). The intra- and inter-assay CV results were 1.05 and 1.97% for glucose, 2.2% and 5.7% for TC, 3.5% and 5.02% for TG, 5.3 and 7.4% for HDL-C, 3.7% and 4.6% for Hcy, and 0% and 1.2% for CRP, respectively. For insulin, the intra-assay CV was 1.28 uU/mL.

2.4. *Vitamin D Deficiency*

VDD was defined as a serum level of 25-OH-D <50 nmol/L (<20 ng/mL), as in most studies in Latin America [3,30].

2.5. *Definitions of Outcome Variables*

T2DM was defined as diabetes previously diagnosed by a physician or a fasting blood glucose level of ≥126 mg/dL [31].

Serum biomarkers. The following were considered abnormal serum concentrations: TC >200 mg/dL, TG >150 mg/dL, and HDL-C ≤50 mg/dL [32]. Hcy >10.4 nmol/L was considered abnormal [33]. Inflammation was determined where CRP was >5 mg/dL [34], and IR was defined when homeostatic model assessment of IR (HOMA-IR) was ≥3.8 [35].

Overweight and obesity were based on the body mass index (BMI) as classified by the WHO guidelines (normal BMI ≤24.9 kg/m^2; overweight 25–29.9 kg/m^2, and obesity >30 kg/m^2) [36].

HBP was defined as a previous diagnosis by a physician of hypertension or a systolic blood pressure >140 mmHg and/or a diastolic blood pressure >90 mmHg [37].

AMI was defined when acute myocardial infarction was self-reported by the subject.

Sedentarism. A lifestyle was defined as sedentary where a woman was classified as having low physical activity according to a validated International Physical Activity Questionnaires (IPAQ) [38].

2.6. *Statistical Analysis*

VDD prevalence rates were reported as proportions with a confidence interval (CI) of 95%; risks were expressed as odds ratios (ORs) with a CI of 95%. The significance level was established at an alpha <0.05, and regression models were adjusted by age, BMI, dwelling (urban/rural), geographical region, ethnicity, WBI, and sedentarism, as well as by the survey design, using the module SVY of STATA SE v14 (College Station, TX, USA, 2013).

Ethical aspects. The ENSANUT 2012 protocol was reviewed and approved by the Research, Ethics and Biosecurity Committees of the National Institute of Public Health in Mexico. Prior informed consent letters were signed by all participants.

3. Results

3.1. *Characteristics of the Sample*

Serum 25-OH-D levels were estimated for 3260 women representing 19 million Mexican women, aged 20–49 years. In this subsample, 33.4% suffered from overweight, 36.4% from obesity and 25% were sedentary. The prevalence rates for T2DM and HPB were 7.6% and 19.5%, respectively. The overall prevalence of cardiovascular risk factors was 48.3%, and within this group, 80.9% had a low HDL-C, 37.1% high TC, 37.1% high TG, 11.8% high Hcy, and 21.6% high CRP (Table 1).

Table 1. Characteristics and distribution of the sample.

Variable	Subgroup	% (95% CI) *
Age (years)	20–29	36.2 (33, 39.6)
	30–39	37.1 (33.8, 40.5)
	40–49	26.8 (24.2, 29.6)
Dwelling	Rural	21.5 (19.7, 23.4)
	Urban	78.6 (76.7, 80.4)
Region of the country	North	22.4 (20.7, 24.2)
	Center	47.7 (45.2, 50.2)
	South	30.1 (27.9, 32.3)
Well-Being Index	Tertile 1 (lower)	25.5 (23.2, 27.9)
	Tertile 2	31.6 (28.8, 34.6)
	Tertile 3 (higher)	43.1 (39.7, 46.6)
Ethnicity	No	94.7 (93.4, 95.7)
	Yes	5.3 (4.3, 6.6)
BMI category	Normal	30.3 (27.2, 33.5)
	Overweight	33.4 (30.4, 36.6)
	Obesity	36.4 (33.4, 39.6)
Sedentarism	No	70.4 (67.2, 73.3)
	Yes	29.6 (26.7, 32.8)
T2DM	No	92.4 (90.4, 94.0)
	Yes	7.6 (6.0, 9.7)
HBP	No	87.9 (85.3, 90.0)
	Yes	19.5 (17.0, 22.3)
TC	<200 mg/dL	75.8 (72.8, 78.6)
	≥200 mg/dL	24.2 (21.5, 27.2)
HDL-C	≥50 mg/dL	19.1 (16.3, 22.2)
	<50 mg/dL	80.9 (77.7, 83.7)
TG	<150 mg/dL	62.9 (59.8, 66.0)
	≥150 mg/dL	37.1 (34.0, 40.3)
AMI	No	98.7 (98.2, 99.1)
	Yes	1.20 (0.81, 1.76)
Hcy	<10.4 nmol/L	87.9 (85.3, 90.0)
	≥10.4 nmol/L	12.1 (9.9, 14.6)
IR	<3.8 HOMA-IR	79.4 (76.2, 82.3)
	≥3.8 HOMA-IR	20.6 (17.7, 23.8)
CRP	<5 g/L	78.4 (75.8, 80.9)
	≥ 5 g/L	21.6 (19.1, 24.2)

N sample = 3260, *n* expanded = 19,336,909. CI: Confidence Interval; BMI: body mass index; T2DM: type 2 diabetes mellitus; HBP: high blood pressure; TC: total cholesterol; HDL-C: high-density lipoprotein; TG: triglycerides; AMI: acute myocardial infarction; Hcy: homocysteine; IR: insulin resistance; CRP: C-reactive protein * Expanded % and 95% CI.

3.2. Prevalence of VDD

The overall prevalence of VDD was 37.2%, significantly higher among women with T2DM compared to women without it (58.6% vs. 34.5%, $p < 0.05$). VDD was also higher among women with obesity (42.5%) vs. normal BMI (29.9%, $p < 0.05$), and with high TC (45.6 vs. 33.9%, $p < 0.05$) and high TG (41.7 vs. 33.8%, $p < 0.09$). No differences emerged regarding the relationships between VDD prevalence and the other cardiovascular risk factors evaluated independently (Figure 1).

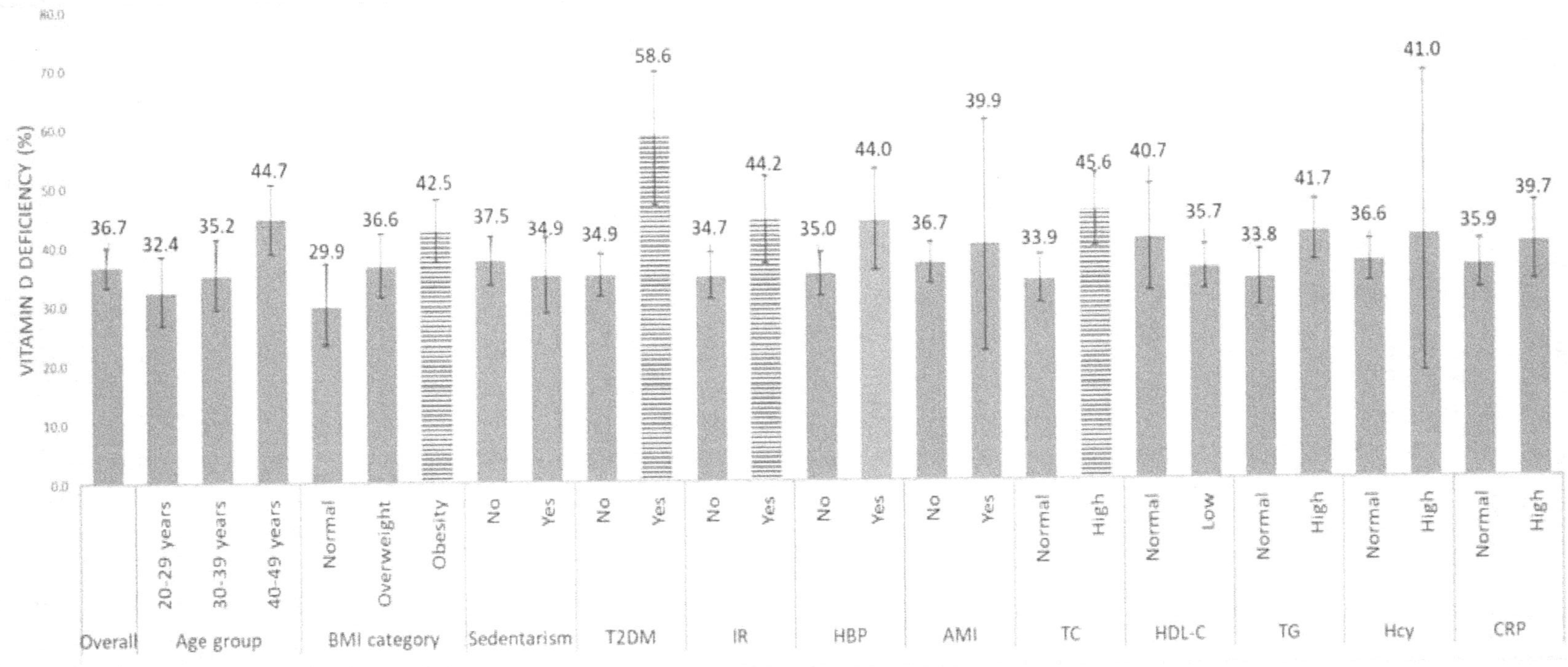

Figure 1. Adjusted prevalence (and 95% confidence interval) of vitamin D deficiency by age group and cardiovascular risk factor among Mexican women aged 20–49 years. BMI: body mass index; T2DM: type 2 diabetes mellitus; IR: insulin resistance; HBP: high blood pressure; TC: total cholesterol; HDL-C: high density lipoprotein; TG: triglycerides; AMI: acute myocardial infarction; Hcy: homocysteine; CRP: C-reactive protein. Horizontal bars indicate a statistical difference (p value < 0.05) among vitamin-D-deficiency prevalence rates in the subcategories. Reference subcategories are 20–29 years for age group; "Normal" for BMI, TC, HDL-C, TG, Hcy, and CRP; and "No" for sedentarism, T2DM, IR, HBP, and AMI. Logistic regression model was adjusted by area (urban/rurality), region of the country, Wellbeing index tertiles, ethnicity and all cardiovascular risk factors.

3.3. Cardiovascular Risk Factors and VDD

We analyzed adjusted logistic models introducing each chronic non-communicable disease and cardiovascular risk factor as dependent variables together with VDD as the independent variable (Figure 2 and Table S1). We found that the risk of obesity was significantly higher in women with VDD (OR: 1.53, $p < 0.05$) than in women without. The risk was also higher when IR (OR: 1.48, $p < 0.05$), T2DM (OR: 2.58, $p < 0.05$) or high TC (OR: 1.45, $p < 0.05$) was present. These models were adjusted by other cardiovascular risk factors as confounding variables. No association was significant between VDD and the rest of the cardiovascular risk factors.

In estimating the prevalence of severe VDD (<20 nmol/L), we found that it was notably low (2.3%, 95% CI 1.3–3.9) and had no significant relationship with cardiovascular outcomes (data not shown). We also tested interactions between VDD and age, BMI and sedentarism, and stratified analysis by oral use of hypoglycemic ($n = 154$), antihypertensive ($n = 129$), and hypolipemic drugs ($n = 210$), as well as by menstrual cycle status, and no impact was observed; therefore, the results were not presented.

4. Discussion

Our study found that VDD was associated with a higher risk for T2DM, obesity, and high TC concentrations in young Mexican women. The major finding of our analysis was the strong association between VDD and a greater risk of T2DM, a result also yielded by other cross-sectional studies [39–42]. On the other hand, some published clinical trials have reported an association between VDD and increased insulin resistance, metabolic syndrome hyperglycemia [43–45], while others have not [12,46].

Several researchers have found an association between intake of VD and calcium and the prevention of T2DM [11]. Other researchers have administered cholecalciferol weekly for six months and found no difference in insulin response or insulin sensitivity in adults at risk of diabetes mellitus [12]. However, for those with prediabetes, VD supplementation has been shown to improve insulin sensitivity [12,47]. Such an effect could be the result of the interaction of calcium fluxes with the VD receptors in the β-cells, needed for the optimal secretion of insulin [48,49]. 25-OH-D induces synchronous Ca^{2+} oscillations with a pattern of pulsatile insulin secretion from the β-cells [50,51]. This may explain the lower level of insulin sensitivity and secretion, as well as all levels of glucose intolerance. Our study showed that IR was significantly associated with VDD and T2DM.

An association between VDD and increased adiposity among Mexican women has previously been demonstrated [22]. Our analysis revealed that VDD was 12.6 percentage points higher in obese women than in those with a normal BMI. We hypothesized that such an association could increase the risk for high rates of TSDM, metabolic syndrome, hypertension, and dyslipidemias found in the Mexican population [52,53]. However, it is not yet known if VDD is a cause or a consequence of obesity in humans, and an ample review of the literature provides evidence for both arguments [54].

Although subjects with a higher BMI had greater skin exposure for VD conversion, an experimental exposure to UV rays produced half the amount of serum VD in women with a high as opposed to a normal BMI [55]. Thus, it is possible that the amount of VD previously contained in the body fat of obese women was large enough to interfere with the conversion or incorporation of 25-OH-D into the serum pool. In a clinical trial involving calcium and VD supplements among overweight and obese individuals, was observed a significant reduction of visceral fat [56]. Obese subjects have greater adipose stores of VD. This enlarged adipose mass in obese individuals serves as a VD reservoir, and the increased amount of VD required to saturate this depot may predispose obese individuals to have an inadequate level of 25-OH-D [57].

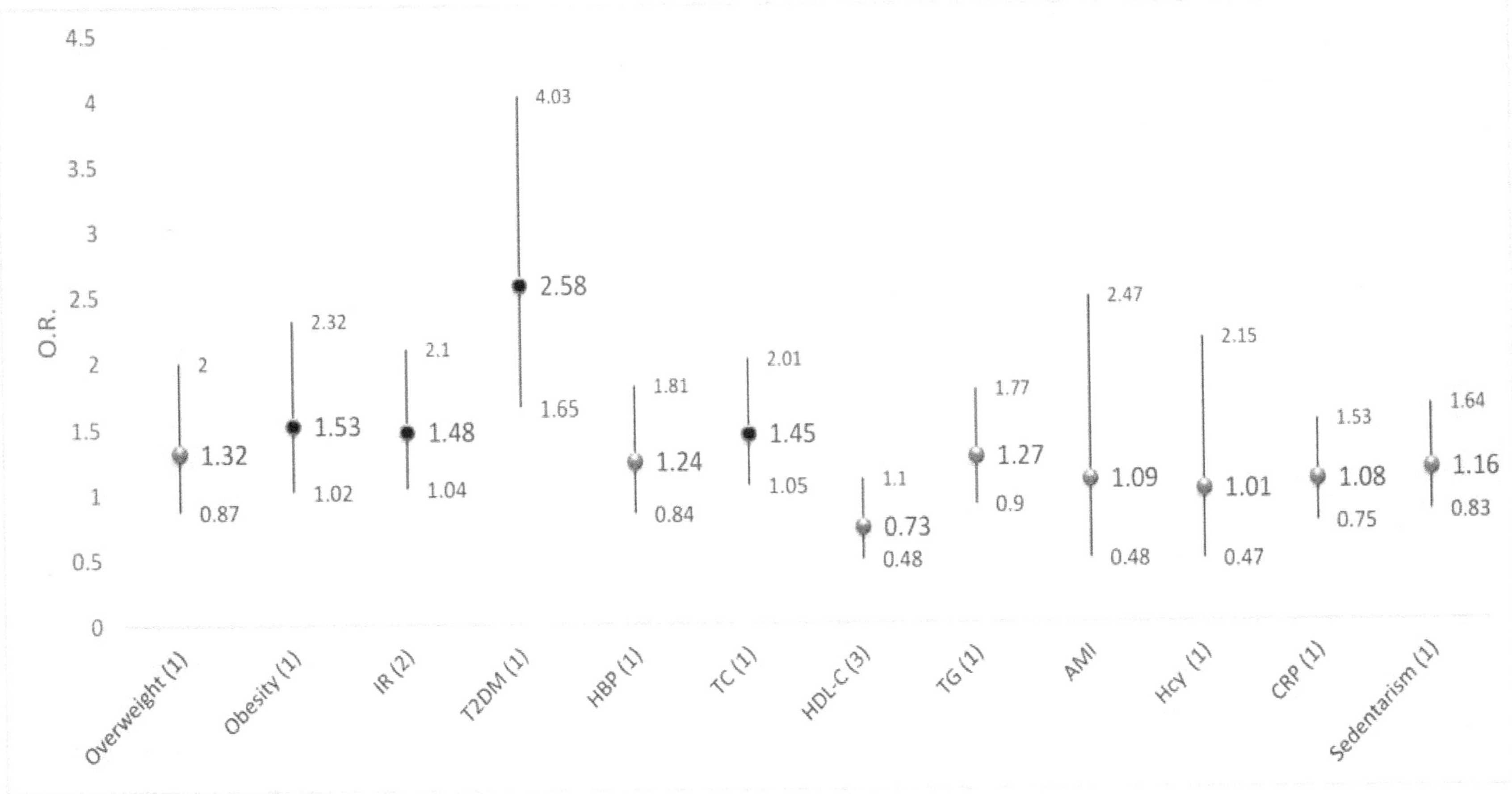

Figure 2. Odds ratios (OR) and 95% confidence interval adjusted for cardiovascular risk factors by vitamin D deficiency in Mexican women aged 20–49 years. BMI: body mass index; PA: physical activity; T2DM: type 2 diabetes mellitus; IR: insulin resistance; HBP: high blood pressure; TC: total cholesterol; HDL-C: high-density lipoprotein; TG: triglycerides; AMI: acute myocardial infarction; Hcy: homocysteine; CRP: C-reactive protein. (1) All models were adjusted by area (urban/rurality), region of the country, Wellbeing index tertiles, ethnicity and the following risk factor variables: HDL-C (<50 mg/dL), TG (<150 mg/dL), TC (<200 mg/dL), HBP, T2DM, CRP (<5 mg/dL), Hcy (<10 umol/L), sedentarism, overweight–obesity, IR, and AMI, except by the risk factor studied in the particular model. (2) Adjusted by all variables in model 1 excluding T2DM. (3) Adjusted by all variables in model 1 excluding TC. Black circle indicate a statistical difference (p value < 0.05).

Our study found that women with VDD had a 1.43 times greater risk (95% CI 1.03–1.99) for high levels of TC compared to women with sufficient VD concentrations ($p = 0.04$). This may be a result of the suppressive effect of VD on the parathyroid hormone (PTH), which reduces lipolysis. Similarly, it has been suggested that VD increases calcium concentrations, reducing the synthesis de novo and releasing hepatic TG [58]. Observational studies have reported that women with VDD have a higher risk of lipid concentration as compared to women with adequate VD status [59–61]. However, in a meta-analysis involving 12 clinical trials with 1346 subjects, VD supplementation was associated with improved LDL-C concentrations, but not with improved TG, HDL-C or TC levels [62]. Meanwhile, a recent randomized controlled trial in postmenopausal women showed positive effects in VD status, bone mineral density, glucose, TC, LDL-C, and apolipoprotein B100 after 24 months of intake of vitamin D-enriched milk [63].

Our study found no association between HBP and VDD, reflecting the findings of other studies [64,65]. However, some observational and randomized clinical trials have found a negative correlation between the two variables [66,67].

The cross-sectional nature of the 2012 ENSANUT makes it difficult to establish causality. However, our results are representative for the entire population of Mexican women aged 20–49 years and for countries with similar socioeconomic characteristics. Another limitation was that data for some variables were collected by means of self-reporting, potentially introducing a degree of measurement bias. Nonetheless, data for all variables were collected in a similar manner; thus, the bias will not affect results for the target population, and the results might even underestimate a potential association. In our analyses, we adjusted results by menstrual cycle status with no significant alteration in the associations, but we were unable to adjust by the current use of estrogen-containing contraception that has been associated with increases in 25-OH-D levels in other populations [19,68]. Nevertheless, in our sample 88% of women had been pregnant and 28% had been sterilized after childbirth. According to the National Survey Report, in 2012 the rate of use of hormonal contraceptives among Mexican women was 12.5% for those aged 20–29 years old, 7.3% among 30–39 year-olds, and 4.6 among 35–49 year-olds, while 42% to 53% reported not using any contraceptive method [69]. Among the strengths of this study is its population-based sample, that allows for representativeness for Mexican women 20–49 years, and the fact that the study includes information on VD serum levels and CVD risk factors.

5. Conclusions

The prevalence of VDD among women 20 to 49 years old is a public health problem in Mexico. Obesity, T2DM, IR, and high TC were found to be associated with VDD. Further research is necessary to assess the biological mechanisms underlying all of these factors and their association with VDD. Also, this study provides scientific evidence supporting the need for public health and nutrition interventions aimed at improving the vitamin D status of Mexican women.

Supplementary Materials:

Table S1: Multivariate logistic regression models for cardiovascular risk factors by Vitamin D Deficiency in Mexican women 20–49 years.

Author Contributions: A.C.-M. and S.V. designed and conducted research; A.C.-M. and C.G.-D. analyzed data; and A.C.-M., S.V., and M.F.-A. wrote the paper. S.V. had primary responsibility for the final content. All authors read and approved the final manuscript.

References

1. Vieth, R. Vitamin D supplementation, 25 hydroxyvitamin D concentrations and safety. *Am. J. Clin. Nutr.* **1999**, *69*, 842–856. [CrossRef] [PubMed]

2. Marwaha, R.K.; Tandon, N.; Reddy, D.R.; Aggarwal, R.; Singh, R.; Sawhney, R.C.; Saluja, B.; Ganie, M.A.; Singh, S. Vitamin D and bone mineral density status of healthy school children in northern India. *Am. J. Clin. Nutr.* **2005**, *82*, 477–482. [CrossRef]
3. Holick, M.F.; Chen, T.C. Vitamin D deficiency: A worldwide problem with health consequences. *N. Engl. J. Med.* **2007**, *357*, 266–281. [CrossRef]
4. Rahmadhani, R.; Zaharan, N.L.; Mohamed, Z.; Moy, F.M.; Jalaludin, M.Y. The associations between VDR BsmI polymorphisms and risk of vitamin D deficiency, obesity and insulin resistance in adolescents residing in a tropical country. *PLoS ONE* **2017**, *12*, e0178695. [CrossRef]
5. Mirhosseini, N.; Vatanparast, H.; Mazidi, M.; Kimball, S.M. The Effect of Improved Serum 25-Hydroxyvitamin D Status on Glycemic Control in Diabetic Patients: A Meta-Analysis. *J. Clin. Endocrinol. Metab.* **2017**, *102*, 3097–3110. [CrossRef] [PubMed]
6. Judd, S.E.; Tangpricha, V. Vitamin D Deficiency and Risk for Cardiovascular Disease. *Am. J. Med. Sci.* **2009**, *338*, 40–44. [CrossRef]
7. Chiu, K.C.; Chu, A.; Go, V.L.; Saad, M.F. Hypovitaminosis D is associated with insulin resistance and B cell disfunction. *Am. J. Clin. Nutr.* **2004**, *79*, 820–825. [CrossRef] [PubMed]
8. Lind, L.; Hanni, A.; Lithell, H.; Hvarfner, A.; Sorensen, O.H.; Ljunghal, S. Vitamin D is related with blood pressure and other cardiovascular risk factors in middle aged men. *Am. J. Hypertens.* **1995**, *8*, 894–901. [CrossRef]
9. Witham, M.D.; Nadir, M.A.; Struthers, A.D. Effect of vitamin D on blood pressure: A systematic review and metaanalysis. *J. Hypertens.* **2009**, *27*, 1948–1954. [CrossRef]
10. Mai, S.; Walker, G.E.; Vietti, R.; Cattaldo, S.; Mele, C.; Priano, L.; Mauro, A.; Bona, G.; Aimaretti, G.; Scacchi, M.; et al. Acute Vitamin D_3 Supplementation in Severe Obesity: Evaluation of Multimeric Adiponectin. *Nutrients* **2017**, *9*, 459. [CrossRef]
11. Pittas, A.G.; Lau, J.; Hue, F.B.; Dowson-Hughs, B. The role of vitamin D and calcium on type 2 diabetes. A systematic review and meta-analyis. *J. Clin. Endocr. Metab.* **2007**, *92*, 2017–2029. [CrossRef]
12. Mousa, A.; Naderpoor, N.; de Courten, M.P.; Teede, H.; Kellow, N.; Walker, K.; Scragg, R.; de Courten, B. Vitamin D supplementation has no effect on insulin sensitivity or secretion in vitamin D-deficient, overweight or obese adults: A randomized placebo-controlled trial. *Am. J. Clin. Nutr.* **2017**, *105*, 1372–1381. [CrossRef]
13. Gómez-Dantés, H.; Fullman, N.; Lamadrid-Figueroa, H.; Cahuana-Hurtado, L.; Darney, B.; Avila-Burgos, L.; Correa-Rotter, R.; Rivera, J.A.; Barquera, S.; González-Pier, E. Dissonant health transition in the states of Mexico, 1990-2013: A systematic analysis for the Global Burden of Disease Study 2013. *Lancet* **2016**, *388*, 2386–2402. [CrossRef]
14. Bodnar, L.M.; Catov, J.M.; Simhan, H.N.; Holick, M.F.; Powers, R.W.; Roberts, J.M. Maternal vitamin D deficiency increases the risk of preeclampsia. *J. Clin. Endocrinol. Metab.* **2007**, *92*, 3517–3522. [CrossRef]
15. Krieger, J.; Cabaset, S.; Canonica, C.; Christoffel, L.; Richard, A.; Schröder, T.; von Wattenwyl, B.L.; Rohrmann, S.; Lötscher, K.Q. Prevalence and determinants of vitamin D deficiency in the third trimester of pregnancy: A multicentre study in Switzerland. *Br. J. Nutr.* **2018**, *119*, 299–309. [CrossRef]
16. Pet, M.A.; Brouwer-Brolsma, E.M. The Impact of Maternal Vitamin D Status on Offspring Brain Development and Function: A Systematic Review. *Adv. Nutr.* **2016**, *7*, 665–678. [CrossRef] [PubMed]
17. Agarwal, S.; Kovilam, O.; Agrawal, D.K. Vitamin D and its impact on maternal-fetal outcomes in pregnancy: A critical review. *Crit Rev. Food Sci. Nutr.* **2018**, *58*, 755–769. [CrossRef]
18. Callegari, E.T.; Garland, S.M.; Gorelik, A.; Reavley, N.; Wark, J.D. Predictors and correlates of serum 25-hydroxyvitamin D concentrations in young women: Results from the Safe-D study. *Br. J. Nutr.* **2017**, *118*, 263–272. [CrossRef]
19. Wagner, C.L.; Taylor, S.N.; Johnson, D.D.; Hollis, B.W. The role of vitamin D in pregnancy and lactation: Emerging concepts. *Women's Health (Lond. Engl.)* **2012**, *8*, 323–340. [CrossRef] [PubMed]
20. Kung, A.W.; Lee, K.K. Knowledge of vitamin D and perceptions and attitudes toward sunlight among Chinese middle-aged and elderly women: A population survey in Hong Kong. *BMC Public Health* **2006**, *6*, 226. [CrossRef] [PubMed]

21. Flores, A.; Flores, M.; Macias, N.; Hernández-Barrera, L.; Rivera, M.; Contreras, A.; Villalpando, S. In Mexican children aged 1–11 years Vitamin D deficiency is common and is associated with overweight. *Public Health Nutr.* **2017**, *28*, 1–9. [CrossRef]
22. Contreras-Manzano, A.; Villalpando, S.; Robledo-Perez, R. Estado de Vitamina D por factores sociodemograficos e índice de masa corporal en mujeres mexicanas en edad reproductiva. *Salud Pública Méx.* **2017**, *59*, 518–525. [CrossRef]
23. Muñoz-Aguirre, P.; Denova-Gutierrez, E.; Flores, M.; Salazar-Martinez, E.; Salmeron, J. High Vitamin D Consumption Is Inversely Associated with Cardiovascular Disease Risk in an Urban Mexican Population. *PLoS ONE* **2016**, *11*, e0166869. [CrossRef]
24. Gutierrez, J.P.; Rivera-Dommarco, J.A.; Shamah-Levy, T.; Villalpando, S.; Franco, A.; Cuevas-Nasu, L. *Encuesta Nacional de Salud y Nutrición 2012 Resultados Nacionales*; Instituto Nacional de Salud Pública: Cuernavaca, Mexico; Available online: https://ensanut.insp.mx/informes/ENSANUT2012ResultadosNacionales.pdf (accessed on 1 April 2019).
25. Romero-Martínez, M.; Shamah-Levy, T.; Franco-Núñez, A.; Villalpando, S.; Cuevas-Nasu, L.; Gutiérrez, J.P.; Rivera-Dommarco, J.A. Encuesta Nacional de Salud y Nutrición 2012: Diseño y cobertura. *Salud Pública Méx.* **2013**, *55* (Suppl. 2), S332–S340. [CrossRef]
26. Gutierrez, J.P. Household socioeconomic classification in the National Health and Nutrition Survey 2012. *Salud Pública Méx.* **2013**, *55* (Suppl. 2), s341–s346.
27. Lohman, T.; Martorell, R.; Roche, A.F. *Anthropometric Reference Standardization Manual*; Human Kinetics: Champaing, IL, USA, 1988.
28. Habicht, J.P. Standardization of quantitative epidemiological methods in the field. *Bol. Oficina. Sanit. Panam* **1974**, *76*, 375–384.
29. National Institute of Standards & Technology. Certificate of Analysis. *Standard Reference Material 968e. Fat-Soluble Vitamins, Carotenoids, and Cholesterol in Human Serum (internet document).* Available online: https://www.aacb.asn.au/documents/item/1233 (accessed on 4 April 2017).
30. Brito, A.; Cori, H.; Ordóñez Pizarro, F.; Mujica, M.; Cediel, G. López de Romaña D. Less than adequate vitamin D status and intake in Latin America and the Caribbean: A problem of unknown magnitude. *Food Nutr. Bull.* **2013**, *34*, 52–64. [CrossRef]
31. American Diabetes Association. Diagnosis and Classification of Diabetes Mellitus. *Diabetes Care* **2013**, *36* (Suppl. 1), 67–74. [CrossRef] [PubMed]
32. Expert panel report on detection evaluation and treatment of high blood cholesterol in adults. Executive summary of the Third report of the national cholesterol education program (NCEP) expert panel on evaluation detection and treatment of high blood cholesterol in adults (adult treatment panel III). *JAMA* **2001**, *285*, 2483–2497.
33. Selhub, J.; Jacqus, P.F.; Rosenberg, I.H.; Rogers, G.; Bowman, B.A.; Gunter, E.W.; Wright, J.D.; Johnson, C.L. Serum total homocysteine concentrations in the third National Health and Nutrition Examination Survey (1991–1994); population reference ranges and contribution of vitamin status to high serum concentrations. *Ann. Intern. Med.* **1999**, *131*, 331–339. [PubMed]
34. Thurnham, D.; McCabe, L.D.; Haldar, S.; Wieringa, F.T.; Northrop-Clewes, C.A.; McCabe, G.P. Adjusting ferritin concentration to remove the effects of subclinical inflammation in the assessment of iron deficiency: A metaanalysis. *Am. J. Clin. Nutr.* **2010**, *92*, 546–555. [CrossRef]
35. Ascaso, J.F.; Romero, P.; Real, J.T.; Priego, A.; Valdecabres, C.; Carmena, R. Insulin resistance quantification by fasting insulin plasma values and HOMA index in a non-diabetic population. *Med. Clin.* **2001**, *117*, 530–533. [CrossRef]
36. WHO. Physical status: The use and interpretation of anthropometry. Report of a WHO Experts Committee. *WHO Tech. Rep. Ser.* **1995**, *854*, 1–452.
37. Chobanian, A.; Bakris, G.; Black, H. The Seventh Report of the Joint National Committee on Prevention, Detection and Evaluation and treatment of High Blood Pressure: The 7 JNC report. *JAMA* **2003**, *289*, 2560–2572. [CrossRef] [PubMed]
38. Medina, C.; Barquera, S.; Janssen, I. Validity and reliability of the International Physical Activity Questionnaire among adults in Mexico. *Rev. Panam Salud Publica* **2013**, *34*, 21–28.
39. Scragg, R.; Holdaway, I.; Metcalf, P.; Baker, J.; Dryson, E. Serum 25-hydroxivitamin D3 decreased impaired glucose tolerance and diabetes mellitus. *Diab. Res. Clin. Pract.* **1985**, *27*, 181–188. [CrossRef]

40. Isaia, G.; Giorgino, R.; Adami, S. High prevalence of hipovitaminosis D in females type 2 diabetic population (letter). *Diabetes Care* **2001**, *24*, 1496. [CrossRef] [PubMed]
41. Scragg, R.; Sower, M.; Bell, C. Serum 25 hydroxyvitamin D, diabetes and ethnicity in the Third National Health and Nutrition Examination Survey. *Diabetes Care* **2004**, *27*, 2813–2818. [CrossRef]
42. Hypönnen, E.; Boucher, E.J.; Berry, D.J.; Power, C. Vitamin D, IFG-1 and metabolic syndrome at 45 years. A cross sectional study in the 1958 British cohort study. *Diabetes* **2008**, *57*, 298–305. [CrossRef]
43. Abbasi, F.; Blasey, B.; Feldman, D.; Cauldfield, M.P.; Hantash, F.M.; Reaven, G.M. Low circulating 25 OH vitamin D concentrations are associated with defects of insulin action and insulin secretion in persons with prediabetes. *J. Nutr.* **2015**, *145*, 714–719. [CrossRef]
44. Kayaniyil, S.; Retnakaran, R.; Harris, S.B.; Vieth, R.; Knight, J.A.; Gerstein, H.C.; Perkins, B.A.; Zinman, B. Prospective Association of vitamin D and β-cell function and glycemia. The PROspective metabolism and Islet cell Evaluation. (PROMISE) cohort study. *Diabetes* **2011**, *60*, 2947–2953. [CrossRef]
45. Dutta, D.; Ali Mondal, S.; Choudhuri, S.; Maisnam, I.; Hasanoor Reza, A.; Bhattacharya, B.; Chowdhury, S.; Mukhopadhyay, S. Vitamin-D supplementation in prediabetes reduced progression to type 2 diabetes and was associated with decreased insulin resistance and systemic inflammation: An open label randomized prospective study from Eastern India. *Diabetes Res. Clin. Pract.* **2014**, *103*, e18–e23. [CrossRef]
46. Mitchell, D.M.; Leder, B.Z.; Cagliero, E.; Mendoza, N.; Henao, M.P.; Hayden, D.L.; Finkelstein, J.S.; Burnett-Bowie, S.M. Insulin secretion and sensitivity in healthy adults with low vitamin D are not affected by high-dose ergocalciferol administration: A randomized controlled trial. *Am. J. Clin. Nutr.* **2015**, *102*, 385–392. [CrossRef]
47. Gagnon, C.; Daly, R.M.; Carpentier, A.; Lu, Z.X.; Shore-Lorenti, C.; Sicaris, K.; Jean, S.; Eveling, P.R. Effect of combined with vitamin D and calcium supplementation on insulin secretion and insulin sensitivity and β-cell function in multiethnic vitamin-D deficient adults at risk of type 2 diabetes: A pilot randomized, placebo controlled trial. *PLoS ONE* **2014**, *9*, e109607. [CrossRef] [PubMed]
48. Zeitz, U.; Weber, K.; Soegiarto, D.W.; Wolf, E.; Balling, R.; Erben, R.G. Impaired insulin secretory capacity in mice lacking a functional vitamin D receptor. *FASEB J.* **2003**, *17*, 509–511. [CrossRef]
49. Sooy, K.; Schermerhorn, T.; Noda, M.; Surana, M.; Rhoten, W.B.; Meyer, M.; Fleischer, N.; Sharp, G.W.; Christakos, S. Calbindin-D(28k) controls [Ca(2+)](i) and insulin release. Evidence obtained from calbindin-d(28k) knockout mice and beta cell lines. *J. Biol. Chem.* **1999**, *274*, 34343–34349. [CrossRef] [PubMed]
50. Sergeev, I.N. Vitamin D-Cellular Ca2+ link to obesity and diabetes. *J. Steroid. Biochem. Mol. Biol.* **2016**, *164*, 326–330. [CrossRef]
51. Sergeev, I.N. 1,25-Dihydroxyvitamin D3 induces Ca^{2+}-mediated apoptosis in adipocytes via activation of calpain and caspase-12. *Biochem. Biophys. Res. Commun.* **2009**, *384*, 18–21. [CrossRef] [PubMed]
52. Barquera, S.; Campos-Nonato, I.; Hernandez-Barrera, L.; Pedroza-Tobias, A.; Rivera Dommarco, J.A. Prevalencia de obesidad en adultos Mexicanos. *Salud Pública Méx.* **2013**, *55* (Suppl. 2), s151–s160. [CrossRef] [PubMed]
53. Villalpando, S.; Shamah-Levy, T.; Rojas, R.; Aguilar-Salinas, C.A. Trends for type 2 diabetes and other cardiovascular risk factors in Mexico from 1993–2006. *Salud Publica Mex.* **2010**, *52* (Suppl. 1), S72–S79. [CrossRef]
54. Dix, C.F.; Barcley, J.L.; Wright, O.R.L. The role of vitamin D in adipogenesis. *Nutr. Rev.* **2018**, *76*, 47–59. [CrossRef]
55. Wortsman, J.; Matsuoka, L.Y.; Chen, T.C.; Lu, Z.; Holick, M.F. Decreased bioavailability of vitamin D in obesity. *Am. J. Clin. Nutr.* **2000**, *72*, 690–693. [CrossRef] [PubMed]
56. Rosenblum, J.L.; Castro, V.M.; Moore, C.E.; Kaplan, L.M. Calcium and vitamin D supplementation is associated with decreased abdominal visceral adipose tissue in overweight and obese adults. *Am. J. Clin. Nutr.* **2012**, *95*, 101–108. [CrossRef]
57. Carrelli, A.; Bucovsky, M.; Horst, R.; Cremers, S.; Zhang, C.; Bessler, M.; Schrope, B.; Evanko, J.; Blanco, J.; Silverberg, S.J.; et al. Vitamin D Storage in Adipose Tissue of Obese and Normal Weight Women. *J. Bone Miner. Res.* **2017**, *32*, 237–242. [CrossRef] [PubMed]
58. Mumford, S.L.; Schisterman, E.F.; Siega-Riz, A.M.; Browne, R.W.; Gaskins, A.J.; Trevisan, M.; Steiner, A.Z.; Daniels, J.L.; Zhang, C.; Perkins, N.J. A Longitudinal Study of Serum Lipoproteins in Relation to Endogenous Reproductive Hormones during the Menstrual Cycle: Findings from the BioCycle Study. *J. Clin. Endocrinol. Metab.* **2010**, *95*, E80–E85. [CrossRef]

59. Tosunbayraktar, G.; Bas, M.; Kut, A.; Buyukkaragoz, A.H. Low serum 25(OH)D levels are associated to higher BMI and metabolic syndrome parameters in adults subjects in Turkey. *Afri. Health Sci.* **2015**, *15*, 1161–1169. [CrossRef] [PubMed]
60. Boteon, E.; Nahas-Neto, J.; Bueloni-Dias, F.; Poloni, P.F.; Orsatti, C.L.; Petri Nahas, E.A. Vitamin D deficiency is associated with metabolic syndrome in postmenopausal women. *Maturitas* **2018**, *107*, 97–102.
61. Jorde, R.; Grimnes, G. Exploring the association between serum 25-hydroxyvitamin D and serum lipids-more than confounding? *Eur. J. Clin. Nutr.* **2018**, *72*, 526–533. [CrossRef] [PubMed]
62. Wang, H.; Xia, N.; Yang, Y.; Peng, D.Q. Influence of vitamin D supplementation on plasma lipids profiles: A metaanalysis of randomized controlled trials. *Lipid Health Dis.* **2012**, *11*, 42. [CrossRef]
63. Reyes-Garcia, R.; Mendoza, N.; Palacios, S.; Salas, N.; Quesada-Charneco, M.; Garcia-Martin, A.; Fonolla, J.; Lara-Villoslada, F.; Muñoz-Torres, M. Effects of Daily Intake of Calcium and Vitamin D-Enriched Milk in Healthy Postmenopausal Women: A Randomized, Controlled, Double-Blind Nutritional Study. *J. Womens Health (Larchmt)* **2018**, *27*, 561–568. [CrossRef] [PubMed]
64. Grübler, M.R.; Gaksch, M.; Kienreich, K.; Verheyen, N.D.; Schmid, J.; Müllner, C.; Richtig, G.; Scharnagl, H.; Trummer, C.; Schwetz, V.; et al. Effects of Vitamin D3 on asymmetric- and symmetric dimethylarginine in arterial hypertension. *J. Steroid. Biochem. Mol. Biol.* **2018**, *175*, 157–163. [CrossRef] [PubMed]
65. Golzarand, M.; Shab-Bidar, S.; Koochakpoor, G.; Speakman, J.R.; Djafarian, K. Effect of vitamin D3 supplementation on blood pressure in adults: An updated meta-analysis. *Nutr. Metab. Cardiovasc. Dis.* **2016**, *26*, 663–673. [CrossRef] [PubMed]
66. Mirhosseini, N.; Vatanparast, H.; Kimball, S.M. The Association between Serum 25(OH)D Status and Blood Pressure in Participants of a Community-Based Program Taking Vitamin D Supplements. *Nutrients* **2017**, *9*, 1244. [CrossRef]
67. Anderesen, L.B.; Pryzybil, L.; Haase, N.; von Bersen-Hoinck, F.; Qadri, F.; Jørgensen, J.S.; Sorensen, G.L.; Fruekilde, P.; Poglitsch, M.; Szijarto, I. Vitamin D depletion aggravates hypertension and target-organ damage. *J. Am. Hearth Assocc.* **2015**, *4*, e001417. [CrossRef]
68. Harmon, Q.E.; Umbach, D.M.; Baird, D.D. Use of Estrogen-Containing Contraception Is Associated With Increased Concentrations of 25-Hydroxy Vitamin D. *J. Clin. Endocrinol Metab.* **2016**, *101*, 3370–3377. [CrossRef]
69. Villalobos, A.; Allen, B.; Serrato, M.; Suárez, L.; De La Vara, E.; Castro, F. Uso de Anticonceptivos y Planificación Familiar Entre Mujeres Adolescentes y Adultas: Cerrando la Breca Entre Metas y Realidades. Available online: https://ensanut.insp.mx/doctos/seminario/M0203.pdf (accessed on 1 April 2019).

9

Polyunsaturated Fatty Acids and Glycemic Control in Type 2 Diabetes

Vibeke H. Telle-Hansen, Line Gaundal and Mari C.W. Myhrstad *

Faculty of Health Sciences, Oslo Metropolitan University, Postbox 4, St. Olavsplass, 0130 Oslo, Norway; vtelle@oslomet.no (V.H.T.-H.); linega@oslomet.no (L.G.)
* Correspondence: mmyhrsta@oslomet.no

Abstract: The impact of dietary fat on the risk of cardiovascular disease (CVD) has been extensively studied in recent decades. Solid evidence indicates that replacing saturated fatty acids (SFAs) with polyunsaturated fatty acids (PUFAs) decreases blood cholesterol levels and prevents CVD and CVD mortality. Studies indicate that fat quality also may affect insulin sensitivity and hence, the risk of type 2 diabetes (T2D). A high intake of SFAs has shown to increase the risk of T2D in prospective studies, while a high intake of PUFAs reduces the risk. Whether PUFAs from marine or vegetable sources affect glycemic regulation differently in T2D remains to be elucidated. The aim of the present review was therefore to summarize research on human randomized, controlled intervention studies investigating the effect of dietary PUFAs on glycemic regulation in T2D. About half of the studies investigating the effect of fish, fish oils, vegetable oils, or nuts found changes related to glycemic control in people with T2D, while the other half found no effects. Even though some of the studies used SFA as controls, the majority of the included studies compared PUFAs of different quality. Considering that both marine and vegetable oils are high in PUFAs and hence both oils may affect glycemic regulation, the lack of effect in several of the included studies may be explained by the use of an inappropriate control group. It is therefore not possible to draw a firm conclusion, and more studies are needed.

Keywords: PUFA; polyunsaturated fatty acids; glycemic control; nuts; fish; fish oil; vegetable oil; type 2 diabetes

1. Introduction

The most important public health challenge in the world today is premature morbidity and mortality from non-communicable diseases (NCDs) like cancer, type 2 diabetes (T2D), and cardiovascular disease (CVD) [1]. Globally, the prevalence of T2D has increased from 108 million in 1980 to 422 million individuals in 2014 [2]. The WHO has estimated that diabetes will be the seventh most important cause of death in the world by 2030 [3]. Relative risk of CVD is increased two to four times in people with T2D compared with non-diabetic subjects, and is the primary cause of death in people with T2D [4].

The health impact of diet is well recognized, and even small dietary changes may contribute to significant health effects [5–7]. Lifestyle and diet can be highly effective in preventing and treating T2D [8–11]. A high intake of saturated fatty acids (SFAs) increases the risk of CVD due to increased low-density lipoprotein (LDL) cholesterol in the blood, while polyunsaturated fatty acids (PUFAs) have the opposite effect [5,12–15]. Studies indicate that dietary fat quality also may affect insulin sensitivity and hence, the risk of T2D. As early as 1959, Kinsell et al. reported on fat quality and insulin regulation [16]. Several studies on fat quality and glycemic regulation have been published since then [17–20]. According to observational studies, both intake of PUFAs and replacement of SFAs with

PUFAs reduce the risk of T2D [21,22]. Imamura and colleagues recently performed a comprehensive meta-analysis and systematic review of dietary fat and glycemic regulation in randomized controlled trials (RCTs). They found that replacing the intake of SFAs with PUFAs improved glycemia and insulin resistance [19]. These results are in accordance with a systematic review from 2014 [13]. However, none of these reviews distinguished between PUFAs derived from marine or vegetable sources, and both people with and without T2D were included.

In addition to the opposing health effects of saturated versus unsaturated fat, specific PUFAs may differ in their health effects. Some studies have indicated that n-6 PUFAs, but not n-3 PUFAs, may improve insulin sensitivity [13]. In a meta-analysis from 2008, n-3 PUFA supplementation in people with T2D had no significant effect on glycemic control [23], whereas vegetable PUFAs were found to reduce fasting insulin and Homeostasis Assessment Model-Insulin Resistance (HOMA-IR) in a more recent meta-analysis in healthy subjects [24]. To what degree PUFAs from different sources affect glycemic regulation in people with T2D remains unknown.

The aim of the present review was therefore to summarize the literature on human intervention studies investigating the effect of marine- and vegetable-derived PUFAs on glycemic regulation in T2D.

2. Materials and Methods

To summarize the effects of PUFAs on glycemic control in people with T2D we performed a literature search in PubMed in August 2018. Only original articles on RCTs in humans were included. Furthermore, only studies with information about glycemic control and/or T2D and/or dietary unsaturated fat were included. The search words were: "glycemic control" AND "type 2 diabetes" AND "PUFA" AND/OR "unsaturated fats" AND/OR "nuts" AND/OR "oils" AND/OR "fatty fish" AND/OR "omega 3" AND/OR "omega 6". We included studies which clearly or possibly fulfilled the following criteria: glycemic control, T2D and dietary interventions, and intake of unsaturated fat. In addition, studies with subjects referred to as non-insulin dependent diabetes mellitus (NIDDM) were also included, and hence these subjects are referred to as NIDDM in the present review. Moreover, we excluded studies that clearly fulfilled at least one of the following criteria: Non original study (for example editorial, review or conference paper), studies that did not compare the criteria measurements to a control group, animal study, articles written in languages other than English, or lack of inclusion criteria measurements (as defined previously). Interventions with ethyl esters and not available articles were excluded, and duplicate articles were removed. In addition to the literature search, two articles were included based on other reviews. In total, 31 articles were identified as eligible and included in the present article. Figure 1 shows the flow chart of the study selection.

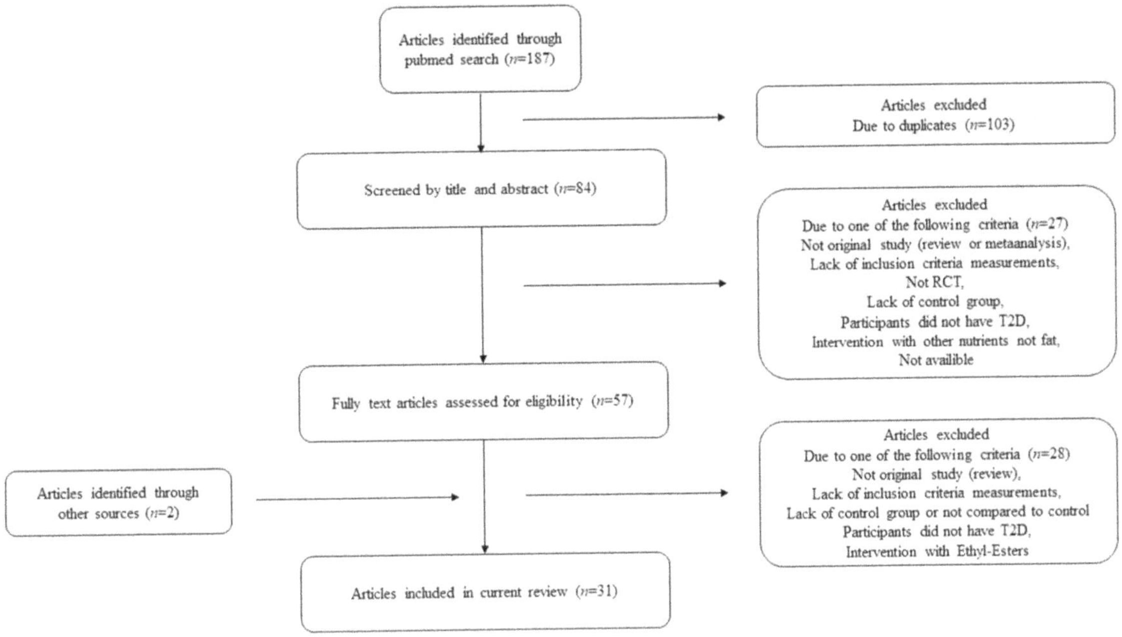

Figure 1. Flow chart of the study selection. RCT: randomized controlled trial; T2D: type 2 diabetes.

3. Results and Discussion

In the present review, we identified 31 RCTs (postprandial and short- and long-term intervention trials (lasting from 30 days to 30 weeks), parallel and crossover design) investigating the effects of PUFAs as dietary components in glycemic regulation in people with T2D or NIDDM (Tables 1–3). Of the 31 included studies, 14 studies investigated the effect of fish, fish oil, eicosapentaenoic acid (EPA) and/or docosahexaenoic acid (DHA) on glycemic regulation [25–38]; 12 studies investigated vegetable oils [39–50]; and five studies investigated the effect of nuts [51–55]. All participants were adults, male and females in the age range between 34 and 84 years (min–max), with T2D or NIDDM.

3.1. Fish and Fish Oil

A relationship between fish and/or marine n-3 fatty acids consumption and reduced risk of CVD was originally suggested by epidemiological studies among Greenland Inuits and Danes [56]. The effects of both the amount and quality of dietary fat and fish oil have since been studied intensively. Suggested mechanisms of the cardiovascular benefits from marine n-3 PUFAs include decreased plasma triglyceride levels and blood pressure, as well as anti-thrombotic, antiarrhythmic, and anti-inflammatory effects [57–59]. The effect of fish oil on glycemic regulation in T2D is less studied. In the present review, 14 intervention studies with fish or fish oil in people with T2D or NIDDM were included (Table 1).

Balfegó and coworkers investigated the effect of a standard diet with sardines on metabolic control [27]. Thirty-five subjects were randomized to follow either a T2D standard diet (control group), or a T2D standard diet enriched with 100 g of sardines per day, 5 days a week (sardine group) for 6 months. The changes in fasting glucose, glycated hemoglobin A1c (HbA1c), fasting insulin and HOMA-IR values were similar between the two groups [27]. The effects of moderate aerobic exercise and the incorporation of fish into a low-fat diet (30 energy (E) % fat) on glycemic control were examined in 49 subjects [34]. The subjects were randomly assigned to a low fat diet (30 E% fat) with or without one fish meal per day (3.6 g n-3 fatty acids) and further randomized to a moderate (55–65% VO_2 max) or light (heart rate <100 bpm) exercise program for eight weeks. While fasting insulin levels decreased in the fish and light exercise group compared with light exercise alone (control), there were no differences in fasting blood glucose concentration after any of the interventions compared with the control group. In the fish and light exercise group, they also demonstrated a significant rise in HbA1c compared with the control group [34].

Table 1. Effects of fish and fish oil on glycemic regulation in type 2 diabetes in randomized controlled trials. Significant results are indicated by an up/down arrow.

Study	Subject Characteristics	Study Design	Intervention	Glucose	Insulin	HbA1c	Other Markers
Wang et al. 2017, European Journal of Nutrition, China	*n* = 99, T2D, 65 years, M/F	6 months Parallel	(1) Corn oil (4 g/day) (2) Fish oil (4 g/day (1.34 g EPA and 1.07 g DHA))	↔	↔	↔	↔ HOMA-IR
Zheng et al. 2016, Mol. Nutr. Food Res, China	*n* = 166, T2D, 59 years, M/F	180 days Parallel	(1) Corn oil (1 g/day) (2) Fish oil (1 g/day (500 mg EPA + DHA, EPA:DHA = 3:2)) (3) Flaxseed oil (1 g/day (630 mg ALA))	↔	↔	(2) ↓ (3) ↔	↔ HOMA-IR
Balfegó et al. 2016, Lipids Health Dis, Spain	*n* = 35, T2D, 60 years, M/F	6 months Parallel	(1) Standard diet (2) Standard diet enriched with sardines 5 days a week (100 g/day)	↔	↔ *Within groups:* (1), (2) ↓	↔ *Within groups:* (1) ↓	↔ HOMA-IR *Within groups:* (1), (2) ↓ HOMA-IR
Sarbolouki et al. 2013, Singapore Med J, Iran	*n* = 67, T2D, 45 years, M/F	3 months Parallel	(1) Corn oil (2 g/day) (2) EPA (2 g/day)	↓	↓	↓	↓ HOMA-IR
Ogawa et al. 2013, Tohoku J Exp Med, Japan	*n* = 30, T2D, 80 years, M/F	3 months Parallel	(1) Liquid diet without EPA/DHA (2) Liquid diet containing EPA (25 mg/100 kcal) and DHA (17 mg/100 kcal)	↓		↓	
Crochemore et al. 2012, Nutr Clin Pract, Brazil	*n* = 41, T2D, 61 years, F	30 days Parallel	(1) Gelatin (500 mg/capsule) (2) Fish oil (2.5 g/day (547.5 mg EPA + 352.5 mg DHA)) (3) Fish oil (1.5 g/day (328.5 mg EPA + 211.5 mg DHA))	↔	↔	↔	↔ HOMA-IR ↔ QUICKI
Pooya et al. 2010, Nutrition, Metabolism & Cardiovascular Disease, Iran	*n* = 81, T2D, Control: 53 years Treatment: 56 years M/F	2 months Parallel	(1) Sunflower oil (2100 mg/day (12% SFA, 71% linoleic acid (LA), 16% MUFA)) (2) n-3 (3 g/day (1584 mg/day EPA, 828 mg/day DHA, 338 mg other n-3))	↔		↓	
Pedersen et al. 2003, EJCN, Denmark	*n* = 44, T2D, 63 years, M/F	8 weeks Parallel	(1) Corn oil (4 g/day) (2) Fish oil (4 g/day (2.6 g EPA + DHA))	↔ *Within groups:* (2) ↑		↔	
Luo et al. 1998, Diabetes Care, France	*n* = 10, T2D, 54 years, M	2 × 2 months Crossover	(1) Sunflower oil (6 g/day(65% n-6, 0,2% n-3, 24% MUFA, 11% SFA)) (2) Fish oil (6 g/day (1.8 g n-3: 18% EPA, 12% DHA, 4% n-6, 36% MUFA, 30% SFA))	↔	↔	↔	↔ euglycemic-hyperinsulinemic clamp

Table 1. *Cont.*

Study	Subject Characteristics	Study Design	Intervention	Glucose	Insulin	HbA1c	Other Markers
Dunstan et al. 1997, Diabetes Care, Australia	n = 49, NIDDM, 52–54 years, M/F	8 weeks parallel	(1) Light exercise (2) Fish (3.6 g n-3/day) and light exercise (3) Fish (3.6 g n-3/day) and moderate exercise (4) Moderate exercise	↔	(2) ↓ (3) (4) ↔	(2) ↑ (3) (4) ↔	
McManus et al. 1996, Diabetes Care, Canada	n = 11, T2D, 62 years, M/F	3 × 3 months Crossover	(1) Linseed oil (35 mg FA/kg body weight/day) (2) Fish oil (35 mg FA/kg body weight/day)	↔	↔	↔	↔ Insulin sensitivity ↔ Glucose effectiveness ↔ Acute insulin response to glucose
Morgan et al. 1995, Diabetes Care, USA	n = 40, NIDDM, 54 years, M/F	12 weeks Parallel	(1) Corn oil (9 g/day) (2) Corn oil (18 g/day) (3) Fish oil (9 g/day) (4) Fish oil (18 g/day)	↔		↔	
Annuzzi et al. 1991, Atherosclerosis, Italy	n = 8, NIDDM, 51 years, M	2 × 2 weeks Crossover	(1) Olive oil (10 g) (2) Fish oil (10 g (1.8 g EPA + 1.2 g DHA))	↔ ↔ daily average	↔ insulin sensitivity		↔ hyperglycemic clamp
Borkman et al. 1989 Diabetes, Austrailia	n = 10, NIDDM, 57 years, M/F	3 × 3 weeks Crossover	(1) Standard diabetic diet (2) Standard diabetic diet + Safflower oil (10 g) (3) Standard diabetic diet + Fish oil (10 g)	(2) (3) ↑	↔		↔ hyperinsulinemic-euglycemic clamp

Significant differences ($p \leq 0.05$) between intervention group(s) and control group are shown with ↑ or ↓, while ↔ indicates no significant difference. When several intervention groups are present, the results for each group are indicated with number. Fasting values are shown, if not otherwise stated. Control group is referred to as (1). DHA: docosahexaenoic acid; EPA: eicosapentaenoic acid; F: female; g: gram; Gr: group; HbA1c: glycated hemoglobin A1c; HOMA-IR: Homeostasis Assessment Model-Insulin Resistance; M: male; mg: milligram; MUFA: monounsaturated fatty acid; n: number; n-3: omega-3; NIDDM: non-insulin dependent diabetes mellitus; PUFA: polyunsaturated fatty acid; SFA: saturated fatty acid; T2D: type 2 diabetes; wt: weight.

Table 2. Effects of vegetable oils on glycemic regulation in type 2 diabetes in randomized controlled trials. Significant results are indicated by an up/down arrow.

Study	Subject Characteristics	Study Design	Intervention	Glucose	Insulin	HbA1c	Other Markers
Zibaeenezhad et al. 2016, Int J Endocrin Metab, Iran	*n* = 90, T2D, 55 years, M/F	3 months Parallel	(1) No oil (2) Walnut oil (15 g/day)	↓		↓	
Foster et al. 2013, Journal of Diabetes Research and Clinical Metabolism, Australia	*n* = 43, T2D, 65 years, F	12 weeks Parallel	(1) Olive oil (2000 mg/day + 40 mg/day zinc) (2) Zink (40 mg/d) (3) Flaxseed oil (2000 mg/day (1200 mg ALA)) (4) Zinc and flaxseed oil (40 mg/day zinc + 2000 mg/day flaxseed oil)	↔	↔ *Within groups:* (1) ↓	↔	↔ HOMA-IR *Within groups:* (1) ↓ HOMA-IR
Jenkins et al. 2014, Diabetes Care, Canada	*n* = 141, T2D, 59 years, M/F	3 months Parallel	(1) whole-wheat bread without canola oil (500 kcal/day) (2) low-GL diet with a canola oil-enriched bread (500 kcal/day)	↔		↓	
Taylor et al. 2010, AJCN, Canada	*n* = 34, T2D, 52 years, M/F	12 weeks Parallel	(1) Bakery products with no flaxseed (2) Bakery products with milled flaxseed (32 g/day) (3) Bakery products with flaxseed oil (13 g/day)	↔	↔	↔	↔ HOMA-IR ↔ QUICKI
Norris et al. 2009, AJCN, United States	*n* = 35, T2D, 60 years, F	2 × 16 weeks crossover	(1) Safflower oil (8 g/day) (2) CLA (*c*9*t*11 and *t*10*c*12) (8 g/day)	↑ *Within groups:* (1) ↓	↔		↑ HOMA-IR *Within groups:* (1) ↓ HOMA-IR
Barre et al. 2008, J Ole Sci, Canada	*n* = 32, T2D, 60 years, M/F	3 months Parallel	(1) Safflower oil 10 g/day (control) (2) Flaxseed oil 10 g/day (60 mg ALA/kg body weight/day)	↔	↔	↔	
Gerhard 2004, AJCN, United States	*n* = 11, T2D, 50 years, M/F	6 weeks Parallel	(1) Low-fat diet (total fat 20 E%, carbohydrates 65 E%, higher in fiber) (2) High MUFA diet (total fat 40 E%, MUFA 26 E%, carbohydrates 45 E%)	↔		↔	↔ Fructosamin

Table 2. *Cont.*

Study	Subject Characteristics	Study Design	Intervention	Glucose	Insulin	HbA1c	Other Markers
Brynes et al. 2000, AJCN, United Kingdom	$n = 9$, T2D, 56 years, M/F	2 × 3 weeks Crossover	(1) high-MUFA isoenergetic diet (olive oil) (2) high-PUFA isoenergetic diet (corn oil)	↔ ↔ iAUC	↔ ↔ iAUC	↔	↔ short insulin tolerance test (SITT)
Tsihlias et al. 2000, AJCN, Canada	$n = 72$, T2D, 42–79 years, M/F	6 months Parallel	(1) High-GI diet (cereals) (10% of energy) (2) Low-GI diet (cereals) (10% of energy) (3) High MUFA diet (margarine and olive oil) (10% of energy)	↔	(3) ↓ mean 8-h insulin (2) ↔ mean 8h insulin	↔	
Christiansen et al. 1997, Diabetes Care, Denmark	$n = 16$, NIDDM, 55 years, M/F	3 × 6 weeks Crossover	(1) SAT diet (20 E% SFA, 5 E% PUFA, 5 E% MUFA) (2) *Cis*-MUFA diet (20 E% *cis*-MUFA, 5 E% PUFA, 5 E% SFA) (3) *Trans*-MUFA diet (20 E% *trans*-MUFA, 5 E% PUFA, 5 E% SFA)	↔ ↔ AUC	↔ (2) ↓ iAUC	↔	(2) ↓ C-peptide iAUC
Lerman-Garber et al., 1994, Diabetes Care, Mexico	$n = 12$, NIDDM, 56 years, F	2 × 4 weeks Crossover	(1) Diet high in MUFA (HMUFA) (olive oil) (2) Diet high in complex carbohydrates (high-CHO)	↔ *Within groups:* (1), (2) ↓	↔ *Within groups:* (1), (2) ↓		↔ Fructosamine
Heine et al. 1989, AJCN, USA	$n = 14$, NIDDM, 52 years, M/F	2 × 30 weeks Crossover	(1) Low P:S diet (P:S ratio 0.3) (2) High P:S diet (P:S ratio 1.0)	↔ ↔ iAUC	↔	↔	↑ Metabolic clearance rate of glucose ↔ C-peptide

Significant differences ($p \leq 0.05$) between intervention group(s) and control group are shown with ↑ or ↓, while ↔ indicates no significant difference. When several intervention groups are present, the results are for each group are indicated with number. Fasting values are shown, if not otherwise stated. Control group is referred to as (1). ALA: alpha-linolenic Acid; CHO: carbohydrates; E%: energy %; F: female; g: gram; GI: glycemic index; GL: glycemic load; HbA1c: glycated hemoglobin A1c; HOMA-%β: HOMA–percentage beta cell function; HOMA-IR: Homeostasis Assessment Model-Insulin Resistance; iAUC: incremental area under the curve; M: male; MUFA: monounsaturated fatty acid; *n*: number; NIDDM: non-insulin dependent diabetes mellitus; P:S: PUFA/SFA ratio; PUFA: polyunsaturated fatty acid; SAT: high saturated fatty acid diet; SFA: saturated fatty acid; T2D: type 2 diabetes; QUICKI: quantitative insulin check.

Table 3. Effects of nuts on glycemic regulation in type 2 diabetes in randomized controlled trials. Significant results are indicated by an up/down arrow.

Study	Subject Characteristics	Study Design	Intervention	Glucose	Insulin	HbA1c	Other Markers
Mohan et al. 2018, J Nutr, India	*n* = 269, T2D, 51 years, M/F	12 weeks Parallel	(1) Standard diabetic diet (2) Standard diabetic diet plus cashew nuts (30 g/day)	↔	↔	↔	↔ HOMA-IR
Sauder et al. 2015, Metabolism, USA	*n* = 30, T2D, 40–74 years, M/F	2 × 4 weeks Crossover	(1) Control diet; based on the American Heart Association's Therapeutic Lifestyle Changes diet (26.9% total fat, 6.7% saturated fat, 186 mg/day cholesterol) (2) Pistachios added to the control diet (20 % of daily energy)	↔	↔	↔	↔ HOMA-IR ↔ Matsuda ↓ Fructosamine
Parham et al. 2014, Rev Diabet Study, Iran	*n* = 48, T2D, 50–53 years, M/F	2 × 12 weeks Crossover	(1) Diet without nuts (2) Pistachio nuts (50 g/day)	↓		↓	
Wien et al. 2014, Nutr Journal, USA	*n* = 60, T2D, 34–84 years, M/F	24 weeks Parallel	(1) ADA meal plan without nuts (2) ADA meal plan with peanuts (20% of total energy (mean 46 g/day))	↔		↔	
Kendall et al. 2011, Nutrition, Metabolism & Cardiovascular Diseases, Canada	*n* = 24 T2D: 68 years Healthy: 36 years M/F	2-h Postprandial Crossover	(1) White bread (50 g available carbohydrate) (2) Mixed nuts (30 g) (3) Mixed nuts (60 g) (4) Mixed nuts (90 g) (5) White bread + mixed nuts (30 g) (6) White bread + mixed nuts (60 g) (7) White bread + mixed nuts (90 g)	(2), (3), (4) ↓ iAUC (healthy and T2D) (6), (7) ↓ iAUC (healthy) (7) ↓ iAUC (T2D)			

Significant differences ($p \leq 0.05$) between intervention group(s) and control group are shown with ↑ or ↓, while ↔ indicates no significant difference. When several intervention groups are present, the results are for each group are indicated with number. Control group is referred to as (1). ADA: American Diabetes Association; d: day; F: female; g: gram; h: hour; HbA1c: glycated hemoglobin A1c; HOMA-IR: Homeostasis Assessment Model-Insulin Resistance; iAUC: incremental area under the curve; M: male; *n*: number; T2D: type 2 diabetes.

The effects of the marine n-3 fatty acids EPA/DHA in a liquid diet on glycemic control was investigated in a multicenter randomized trial with 30 elderly [29]. The subjects were divided into two groups receiving either an EPA/DHA-rich diet (EPA 25 mg/100 kcal and DHA 17 mg/100 kcal) or a diet without EPA/DHA (control group). A significant reduction in fasting blood glucose and HbA1c was observed after intake of EPA/DHA compared with the control diet [29]. Sarbolouki et al. included 67 men and women in a double blind, placebo-controlled randomized study to investigate the effects of EPA on glycemic regulation [28]. The participants received either EPA (2 g/day, 95% pure EPA) or placebo (2 g corn oil/day) for three months. EPA treatment reduced fasting plasma glucose, HbA1c, and HOMA-IR compared with the control group [28]. In a randomized, double blind, placebo-controlled trial, Wang and colleagues investigated the effect of 4 g fish oil per day (1.34 g EPA and 1.07 g DHA) or corn oil (control) on glucose metabolism in 99 subjects [25]. There were no significant effects on fasting serum glucose, insulin, HbA1c, or HOMA-IR after fish oil treatment for six months compared with corn oil [25]. Zhen et al. investigated the effects of n-3 PUFA from marine or vegetable sources on glycemic control in 166 subjects [26]. The study was a double blind RCT and the participants received either fish oil (2 g/day EPA + DHA), flaxseed oil (2.5 g/day alpha linolenic acid (ALA)), or corn oil (control group) for 180 days. Intake of fish oil, but not flaxseed oil, reduced HbA1c compared with corn oil. There were no effect on fasting insulin or glucose [26]. In order to determine the effects of n-3 fatty acids, a randomized, double blind, placebo-controlled trial was conducted in 81 subjects [31]. The subjects received capsules with either n-3 fatty acids (1.6 g/day EPA and 0.8 g/day DHA) or sunflower oil (control group) for two months. Treatment with n-3 fatty acids significantly decreased HbA1c, while fasting blood glucose was not significantly altered [31]. In line with these results, 6 g/day of either fish oil (1.8 g n-3 PUFAs) or sunflower oil (control) given to 10 men for two months did not show any significant changes in fasting blood glucose, insulin, or HbA1c between the groups [33]. The study had a randomized, double blind crossover design. In the same study, supplementation with fish oil did not alter basal hepatic glucose production and there were no difference in insulin suppression of hepatic glucose production nor in insulin stimulation of whole-body glucose disposal measured by the euglycemic-hyperinsulinemic clamp between the groups [33]. In a double blind RCT, Pedersen and colleagues investigated the impact of vitamin E-enriched fish oil in 44 subjects [32]. The participants received a daily dose of 4 g of either fish oil (2.6 g/day EPA + DHA) or corn oil (control) for eight weeks, in addition to an equal amount of vitamin E (53.6 g/day). There were no significant changes in fasting blood glucose or HbA1c between the groups. However, within the fish oil group, fasting blood glucose was increased [32]. In a double blind, randomized crossover study, 10 g of fish oil (1.8 g EPA + 1.2 g DHA) or olive oil (control) were given daily to eight male subjects for two weeks [37]. There were no significant changes in fasting blood glucose, average daily blood glucose, hyperglycemic clamp, nor insulin sensitivity [37]. In a double blind, randomized, crossover study, 11 subjects received supplements with fish oil, linseed oil, or olive oil (control) for three months in a dose corresponding to 35 mg fatty acids per kilogram body weight [35]. Neither fish oil nor linseed oil modulated glycemic control (fasting glucose and insulin, HbA1c, insulin sensitivity, glucose effectiveness, acute insulin response to glucose) compared with the control group [35]. Morgan and colleagues gave 40 subjects (18 men and 22 women) 9 g of fish oil, 18 g of fish oil, 9 g of corn oil, or 18 g of corn oil daily as a supplement for 12 weeks [36]. They did not detect any effect within (9 g versus 18 g) nor between (fish oil groups combined versus corn oil groups combined) the intervention groups on fasting glucose or HbA1c [36]. In a study by Borkman et al., 10 subjects were included in a three week blinded crossover study [38]. Subjects were given a standard diabetic diet supplemented with a daily dose of 10 g fish oil concentrate (30% n-3 fatty acids), 10 g safflower oil, or no supplementation (control). Fasting blood glucose increased with 14% during fish oil and 11% during safflower oil supplementation compared with control, whereas fasting insulin level remained unchanged [38].

Taken together, about half of the included studies (eight out of 14) found no significant changes related to markers of glycemic regulation such as fasting glucose, insulin, HbA1c or markers related to insulin resistance or sensitivity [25,27,30,32,33,35–37] after intervention with fish or fish oil when compared with a control group. In five of the studies a reduction in glucose [28,29], insulin [28,34] and/or HbA1c [26,28,29,31] was observed. Impaired glycemic regulation was observed in two studies, where intake of fish or fish oil increased fasting glucose [38] and an increase in HbA1c [34] was observed after intake of fish in combination with light exercise. In addition to the between groups effects, two of the studies found an additional effect on glycemic regulation within groups, in which Dunstan et al. observed increased HbA1c [34], while Balfego et al. found decreased effect on fasting insulin, HbA1c, and HOMA-IR [27]. In a recent meta-analysis of 11 RCTs including people with T2D, overweight individuals, or healthy individuals, Akinkuolie et al. showed that consumption of n-3 PUFAs did not affect insulin [60]. In line with this, a lack of association between n-3 PUFAs in blood and risk of T2D was the conclusion in the Uppsala Longitudinal Study of Adult Men (ULSAM) [61].

Since about half of the studies in the present review reported improved glycemic regulation while the other half reported no or impaired effects, it is difficult to draw a firm conclusion about fish and fish oil and glycemic regulation.

3.2. *Vegetable Oils*

Vegetable oils are rich in PUFAs, the main constituent being n-6 fatty acids, and in particular linoleic acid (LA). There is convincing evidence that partial replacement of SFAs with monounsaturated fatty acids (MUFAs) or PUFAs lowers fasting blood total- and LDL-cholesterol [5,13–15] and thereby reduces the risk of developing CVDs [5,6,13,14,62–64]. In addition to the cholesterol-lowering effects of PUFAs, some studies indicate that PUFAs may improve glycemic regulation [13,19]. Twelve studies investigating the effect of vegetable oils on glycemic control in people with T2D or NIDDM were included in this review (Table 2).

Foster and colleagues examined markers of glycemic control in 43 postmenopausal women after intake of flaxseed oil (high in alpha-linolenic acid (ALA)) for 12 weeks [40]. The study was a randomized, double blind, placebo-controlled trial, and the participants received either 40 mg/day zinc, 2 g/day flaxseed oil, both zinc and flaxseed oil, or olive oil (control). There were no significant changes in blood glucose, insulin, HbA1c or HOMA-IR between the intervention groups after 12 weeks. However, insulin and HOMA-IR decreased within the control group [40]. In a study by Jenkins et al., the combined effect of ALA, MUFAs, and low glycemic load on glycemic control and CVD risk factors were investigated in 141 subjects [41]. The study was a RCT with a parallel design and the subjects were provided daily with canola oil-enriched whole-wheat bread (500 kcal/day or 31 g canola oil per 2000 kcal) or whole-wheat bread without canola oil (500 kcal) (control diet). The test diet significantly reduced HbA1c compared with the control diet and the result remained statistically significant after adjustment for body weight change [41]. Barre and coworkers investigated the effect of flaxseed oil on glycemic control in 32 subjects [44]. The subjects were randomly assigned to receive 10 g/day of flaxseed oil or safflower oil for three months. The amount of ALA was approximately 60 mg/kg body weight/day in the flaxseed oil group. Flaxseed oil had no impact on fasting blood glucose, insulin, or HbA1c compared with the control group [44]. Conjugated linoleic acid (CLA), the *trans* fatty acid of LA, was compared with safflower oil high in *cis*-LA in 35 obese, postmenopausal women [43]. The participants consumed 8 g oil per day for 16 weeks in a crossover study, with four weeks washout in between the intervention periods, giving a total of 36 weeks. The aim of the study was to investigate weight reduction, and they found a significant reduction in BMI after CLA oil intake but not after safflower oil intake. Nevertheless, even though a weight reduction is associated with improved glycemic regulation, there was a significant reduction in fasting blood glucose only within the safflower oil group [43]. To investigate the long-term effects of a diet enriched in LA on insulin sensitivity, Heine and colleagues conducted a randomized, crossover study in 14 subjects [50]. The PUFA to SFA ratio (P:S ratio) of the diets were altered by substituting LA-rich fats and oils for products rich in saturated fats. The participants received a diet (total fat content of 38–39 E%) with a P:S ratio of 0.3 (low P:S diet) or 1.0 (high P:S diet) in a randomized order for 30 weeks each. Fasting blood glucose, insulin, HbA1c, glucose incremental area under the curve (iAUC), C-peptide, and insulin responses did not differ between the groups after intervention. However, the metabolic clearance rate of glucose was higher in the high P:S diet compared with the control group. This difference was only observed at the lowest infusion rate (6 mg/kg/min) [50]. A 12-week intervention with bakery products containing flaxseed oil (13 g/day), milled flaxseed (32 g/day), or no flaxseed (control group) investigated the effects on fasting blood glucose, insulin, and HbA1c in 34 adult males and females [42]. The flaxseed and flaxseed oil groups received equivalent amounts of 7.4 g ALA per day. There were no differences in fasting HbA1c, glucose and insulin after the intervention period [42]. Isocaloric diets with different fatty acid composition was investigated in a randomized crossover trial with 16 obese subjects for six weeks [48]. The energy content of carbohydrate, protein and fats were kept constant, but the diets differed in fat composition. There were no significant changes between the diets in HbA1c, fasting blood glucose, insulin, or postprandial glycemic response. However, serum insulin and C-peptide responses increased following the *trans*-MUFA and SAT diets compared with the *cis*-MUFA diet [48]. In a study by Gerhard et al., the effect of two ad libitum diets on glycemic control was investigated [45]. Eleven subjects were randomly assigned to receive an ad libitum low-fat, high-carbohydrate diet (20 E% total fat, 65 E% carbohydrates, higher in fiber), or a high-MUFA diet (40 E% total fat, 26 E% MUFAs, 45 E% carbohydrates), each for six weeks. There were no effect on fasting glucose or HbA1c after the high-MUFA diet compared with low-fat diet [45]. Brynes and coworkers investigated the effect of an isoenergetic high-MUFA diet (olive oil) compared with high-PUFA diet (corn oil), on glycemic regulation in nine overweight subjects [46]. Glycemic control remained stable throughout the study and there were no change in fasting or postprandial iAUC for glucose or insulin in response to an identical standard meal after 24 days of intervention [46]. Instead of comparing fat quality, intake of MUFAs from oil or margarine was compared with intake of carbohydrates from breakfast cereals with either a high or low glycemic index [47]. After a six-month intervention with 72 subjects there were no differences in fasting blood glucose or HbA1c between the groups. After a standard breakfast and lunch, a reduction in mean 8-h plasma insulin in the group given MUFAs compared with the cereal group was however observed [47]. During a four-week period, 12 women received an isocaloric diet high in either MUFAs (HMUFA) or complex carbohydrates (high-CHO). This crossover study had a four-week washout period during which the subjects followed the American Diabetes Association (ADA) isocaloric diet. Glycemic control, including fasting blood glucose, insulin and fructosamine did not significantly change with the different intervention diets. However, fasting blood glucose and insulin were reduced within both groups after intervention [49]. The effect of walnut oil on blood glucose in 90 subjects was investigated in a RCT, lasting for three months [39]. In the experimental group, walnut oil (15 g/day) was added to the diet, while the control group did not undergo any intervention. HbA1c level and fasting blood glucose decreased significantly in the experiment group compared with the control group [39].

In summary, six of the 12 studies investigating vegetable oils on glycemic regulation such as fasting glucose, insulin, HbA1c or markers related to insulin resistance or insulin sensitivity did not find any effects in people with T2D [40,42,44–46,49], although two of the studies found within group changes [40,49]. In the other six studies however, there were changes in glycemic regulation either between or within groups [39,41,43,47,49,50]. In contrast to the studies showing a decreasing effect on glycemic regulation after intervention, the study by Norris et al. found increased fasting glucose levels and HOMA-IR after intervention with CLA compared with safflower oil (control group). However, safflower oil reduced both fasting glucose levels and HOMA-IR within the control group [43]. Even though CLA, a *trans* fatty acid, is debated for its possible health effects [65], *trans* fatty acids in general are well known for their cholesterol increasing effects [66] and may explain the impaired effects related to glycemic regulation. Vegetable oils mainly consist of n-6 PUFAs and in particular LA, and other studies have shown a beneficial effect of n-6 PUFAs on glycemic regulation. A recent pooled analysis from prospective cohort studies demonstrated that higher levels of LA in blood were associated with a 43% reduced relative risk for T2D [67]. This is in line with the results from the ULSAM study. Men who developed T2D had a lower proportion of LA and a higher proportion of SFAs (C:14 and C:16) in serum cholesterol esters compared with those who did not develop T2D [61]. Summers et al. showed that switching from a diet rich in SFAs to a diet rich in PUFAs for 5 weeks improved insulin sensitivity in people with T2D, non-obese and obese subjects [68]. Even though others have found improved glycemic regulation after intervention with PUFAs, we are not able to draw firm conclusions based on the studies included in the present review.

3.3. *Nuts*

Nuts are high-energy, nutrient-dense foods that are rich in PUFAs and other bioactive components, including fiber, antioxidants, vitamins and minerals [69]. Epidemiological studies have found an inverse relationship between nut consumption and reduced risk of T2D [70,71]. In the present review, five RCTs intervening with different nuts (cashew, pistachio, peanuts or mixed nuts) in people with T2D were included (Table 3).

In the study by Mohan and coworkers, they investigated the effect of a standard diabetic diet with 30 g cashew nuts per day for 12 weeks on glycemic regulation in 300 subjects [51]. They did not find any significant differences in glycemic regulation (fasting blood glucose, insulin, HbA1c, and HOMA-IR) after the intervention [51]. In another study, by Parham et al., the effect of pistachio nut supplementation on glycemic control and inflammatory markers was investigated [53]. The study included 48 subjects in a double blind, randomized, placebo-controlled crossover trial. The subjects received either 25 g pistachio nuts twice a day or a control diet without nuts for 12 weeks, followed by an eight-week washout period, before switching interventions. A decrease in HbA1c and fasting blood glucose was observed after intake of pistachio nuts compared with the control group. There were no effects on HOMA-IR after intake of pistachio nuts [53]. Also, Sauder and coworkers investigated the effect of pistachio nuts on glycemic control [52]. They included 30 subjects in a randomized, controlled, crossover study. After a two-week run-in period, participants consumed diets with pistachio nuts (contributing with 20% of total energy) or without pistachio nuts (control group) for four weeks each, separated by a two-week washout period. Glycemic measures were assessed both fasted and during a 75-g oral glucose tolerance test. There were no effect on fasting glucose, insulin, HbA1c, HOMA-IR or glucose area under the curve (AUC) or insulin AUC after intake of nuts compared with control group [52]. Wien and colleagues investigated the effect of incorporating peanuts into the American Diabetes Association (ADA) meal plan on cardio-metabolic parameters [54]. They performed a 24-week parallel RCT with 60 subjects. The intervention group received an ADA meal plan containing about 20% of energy from peanuts, while the control group followed a peanut-free ADA meal plan. After 24 weeks of intervention, there were no differences in fasting blood glucose or HbA1c between the groups. [54]. In a study by Kendall and colleagues, the effect of nut consumption alone or in combination with white bread on postprandial glycaemia in 14 healthy compared with 10 people with T2D were examined [55]. The participants consumed 30, 60, and 90 g of mixed nuts alone or in combination with white bread (50 g available carbohydrate). All three doses of mixed nuts consumed alone significantly reduced the glycemic response compared with the control group. Adding nuts (60 g and 90 g) to white bread significantly reduced the glycemic response in healthy subjects however, significant reduction in glycemic response were only observed after adding 90 g nuts to white bread in people with T2D [55].

Taken together, three of the five studies investigating intake of nuts and glycemic regulation such as fasting blood glucose, insulin, HbA1c or markers related to insulin resistance or sensitivity found beneficial effects in T2D. Pistachio nuts reduced both fasting blood glucose levels and HbA1c [53] or fructosamine [52], and intervention with mixed nuts led to reduction in postprandial glycemic response [55]. In these studies, nut consumption benefits glycemic regulation regardless of the type of nuts, study design or duration. These results are in line with the The Prevención con Dieta Mediterránea (PREDIMED)-study, in which 30 g nuts per day (almonds, hazelnuts, and walnuts), given as supplements to a Mediterranean diet, significantly reduced the incidence of T2D compared with a low-fat diet without nut supplementation in high risk subjects [72].

4. Discussion

In the present summary, improvements related to glycemic control in people with T2D were observed in about half of the studies investigating the effect of fish, fish oil, or vegetable oil. Intake of nuts may however indicate a more beneficial effect, even though the number of studies are limited. The present review also demonstrates that the studies investigating the effect of PUFAs on glycemic control in subjects with T2D or NIDDM are quite different in design with respect to type of dietary intervention, study duration, and measurements of glycemic control, and hence the results are difficult to compare. Most importantly, the intervention and the control food differ largely between the studies. Of the included studies, mainly vegetable oils (corn, sunflower, linseed, and olives) functioned as control for both fish and fish oil interventions, and for different vegetable oils. Hence, the studies are comparing PUFAs of different quality. Considering that vegetable oils are high in PUFAs and therefore may affect glycemic regulation, the lack of effect in several of the included studies may be explained by the use of an inappropriate control group. It is therefore not possible to conclude whether intake of marine- or vegetable-derived PUFAs will have a positive effect on glycemic regulation in people with T2D. In the previous mentioned meta-analysis performed by Imamura et al., intake of PUFAs was compared with intake of SFAs. Changing the intake of SFAs with PUFAs improved glycaemia and insulin resistance [19]. SFAs may therefore represent a better control group when investigating the effect of PUFAs on glycemic regulation. The study by Imamura et al. was however not unique to T2D, as both healthy and people with T2D were included. This may explain the discrepant findings between previous studies and the present review. In addition, Coelho et al. conclude that supplementation of 0.42–5.2 g PUFAs per day for at least eight weeks may become an alternative treatment for T2D. However, only six studies were included in the review [20]. In contrast, a meta-analysis from 2011 did not find any effect of n-3 PUFA consumption on insulin sensitivity. The study included 11 studies investigating the effect in both healthy and people with T2D [60]. In addition, ALA-enriched diets did not affect HbA1c, fasting blood glucose, or insulin in a meta-analysis conducted in people with T2D. The study included eight interventions [73]. In conclusion, the reported discrepancies between other studies and this review regarding PUFAs and glycemic control are probably due to the heterogeneity of the studies.

Even though fat quality has been shown to affect glycemic regulation, it is possible that also fat quantity will be of importance. Vessby and coworkers reported that a total fat intake of more than 37 E% increases the risk of insulin resistance independent of fat quality [74]. Total fat intake were not consistently reported in the present reviewed studies, and hence we cannot rule out that a high total fat intake may have affected the results.

Limitations of the current review includes the search strategy. To ensure that the included studies had focus on glycemic regulation, the search words "glycemic control" were used. This may have affected the number of articles and we cannot rule out the possibility that some relevant studies have not been included. We did however include two studies from other reviews.

5. Conclusions

In the present review, we have identified studies that show beneficial effects of both marine and vegetable-derived PUFAs on glycemic control in people with T2D. The studies are however different in design and no firm conclusions can be drawn. In order to understand the role of PUFAs in the management of T2D, we suggest more well designed RCTs where the effect of PUFAs specifically is compared with the effect of SFAs.

Author Contributions: All authors contributed to the review. Literature search, V.H.T.-H., L.G., M.C.W.M.; Writing—Original Draft Preparation, V.H.T.-H.; Writing—Review and Editing, V.H.T.-H., L.G., M.C.W.M.

References

1. World Health Organization. The Top 10 Causes of Death. 2018. Available online: https://www.who.int/news-room/fact-sheets/detail/the-top-10-causes-of-death (accessed on 30 March 2019).
2. World Health Organization. *Global Report on Diabetes*; WHO: Geneva, Switzerland, 2016.
3. World Health Organization. Diabetes. 2018. Available online: https://www.who.int/en/news-room/fact-sheets/detail/diabetes (accessed on 30 March 2019).
4. Yoo, J.Y.; Kim, S.S. Probiotics and Prebiotics: Present Status and Future Perspectives on Metabolic Disorders. *Nutrients* **2016**, *8*, 173. [CrossRef] [PubMed]
5. Ulven, S.M.; Leder, L.; Elind, E.; Ottestad, I.; Christensen, J.J.; Telle-Hansen, V.H.; Skjetne, A.J.; Raael, E.; Sheikh, N.A.; Holck, M.; et al. Exchanging a few commercial, regularly consumed food items with improved fat quality reduces total cholesterol and LDL-cholesterol: A double-blind, randomised controlled trial. *Br. J. Nutr.* **2016**, *116*, 1383–1393. [CrossRef]
6. Estruch, R.; Ros, E.; Salas-Salvadó, J.; Covas, M.I.; Corella, D.; Arós, F.; Gómez-Gracia, E.; Ruiz-Gutiérrez, V.; Fiol, M.; Lapetra, J.; et al. Primary Prevention of Cardiovascular Disease with a Mediterranean Diet Supplemented with Extra-Virgin Olive Oil or Nuts. *N. Engl. J. Med.* **2018**, *379*, 1387–1389. [PubMed]
7. GBD 2015 Risk Factors Collaborators. Global, regional, and national comparative risk assessment of 79 behavioural, environmental and occupational, and metabolic risks or clusters of risks, 1990–2015: A systematic analysis for the Global Burden of Disease Study 2015. *Lancet* **2016**, *388*, 1659–1724. [CrossRef]
8. Knowler, W.C.; Barrett-Connor, E.; Fowler, S.E.; Hamman, R.F.; Lachin, J.M.; Walker, E.A.; Nathan, D.M. Reduction in the incidence of type 2 diabetes with lifestyle intervention or metformin. *N. Engl. J. Med.* **2002**, *346*, 393–403.
9. Lim, E.L.; Hollingsworth, K.G.; Aribisala, B.S.; Chen, M.J.; Mathers, J.C.; Taylor, R. Reversal of type 2 diabetes: Normalisation of beta cell function in association with decreased pancreas and liver triacylglycerol. *Diabetologia* **2011**, *54*, 2506–2514. [CrossRef] [PubMed]
10. Barnard, N.D.; Katcher, H.I.; Jenkins, D.J.; Cohen, J.; Turner-McGrievy, G. Vegetarian and vegan diets in type 2 diabetes management. *Nutr. Rev.* **2009**, *67*, 255–263. [CrossRef] [PubMed]
11. Barnard, R.J.; Jung, T.; Inkeles, S.B. Diet and exercise in the treatment of NIDDM. The need for early emphasis. *Diabetes Care* **1994**, *17*, 1469–1472. [CrossRef] [PubMed]
12. O'Flaherty, M.; Flores-Mateo, G.; Nnoaham, K.; Lloyd-Williams, F.; Capewell, S. Potential cardiovascular mortality reductions with stricter food policies in the United Kingdom of Great Britain and Northern Ireland. *Bull. World Health Organ.* **2012**, *90*, 522–531. [CrossRef]
13. Schwab, U.; Lauritzen, L.; Tholstrup, T.; Haldorsson, T.I.; Risérus, U.; Uusitupa, M.; Becker, W. Effect of the amount and type of dietary fat on cardiometabolic risk factors and risk of developing type 2 diabetes, cardiovascular diseases, and cancer: A systematic review. *Food Nutr. Res.* **2014**, *58*, 25145. [CrossRef] [PubMed]
14. Mozaffarian, D.; Micha, R.; Wallace, S. Effects on Coronary Heart Disease of Increasing Polyunsaturated Fat in Place of Saturated Fat: A Systematic Review and Meta-Analysis of Randomized Controlled Trials. *PLoS Med.* **2010**, *7*, e1000252. [CrossRef] [PubMed]
15. Jakobsen, M.U.; O'Reilly, E.J.; Heitmann, B.L.; Pereira, M.A.; Bälter, K.; Fraser, G.E.; Goldbourt, U.; Hallmans, G.; Knekt, P.; Liu, S.; et al. Major types of dietary fat and risk of coronary heart disease: A pooled analysis of 11 cohort studies123. *Am. J. Clin. Nutr.* **2009**, *89*, 1425–1432. [CrossRef]
16. Kinsell, L.W.; Michaels, G.D.; Olson, F.E.; Coelho, M.; McBride, Y.; Fukayama, G.; Conklin, J.; Walker, G. Dietary Fats and the Diabetic Patient. *N. Engl. J. Med.* **1959**, *261*, 431–434. [CrossRef] [PubMed]
17. Mann, J. Nutrition Recommendations for the Treatment and Prevention of Type 2 Diabetes and the Metabolic Syndrome: An Evidenced-Based Review. *Nutr. Rev.* **2006**, *64*, 422–427. [CrossRef]
18. Riserus, U.; Willett, W.C.; Hu, F.B. Dietary fats and prevention of type 2 diabetes. *Prog. Lipid Res.* **2009**, *48*, 44–51. [CrossRef] [PubMed]
19. Imamura, F.; Micha, R.; Wu, J.H.Y.; Otto, M.C.D.O.; Otite, F.O.; Abioye, A.I.; Mozaffarian, D. Effects of Saturated Fat, Polyunsaturated Fat, Monounsaturated Fat, and Carbohydrate on Glucose-Insulin Homeostasis: A Systematic Review and Meta-analysis of Randomised Controlled Feeding Trials. *PLoS Med.* **2016**, *13*, 1002087. [CrossRef]

20. Coelho, O.G.L.; da Silva, B.P.; Rocha, D.M.U.P.; Lopes, L.L.; Alfenas, R.C.G. Polyunsaturated fatty acids and type 2 diabetes: Impact on the glycemic control mechanism. *Crit. Rev. Food Sci. Nutr.* **2017**, *57*, 3614–3619. [CrossRef]
21. Meyer, K.A.; Kushi, L.H.; Jacobs, D.R.; Folsom, A.R. Dietary Fat and Incidence of Type 2 Diabetes in Older Iowa Women. *Diabetes Care* **2001**, *24*, 1528–1535. [CrossRef]
22. Salmerón, J.; Hu, F.B.; Manson, J.E.; Stampfer, M.J.; Colditz, G.A.; Rimm, E.B.; Willett, W.C. Dietary fat intake and risk of type 2 diabetes in women. *Am. J. Clin. Nutr.* **2001**, *73*, 1019–1026. [CrossRef] [PubMed]
23. Hartweg, J.; Perera, R.; Montori, V.M.; Dinneen, S.F.; Neil, A.H.; Farmer, A.J. Omega-3 polyunsaturated fatty acids (PUFA) for type 2 diabetes mellitus. *Cochrane Database Syst. Rev.* **2008**. [CrossRef] [PubMed]
24. Wanders, A.J.; Blom, W.A.M.; Zock, P.L.; Geleijnse, J.M.; Brouwer, I.A.; Alssema, M. Plant-derived polyunsaturated fatty acids and markers of glucose metabolism and insulin resistance: A meta-analysis of randomized controlled feeding trials. *BMJ Open Diabetes Res. Care* **2019**, *7*, e000585. [CrossRef]
25. Wang, F.; Wang, Y.; Zhu, Y.; Liu, X.; Xia, H.; Yang, X.; Sun, G. Treatment for 6 months with fish oil-derived n-3 polyunsaturated fatty acids has neutral effects on glycemic control but improves dyslipidemia in type 2 diabetic patients with abdominal obesity: A randomized, double-blind, placebo-controlled trial. *Eur. J. Nutr.* **2017**, *56*, 2415–2422. [CrossRef] [PubMed]
26. Zheng, J.S.; Lin, M.; Fang, L.; Yu, Y.; Yuan, L.; Jin, Y.; Feng, J.; Wang, L.; Yang, H.; Chen, W.; et al. Effects of n-3 fatty acid supplements on glycemic traits in Chinese type 2 diabetic patients: A double-blind randomized controlled trial. *Mol. Nutr. Food Res.* **2016**, *60*, 2176–2184. [CrossRef]
27. Balfegó, M.; Canivell, S.; Hanzu, F.A.; Sala-Vila, A.; Martínez-Medina, M.; Murillo, S.; Mur, T.; Ruano, E.G.; Linares, F.; Porras, N.; et al. Effects of sardine-enriched diet on metabolic control, inflammation and gut microbiota in drug-naïve patients with type 2 diabetes: A pilot randomized trial. *Lipids Heal.* **2016**, *15*, 78. [CrossRef] [PubMed]
28. Sarbolouki, S.; Javanbakht, M.; Derakhshanian, H.; Hosseinzadeh, P.; Zareei, M.; Hashemi, S.; Dorosty, A.; Eshraghian, M.; Djalali, M. Eicosapentaenoic acid improves insulin sensitivity and blood sugar in overweight type 2 diabetes mellitus patients: A double-blind randomised clinical trial. *Singap. Med. J.* **2013**, *54*, 387–390. [CrossRef]
29. Ogawa, S.; Abe, T.; Nako, K.; Okamura, M.; Senda, M.; Sakamoto, T.; Ito, S. Eicosapentaenoic Acid Improves Glycemic Control in Elderly Bedridden Patients with Type 2 Diabetes. *Tohoku J. Exp. Med.* **2013**, *231*, 63–74. [CrossRef]
30. Crochemore, I.C.C.; Souza, A.F.; de Souza, A.C.; Rosado, E.L. Omega-3 polyunsaturated fatty acid supplementation does not influence body composition, insulin resistance, and lipemia in women with type 2 diabetes and obesity. *Nutr. Clin. Pract.* **2012**, *27*, 553–560. [CrossRef]
31. Pooya, S.; Jalali, M.D.; Jazayery, A.D.; Saedisomeolia, A.; Eshraghian, M.R.; Toorang, F. The efficacy of omega-3 fatty acid supplementation on plasma homocysteine and malondialdehyde levels of type 2 diabetic patients. *Nutr. Metab. Cardiovasc. Dis.* **2010**, *20*, 326–331. [CrossRef] [PubMed]
32. Pedersen, H.; Petersen, M.; Major-Pedersen, A.; Jensen, T.; Nielsen, N.S.; Lauridsen, S.T.; Marckmann, P. Influence of fish oil supplementation on in vivo and in vitro oxidation resistance of low-density lipoprotein in type 2 diabetes. *Eur. J. Clin. Nutr.* **2003**, *57*, 713–720. [CrossRef]
33. Luo, J.; Rizkalla, S.W.; Vidal, H.; Oppert, J.-M.; Colas, C.; Boussairi, A.; Guerre-Millo, M.; Chapuis, A.-S.; Chevalier, A.; Durand, G.; et al. Moderate Intake of n-3 Fatty Acids for 2 Months Has No Detrimental Effect on Glucose Metabolism and Could Ameliorate the Lipid Profile in Type 2 Diabetic Men: Results of a controlled study. *Diabetes Care* **1998**, *21*, 717–724. [CrossRef]
34. Dunstan, D.W.; Mori, T.A.; Puddey, I.B.; Beilin, L.J.; Burke, V.; Morton, A.R.; Stanton, K.G. The Independent and Combined Effects of Aerobic Exercise and Dietary Fish Intake on Serum Lipids and Glycemic Control in NIDDM: A randomized controlled study. *Diabetes Care* **1997**, *20*, 913–921. [CrossRef]
35. McManus, R.M.; Jumpson, J.; Finegood, D.T.; Clandinin, M.T.; Ryan, E.A. A Comparison of the Effects of n-3 Fatty Acids from Linseed Oil and Fish Oil in Well-Controlled Type II Diabetes. *Diabetes Care* **1996**, *19*, 463–467. [CrossRef]
36. Morgan, W.A.; Raskin, P.; Rosenstock, J. A Comparison of Fish Oil or Corn Oil Supplements in Hyperlipidemic Subjects with NIDDM. *Diabetes Care* **1995**, *18*, 83–86. [CrossRef]

37. Annuzzi, G.; Rivellese, A.; Capaldo, B.; Di Marino, L.; Iovine, C.; Marotta, G.; Riccardi, G. A controlled study on the effects of n − 3 fatty acids on lipid and glucose metabolism in non-insulin-dependent diabetic patients. *Atherosclerosis* **1991**, *87*, 65–73. [CrossRef]
38. Borkman, M.; Chisholm, D.J.; Furler, S.M.; Storlien, L.H.; Kraegen, E.W.; Simons, L.A.; Chesterman, C.N. Effects of Fish Oil Supplementation on Glucose and Lipid Metabolism in NIDDM. *Diabetes* **1989**, *38*, 1314–1319. [CrossRef]
39. Zibaeenezhad, M.; Aghasadeghi, K.; Hakimi, H.; Yarmohammadi, H.; Nikaein, F. The Effect of Walnut Oil Consumption on Blood Sugar in Patients with Diabetes Mellitus Type 2. *Int. J. Endocrinol. Metab.* **2016**, *14*, e34889.
40. Foster, M.; Petocz, P.; Caterson, I.D.; Samman, S. Effects of zinc and α-linolenic acid supplementation on glycemia and lipidemia in women with type 2 diabetes mellitus: A randomized, double-blind, placebo-controlled trial. *J. Diabetes Res. Clin. Metab.* **2013**, *2*, 3–9. [CrossRef]
41. Jenkins, D.J.; Kendall, C.W.; Vuksan, V.; Faulkner, D.; Augustin, L.S.; Mitchell, S.; Ireland, C.; Srichaikul, K.; Mirrahimi, A.; Chiavaroli, L.; et al. Effect of Lowering the Glycemic Load With Canola Oil on Glycemic Control and Cardiovascular Risk Factors: A Randomized Controlled Trial. *Diabetes Care* **2014**, *37*, 1806–1814. [CrossRef]
42. Taylor, C.G.; Noto, A.D.; Stringer, D.M.; Froese, S.; Malcolmson, L. Dietary Milled Flaxseed and Flaxseed Oil Improve N-3 Fatty Acid Status and Do Not Affect Glycemic Control in Individuals with Well-Controlled Type 2 Diabetes. *J. Am. Nutr.* **2010**, *29*, 72–80. [CrossRef]
43. Norris, L.E.; Collene, A.L.; Asp, M.L.; Hsu, J.C.; Liu, L.-F.; Richardson, J.R.; Li, D.; Bell, D.; Osei, K.; Jackson, R.D.; et al. Comparison of dietary conjugated linoleic acid with safflower oil on body composition in obese postmenopausal women with type 2 diabetes mellitus1234. *Am. J. Clin. Nutr.* **2009**, *90*, 468–476. [CrossRef]
44. Barre, D.E.; Mizier-Barre, K.A.; Griscti, O.; Hafez, K. High Dose Flaxseed Oil Supplementation May Affect Fasting Blood Serum Glucose Management in Human Type 2 Diabetics. *J. Oleo Sci.* **2008**, *57*, 269–273. [CrossRef]
45. Gerhard, G.T.; Ahmann, A.; Meeuws, K.; McMurry, M.P.; Duell, P.B.; Connor, W.E. Effects of a low-fat diet compared with those of a high-monounsaturated fat diet on body weight, plasma lipids and lipoproteins, and glycemic control in type 2 diabetes. *Am. J. Clin. Nutr.* **2004**, *80*, 668–673. [CrossRef] [PubMed]
46. Brynes, A.E.; Edwards, C.M.; Jadhav, A.; Ghatei, M.A.; Bloom, S.R.; Frost, G.S. Diet-induced change in fatty acid composition of plasma triacylglycerols is not associated with change in glucagon-like peptide 1 or insulin sensitivity in people with type 2 diabetes. *Am. J. Clin. Nutr.* **2000**, *72*, 1111–1118. [CrossRef]
47. Tsihlias, E.B.; Gibbs, A.L.; McBurney, M.I.; Wolever, T.M. Comparison of high- and low-glycemic-index breakfast cereals with monounsaturated fat in the long-term dietary management of type 2 diabetes. *Am. J. Clin. Nutr.* **2000**, *72*, 439–449. [CrossRef] [PubMed]
48. Christiansen, E.; Schnider, S.; Palmvig, B.; Tauber-Lassen, E.; Pedersen, O. Intake of a Diet High in Trans Monounsaturated Fatty Acids or Saturated Fatty Acids: Effects on postprandial insulinemia and glycemia in obese patients with NIDDM. *Diabetes Care* **1997**, *20*, 881–887. [CrossRef]
49. Lerman-Garber, I.; Ichazo-Cerro, S.; Cardoso-Saldaña, G.; Posadas-Romero, C.; Zamora-Gonzalez, J. Effect of a High-Monounsaturated Fat Diet Enriched With Avocado in NIDDM Patients. *Diabetes Care* **1994**, *17*, 311–315. [CrossRef]
50. Heine, R.J.; Mulder, C.; Popp-Snijders, C.; Van Der Meer, J.; Van Der Veen, E.A. Linoleic-acid-enriched diet: Long-term effects on serum lipoprotein and apolipoprotein concentrations and insulin sensitivity in noninsulin-dependent diabetic patients. *Am. J. Clin. Nutr.* **1989**, *49*, 448–456. [CrossRef]
51. Mohan, V.; Gayathri, R.; Lakshmipriya, N.; Anjana, R.M.; Spiegelman, D.; Jeevan, R.G.; Balasubramaniam, K.K.; Jayanthan, M.; Gopinath, V.; Divya, S.; et al. Cashew Nut Consumption Increases HDL Cholesterol and Reduces Systolic Blood Pressure in Asian Indians with Type 2 Diabetes: A 12-Week Randomized Controlled Trial. *J. Nutr.* **2018**, *148*, 63–69. [CrossRef]
52. Sauder, K.A.; McCrea, C.E.; Ulbrecht, J.S.; Kris-Etherton, P.M.; West, S.G.; Kris-Ethertonb, S.G.W.P.M. Effects of pistachios on the lipid/lipoprotein profile, glycemic control, inflammation, and endothelial function in type 2 diabetes: A randomized trial. *Metab. Clin. Exp.* **2015**, *64*, 1521–1529. [CrossRef]

53. Parham, M.; Heidari, S.; Khorramirad, A.; Hozoori, M.; Hosseinzadeh, F.; Bakhtyari, L.; Vafaeimanesh, J. Effects of Pistachio Nut Supplementation on Blood Glucose in Patients with Type 2 Diabetes: A Randomized Crossover Trial. *Diabetes Stud.* **2014**, *11*, 190–196. [CrossRef]
54. Wien, M.; Oda, K.; Sabaté, J. A randomized controlled trial to evaluate the effect of incorporating peanuts into an American Diabetes Association meal plan on the nutrient profile of the total diet and cardiometabolic parameters of adults with type 2 diabetes. *Nutr. J.* **2014**, *13*, 10. [CrossRef] [PubMed]
55. Kendall, C.; Esfahani, A.; Josse, A.; Augustin, L.; Vidgen, E.; Jenkins, D. The glycemic effect of nut-enriched meals in healthy and diabetic subjects. *Nutr. Metab. Cardiovasc. Dis.* **2011**, *21*, S34–S39. [CrossRef]
56. Bang, H.O.; Dyerberg, J. Plasma lipids and lipoproteins in Greenlandic west coast Eskimos. *Acta Med. Scand.* **1972**, *192*, 85–94. [CrossRef] [PubMed]
57. Mozaffarian, D.; Wu, J.H. Omega-3 fatty acids and cardiovascular disease: Effects on risk factors, molecular pathways, and clinical events. *J. Am. Coll. Cardiol.* **2011**, *58*, 2047–2067. [CrossRef]
58. Delany, J.P.; Vivian, V.M.; Snook, J.T.; Anderson, P.A. Effects of fish oil on serum lipids in men during a controlled feeding trial. *Am. J. Clin. Nutr.* **1990**, *52*, 477–485. [CrossRef]
59. Saynor, R.; Verel, D.; Gillott, T. The long-term effect of dietary supplementation with fish lipid concentrate on serum lipids, bleeding time, platelets and angina. *Atherosclerosis* **1984**, *50*, 3–10. [CrossRef]
60. Akinkuolie, A.O.; Ngwa, J.S.; Meigs, J.B.; Djoussé, L. Omega-3 polyunsaturated fatty acid and insulin sensitivity: A meta-analysis of randomized controlled trials. *Clin. Nutr.* **2011**, *30*, 702–707. [CrossRef]
61. Vessby, B.; Aro, A.; Skarfors, E.; Berglund, L.; Salminen, I.; Lithell, H. The Risk to Develop NIDDM Is Related to the Fatty Acid Composition of the Serum Cholesterol Esters. *Diabetes* **1994**, *43*, 1353–1357. [CrossRef]
62. Sacks, F.M.; Campos, H. Polyunsaturated Fatty Acids, Inflammation, and Cardiovascular Disease: Time to Widen Our View of the Mechanisms. *J. Clin. Endocrinol. Metab.* **2006**, *91*, 398–400. [CrossRef]
63. Farvid, M.S.; Ding, M.; Pan, A.; Sun, Q.; Chiuve, S.E.; Steffen, L.M.; Willett, W.C.; Hu, F.B. Dietary Linoleic Acid and Risk of Coronary Heart Disease: A Systematic Review and Meta-Analysis of Prospective Cohort Studies. *Circulation* **2014**, *130*, 1568–1578. [CrossRef]
64. Warensjö, E.; Sundström, J.; Vessby, B.; Cederholm, T.; Risérus, U. Markers of dietary fat quality and fatty acid desaturation as predictors of total and cardiovascular mortality: A population-based prospective study. *Am. J. Clin. Nutr.* **2008**, *88*, 203–209. [CrossRef]
65. Kim, J.H.; Kim, Y.; Kim, Y.J.; Park, Y. Conjugated Linoleic Acid: Potential Health Benefits as a Functional Food Ingredient. *Annu. Rev. Food Sci. Technol.* **2016**, *7*, 221–244. [CrossRef]
66. Brouwer, I.A.; Wanders, A.J.; Katan, M.B. Trans fatty acids and cardiovascular health: Research completed? *Eur. J. Clin. Nutr.* **2013**, *67*, 541–547. [CrossRef]
67. Wu, J.H.Y.; Marklund, M.; Imamura, F.; Tintle, N.; Korat, A.V.A.; De Goede, J.; Zhou, X.; Yang, W.-S.; Otto, M.C.D.O.; Kröger, J.; et al. Omega-6 fatty acid biomarkers and incident type 2 diabetes: Pooled analysis of individual-level data for 39 740 adults from 20 prospective cohort studies. *Lancet Diabetes Endocrinol.* **2017**, *5*, 965–974. [CrossRef]
68. Summers, L.K.M.; Fielding, B.A.; Bradshaw, H.A.; Ilic, V.; Beysen, C.; Clark, M.L.; Moore, N.R.; Frayn, K.N. Substituting dietary saturated fat with polyunsaturated fat changes abdominal fat distribution and improves insulin sensitivity. *Diabetologia* **2002**, *45*, 369–377. [CrossRef]
69. Ros, E. Nuts and CVD. *Br. J. Nutr.* **2015**, *113* (Suppl. 2), S111–S120. [CrossRef]
70. Luo, C.; Zhang, Y.; Ding, Y.; Shan, Z.; Chen, S.; Yu, M.; Hu, F.B.; Liu, L. Nut consumption and risk of type 2 diabetes, cardiovascular disease, and all-cause mortality: A systematic review and meta-analysis. *Am. J. Clin. Nutr.* **2014**, *100*, 256–269. [CrossRef]
71. Jiang, R.; Manson, J.E.; Stampfer, M.J.; Liu, S.; Willett, W.C.; Hu, F.B. Nut and Peanut Butter Consumption and Risk of Type 2 Diabetes in Women. *JAMA* **2002**, *288*, 2554–2560. [CrossRef]
72. Salas-Salvadó, J.; Bulló, M.; Babio, N.; Martínez-González, M.Á.; Ibarrola-Jurado, N.; Basora, J.; Estruch, R.; Covas, M.I.; Corella, D.; Arós, F.; et al. Reduction in the incidence of type 2 diabetes with the Mediterranean diet: Results of the PREDIMED-Reus nutrition intervention randomized trial. *Diabetes Care* **2011**, *34*, 14–19. [CrossRef]

73. Jovanovski, E.; Li, D.; Ho, H.V.T.; Djedovic, V.; Marques, A.D.C.R.; Shishtar, E.; Mejia, S.B.; Sievenpiper, J.L.; De Souza, R.J.; Duvnjak, L.; et al. The effect of alpha-linolenic acid on glycemic control in individuals with type 2 diabetes: A systematic review and meta-analysis of randomized controlled clinical trials. *Medicine* **2017**, *96*, e6531. [CrossRef]
74. Vessby, B.; Uusitupa, M.; Hermansen, K.; Riccardi, G.; Rivellese, A.A.; Tapsell, L.C.; Nälsén, C.; Berglund, L.; Louheranta, A.; Rasmussen, B.M.; et al. Substituting dietary saturated for monounsaturated fat impairs insulin sensitivity in healthy men and women: The KANWU study. *Diabetologia* **2001**, *44*, 312–319. [CrossRef] [PubMed]

10

Serum Magnesium Concentrations in the Canadian Population and Associations with Diabetes, Glycemic Regulation and Insulin Resistance

Jesse Bertinato [1,2,*], Kuan Chiao Wang [3] and Stephen Hayward [3]

1 Nutrition Research Division, Food Directorate, Health Products and Food Branch, Health Canada, Sir Frederick G. Banting Research Centre, 251 Sir Frederick Banting Driveway, Ottawa, ON K1A 0K9, Canada

2 Department of Biochemistry, Microbiology and Immunology, University of Ottawa, Ottawa, ON K1H 8M5, Canada

3 Bureau of Food Surveillance and Science Integration, Food Directorate, Health Products and Food Branch, Health Canada, Ottawa, ON K1A 0K9, Canada; kuan.chiao.wang@hc-sc.gc.ca (K.C.W.); stephen.hayward@hc-sc.gc.ca (S.H.)

* Correspondence: jesse.bertinato@hc-sc.gc.ca

Abstract: Total serum magnesium (Mg) concentration (SMC) is commonly used to assess Mg status. This study reports current SMCs of Canadians and their associations with demographic factors, diabetes, and measures of glycemic control and insulin resistance using results from the Canadian Health Measures Survey cycle 3 (2012–2013). Associations were examined in adults aged 20–79 years using linear mixed models. Mean SMCs and percentile distributions for 11 sex-age groups between 3 and 79 years ($n = 5561$) are reported. SMCs were normally distributed and differences ($p < 0.05$) among sex and age groups were small. Between 9.5% and 16.6% of adult sex-age groups had a SMC below the lower cut-off of a population-based reference interval (0.75–0.955 mmol·L^{-1}) established in the United States population as part of the NHANES I conducted in 1971–1974. Having diabetes was associated with 0.04 to 0.07 mmol·L^{-1} lower SMC compared to not having diabetes in the various models. Body mass index, glycated hemoglobin, serum glucose and insulin concentrations, and homeostatic model assessment of insulin resistance were negatively associated with SMC. This is the first study to report SMCs in a nationally representative sample of the Canadian population. A substantial proportion of Canadians are hypomagnesaemic in relation to a population-based reference interval, and SMC was negatively associated with diabetes and indices of glycemic control and insulin resistance.

Keywords: Canada; diabetes; glycemic regulation; homeostatic model assessment of insulin resistance; serum magnesium concentration

1. Introduction

Magnesium (Mg) is a mineral nutrient that functions as a catalytic co-factor and structural component of enzymes and plays an important role as a calcium antagonist [1]. Mg is essential for many biological processes including the synthesis of organic molecules, cell proliferation, energy production, muscle contraction and relaxation, bone development, mineral metabolism, and glucose homeostasis [1–4]. In North America, Mg intakes fall short of dietary recommendations for a large segment of the population [5–7]. However, the extent of Mg deficiency in the general population and related health risks are unclear because of the uncertainty regarding Mg intakes needed for optimal health. This is underscored by the large differences in recommended intakes for

Mg established by different scientific bodies [8–10]. In addition, current information on Mg status of the North American population is lacking.

Total serum Mg concentration is the most widely used nutritional biomarker for assessing Mg status [1,11,12]. A recent meta-analysis of randomized controlled trials showed that serum (or plasma) Mg concentrations were significantly increased by oral Mg supplementation in a dose- and time-dependent manner [13]. Notably, little or no change in serum Mg was observed with higher baseline circulating Mg concentrations. Together, these results suggest that serum Mg concentrations can provide meaningful information on Mg status.

Information on serum Mg concentrations in the Canadian or United States populations from nationally-representative health surveys is limited. The last national estimates were based on data collected over 40 years ago in the first National Health and Nutrition Examination Survey (NHANES I) conducted in the United States between 1971 and 1974 [14]. These estimates were used to establish a population-based reference interval for adults of 0.75–0.955 mmol·L^{-1}. Based on this reference interval, a serum Mg concentration below 0.75 mmol·L^{-1} is usually defined as hypomagnesaemia (low serum Mg concentration).

Low Mg intakes and/or serum Mg concentrations have been associated with a number of diseases and health conditions including hypertension [15,16], sudden cardiac death [17,18], reduced bone mineral density [19], cardiovascular disease events [20,21], and colorectal cancer [22,23]. Poor Mg status may also impair growth of lean body mass [24] and decrease physical performance [25]. Diabetes (both type 1 and type 2) is the most common metabolic disorder associated with Mg deficiency [26–30], with reported incidence rates of hypomagnesaemia in diabetics as high as 13.5%–47.7% [27]. Multiple factors likely contribute to the hypomagnesaemia, including increased Mg loss through excretion by the kidneys. The higher renal Mg excretion is caused by reduced tubular Mg reabsorption resulting from glucose-induced osmotic diuresis and possibly insulin resistance [27,31]. Serum Mg has been negatively associated with fasting glucose and insulin concentrations and glycated hemoglobin (HbA_{1c}), a measure of long-term glycemic control [32–34]. Negative associations have also been reported with indirect indices of insulin resistance including quantitative insulin sensitivity check index (QUICKI), homeostatic model assessment of insulin resistance (HOMA-IR), and McAuley's index [32,35].

Nationally-representative data are preferred over non-national data for the development of nutrition policies and regulations. National estimates of serum Mg concentrations have never been reported for Canadians. The primary objective of this study was to report current national estimates of serum Mg concentrations for the Canadian population for ages 3–79 years using results from the Canadian Health Measures Survey (CHMS) cycle 3 conducted between 2012 and 2013. In Canada, the high prevalence of obesity [36] and co-morbidities such as insulin resistance and diabetes [37] may have a negative effect on the Mg status of the population. Thus, secondary analyses were performed to examine population-level associations between serum Mg concentrations and demographic factors, diabetes, and measures of glycemic regulation and insulin resistance in adults in order to add to our understanding of subpopulations at increased risk for Mg deficiency.

2. Materials and Methods

2.1. *Survey Design*

The CHMS is a cross-sectional, population-based survey that collects health information through a household interview and direct physical measures. The CHMS used a multi-stage sampling design. For cycle 3 of the survey, anthropometric measurements and biological samples were collected in a mobile examination centre (MEC) over 2 years from January 2012 to December 2013. Samples were collected from ~5700 volunteers aged 3 to 79 years from 16 collection sites stratified in five regions across Canada: Atlantic, Quebec, Ontario, Prairies, and British Columbia. The survey was designed to provide national estimates for children 3–5 years and for ages 6–11, 12–19, 20–39, 40–59, and 60–79 years for both sexes. Cycle 3 included members of the populations of the 10 provinces. Persons living in the territories, living on reserves and other aboriginal settlements in the provinces, full-time members of the Canadian Forces, the institutionalized, and persons living in certain remote areas were excluded from the survey. Altogether, these exclusions represent ~4% of the target population. The CHMS cycle 3 was approved by the Health Canada and Public Health Agency of Canada Research Ethics Board. Informed written consent was obtained from all participants older than 14 years of age. Parents or legal guardians provided written consent for younger children and the child gave assent. More detailed information on the aims of the CHMS, target population, and methodologies can be found elsewhere [38].

2.2. Biochemical Measurements

Fasted ($\geq$12 h) and nonfasted blood samples were collected and processed in a MEC. Whole blood was collected in 10 mL K_2EDTA tubes (CABD366643L, VWR International, Mississauga, ON, Canada). Serum was isolated from blood collected in 4 mL serum tubes (CABD367812L, VWR International). Whole blood and serum samples were shipped to the Nutrition Laboratory, Health Canada for measurement of HbA_{1c} (whole blood) and serum Mg, albumin, triglyceride, and glucose concentrations using the Vitros 5.1 FS clinical chemistry analyzer (Ortho Clinical Diagnostics, Mississauga, ON, Canada). Serum insulin concentration was measured using the Advia Centaur XP immunoassay analyzer (Siemens Healthcare Diagnostics, Mississauga, ON, Canada). The inter-assay (within lab precision) coefficients of variability (low–high concentration range) for HbA_{1c}, Mg, albumin, triglycerides, glucose and insulin were 1.9%–3.1%, 1.7%–0.9%, 1.7%–0.9%, 1.4%–0.9%, 1.5%–1.2%, and 5.9%–4.8%, respectively. Triglycerides and insulin were only measured in fasted participants. Results from samples with degree of hemolysis exceeding the threshold value for the assay were excluded from the analyses.

2.3. Collection of Demographic Information

Information on age, sex, race (i.e., white, South Asian, Chinese, black, Filipino, Latin American, Arab, Southeast Asian, West Asian, Korean, Japanese, other), diabetes, and yearly household income was collected at a household interview with the participants. The interview was conducted by trained interviewers using a computer-assisted interviewing method [38].

2.4. Calculations

QUICKI, HOMA-IR, and McAuley's index were calculated using the following equations: QUICKI, $(\log \text{insulin } (\mu\text{IU}\cdot\text{mL}^{-1}) + \log \text{glucose } (\text{mg}\cdot\text{dL}^{-1}))^{-1}$; HOMA-IR, $(\text{glucose } (\text{mmol}\cdot\text{L}^{-1}) \times \text{insulin } (\mu\text{IU}\cdot\text{mL}^{-1}))\ 22.5^{-1}$; and McAuley's index, $\exp(2.63 - 0.28 \ln \text{insulin } (\mu\text{IU mL}^{-1}) - 0.31 \ln \text{triglycerides } (\text{mmol}\cdot\text{L}^{-1}))$. BMI was calculated from weight and height measurements.

2.5. Statistical Analyses

The CHMS cycle 3 sampling design yields national estimates when survey weights are applied. Bootstrap weights were used for all variance estimations to account for the complex sampling design [39]. The 16 collection sites from five regional strata restricted the statistical analyses to 11 degrees of freedom. Descriptive statistics are presented as arithmetic means and percentiles with 95% confidence intervals. A *t*-test or ANOVA followed by Tukey's test was used for pairwise comparison of means. Association of serum Mg concentration with demographic and biochemical characteristics were assessed via linear mixed models. Age, sex, race (white or non-white), diabetes (type 1 and type 2 combined), BMI, and yearly household income were designated as fixed effects. HbA_{1c}, QUICKI, HOMA-IR, McAuley's index, and serum albumin, glucose, insulin, and triglyceride concentrations were modeled as random effects to account for the inherent variability associated with these measurements during sampling. Model 1 included the full adult sample set (fasted and nonfasted participants), and associations between Mg concentrations and age, sex, race, diabetes, BMI, household income, albumin, and HbA_{1c} were examined. Two additional models were developed using the fasted subsample. In model 2, associations with glucose, insulin, and triglycerides were investigated in addition to the variables examined in Model 1. In Model 3, associations with the indirect indices of insulin resistance QUICKI, HOMA-IR, and McAuley's index were examined instead of the direct measures glucose, insulin, and triglycerides. The SURVEYREG procedure with backwards elimination was used to develop the final models. For the purpose of interpretation, estimates for the continuous variables were also determined after a transformation using the 5th and 95th percentiles:

$$Y = (X - \text{5th percentile of } X) \div (\text{95th percentile of } X - \text{5th percentile of } X) \quad (1)$$

Pregnant women ($n = 19$) and participants with a missing or invalid value were excluded from the analyses. The coefficients of variation for all estimates were <16.6% and considered acceptable for unrestricted release based on the CHMS sampling variability guidelines [40]. Statistical significance was set a $p < 0.05$. Statistical analyses were performed using SAS/STAT® 9.3 software (SAS Institute Inc., Cary, NC, USA).

3. Results

Means and percentile distributions for total serum Mg concentration for 11 sex-age groups between 3 and 79 years are presented in Table 1. Distributions were symmetrical and thus arithmetic means were reported. In general, differences ($p < 0.05$) among sex and age groups were small. For ages 6–11 years, 20–39 years and 40–59 years females had lower means compared to males. Estimations for adolescents and adults at the 10th percentile were below a population-based reference interval for adults of 0.75–0.955 mmol·L^{-1} [14]. Between 9.5% and 16.6% of the adult sex-age groups had a serum Mg concentration below 0.75 mmol·L^{-1} (Figure 1). Estimates for the 25th and 95th percentiles for all sex-age groups were within the reference interval (Table 1). Boxplots show a greater number of older adults of both sexes with serum Mg concentration below the lower fence (i.e., 1.5 × interquartile range) (Figure S1).

Mean serum Mg concentration between fasted and nonfasted participants were similar ($p \geq 0.05$) for most sex-age groups (Table S1). However, fasted males and females 6–11 years had lower means than corresponding nonfasted participants. Conversely, fasted females aged 60–79 years had a higher mean compared to non-fasting females of the same age range.

Association of serum Mg concentration with demographic factors, diabetes and measures of glycemic control and insulin resistance were examined in adults aged 20–79 years using mixed models (data for children and adolescents aged 3–19 years were excluded from these analyses). Serum albumin concentration was included in the models because of a linear relationship with serum Mg at high and low concentrations [41]. For continuous variables associations were estimated for a defined unit change and after transformation using the 5th and 95th percentiles. After transformation the estimated change in serum Mg corresponds to the change in the continuous variable from the 5th to the 95th percentile in the population. This is a better indication of the relative strengths of the associations among variables since the magnitudes of associations are compared without confounding by their scales. Estimates of the 5th and 95th percentiles for each continuous variable are presented for each model.

In Model 1, associations were estimated in fasted and nonfasted adults (Table 2). Being male was associated with higher serum Mg, whereas white race (compared to non-white) or having diabetes (type 1 or type 2) was associated with lower Mg concentrations. Age, household income, and serum albumin concentration were positively associated with serum Mg, while BMI and HbA_{1c} showed a negative association.

In Models 2 and 3, associations were examined in fasted adults. In Model 2, serum Mg was positively associated with age and household income and negatively associated with diabetes and serum glucose and insulin concentrations (Table 3). In Model 3, age and household income showed positive associations, whereas diabetes and HOMA-IR showed negative associations (Table 4).

Table 1. Means and distributions of serum magnesium concentrations by sex and age in the Canadian population.

Sex and Age	n	Serum Magnesium		Distribution of Serum Magnesium Concentrations													
				5th		10th		25th		50th		75th		90th		95th	
		Arithmetic Mean [1]	95% CI	Estimate	95% CI	Estimate	95% CI	Estimate	95% CI	Estimate	95% CI	Estimate	95% CI	Estimate	95% CI	Estimate	95% CI
		mmol·L^{-1}															
All [2]																	
3–5 years	505	0.83	0.82, 0.84	0.74	0.72, 0.76	0.76	0.74, 0.77	0.78	0.77, 0.80	0.82	0.80, 0.84	0.86	0.84, 0.88	0.90	0.87, 0.93	0.92	0.90, 0.95
Male [3]																	
6–11 years	493	0.83 [a,*]	0.82, 0.84	0.73	0.71, 0.76	0.76	0.73, 0.78	0.79	0.78, 0.81	0.83	0.82, 0.84	0.86	0.85, 0.88	0.88	0.86, 0.91	0.91	0.88, 0.94
12–19 years	490	0.80 [c]	0.78, 0.81	0.71	0.68, 0.74	0.73	0.70, 0.75	0.76	0.72, 0.79	0.79	0.77, 0.81	0.83	0.80, 0.85	0.87	0.84, 0.89	0.88	0.87, 0.90
20–39 years	510	0.81 [b,c,*]	0.80, 0.82	0.69	0.64, 0.74	0.73	0.70, 0.76	0.77	0.74, 0.79	0.80	0.79, 0.82	0.84	0.83, 0.86	0.87	0.86, 0.89	0.90	0.87, 0.92
40–59 years	538	0.82 [a,b,*]	0.81, 0.83	0.71	0.68, 0.73	0.74	0.71, 0.77	0.78	0.76, 0.80	0.82	0.80, 0.84	0.86	0.84, 0.88	0.90	0.88, 0.92	0.91	0.88, 0.94
60–79 years	509	0.81 [b]	0.81, 0.82	0.69	0.67, 0.71	0.72	0.71, 0.74	0.77	0.75, 0.79	0.82	0.80, 0.84	0.86	0.84, 0.87	0.89	0.88, 0.91	0.91	0.89, 0.93
Female [3]																	
6–11 years	455	0.82 [a]	0.81, 0.83	0.74	0.72, 0.76	0.75	0.73, 0.78	0.78	0.77, 0.80	0.82	0.80, 0.84	0.85	0.83, 0.86	0.88	0.86, 0.89	0.89	0.88, 0.90
12–19 years	486	0.79 [d]	0.78, 0.80	0.70	0.68, 0.72	0.72	0.70, 0.73	0.75	0.73, 0.77	0.78	0.77, 0.80	0.82	0.80, 0.83	0.86	0.84, 0.87	0.88	0.86, 0.90
20–39 years	511	0.80 [c,d]	0.79, 0.80	0.71	0.70, 0.72	0.73	0.71, 0.75	0.76	0.74, 0.78	0.79	0.77, 0.80	0.82	0.80, 0.84	0.85	0.82, 0.88	0.87	0.85, 0.89
40–59 years	532	0.81 [b,c]	0.80, 0.82	0.69	0.64, 0.74	0.72	0.69, 0.76	0.76	0.74, 0.78	0.81	0.79, 0.82	0.85	0.83, 0.87	0.88	0.86, 0.89	0.89	0.87, 0.92
60–79 years	532	0.82 [a,b]	0.81, 0.83	0.67	0.65, 0.69	0.71	0.69, 0.73	0.77	0.75, 0.79	0.82	0.80, 0.83	0.86	0.84, 0.88	0.90	0.88, 0.92	0.93	0.90, 0.97

[1] Values in a column and within a sex group without a common superscript letter differ, $p < 0.05$. * Different compared to females in the same age group, $p < 0.05$; [2] Includes nonfasted males and females; [3] Includes fasted and nonfasted participants.

Table 2. Association of serum Mg with demographic factors, diabetes and biochemical measures [1].

IV	Estimate (95% CI) [2,3]	Estimate (95% CI) [3,4]	p	Distribution of Continuous IV	
	mmol·L^{-1}			5th (95% CI)	95th (95% CI)
Male [5]	0.01 (0.00, 0.01)	-	<0.01	-	-
White race [6]	−0.01 (−0.02, −0.00)	-	<0.001	-	-
Diabetes [7]	−0.04 (−0.05, −0.02)	-	<0.001	-	-
Age, year	0.01 (0.01, 0.01)	0.05 (0.04, 0.05)	<0.001	21.1 (18.3, 23.9)	71.7 (70.1, 73.3)
BMI, kg·m^{-2}	−0.002 (−0.002, −0.001)	−0.03 (−0.03, −0.02)	<0.001	19.7 (19.1, 20.3)	36.3 (34.7, 38.0)
Household income, K	0.0005 (0.0001, 0.0008)	0.01 (0.00, 0.01)	<0.01	15.0 (11.5, 18.5)	196.7 (166.2, 227.2)
Serum albumin, g·L^{-1}	0.002 (0.001, 0.003)	0.02 (0.01, 0.03)	<0.001	37.8 (36.3, 39.3)	48.9 (47.4, 50.5)
HbA_{1c}, %	−0.01 (−0.02, −0.01)	−0.02 (−0.03, −0.02)	<0.001	4.8 (4.6, 5.0)	6.5 (6.1, 6.9)

[1] Results from fasted and nonfasted adults aged 20–79 years, $n = 2838$ (Model 1). Sex, race, diabetes, age, BMI, household income, serum albumin concentration and HbA_{1c} were tested in the model. All variables were statistically significant ($p < 0.05$) and retained in the final model. HbA_{1c}, glycated hemoglobin; IV, independent variables; Mg, magnesium; [2] Changes in serum Mg concentrations associated with being male (compared to female), white race (compared to non-white race), diabetes, a 10 years increment in age, a 1 kg·m^{-2} increment in BMI, a $10 K increment in yearly household income, a 1 g·L^{-1} increment in serum albumin concentration and a 1% increment in HbA_{1c}; [3] Estimates are adjusted for all IV in the model; [4] Continuous variables were transformed using the 5th and 95th percentiles prior to analysis; [5] Males, $n = 1438$; [6] Whites, $n = 2331$; [7] Diabetics, $n = 217$.

Table 3. Association of serum Mg with demographic factors, diabetes and serum glucose and insulin concentrations [1].

IV	Estimate (95% CI) [2,3]	Estimate (95% CI) [3,4]	p	Distribution of Continuous IV	
	mmol·L^{-1}			5th (95% CI)	95th (95% CI)
Diabetes [5]	−0.06 (−0.07, −0.04)	-	<0.001	-	-
Age, year	0.01 (0.01, 0.01)	0.04 (0.03, 0.05)	<0.001	20.6 (17.9, 23.3)	70.8 (69.1, 72.4)
Household income, K	0.0008 (0.0004, 0.0012)	0.02 (0.01, 0.02)	<0.001	14.5 (10.3, 18.7)	199.0 (162.5, 235.6)
Serum glucose, mmol·L^{-1}	−0.01 (−0.01, −0.00)	−0.01 (−0.02, −0.01)	<0.001	4.3 (4.1, 4.4)	6.6 (5.9, 7.4)
Serum insulin, pmol·L^{-1}	−0.00008 (−0.00013, −0.00004)	−0.01 (−0.02, −0.00)	<0.001	25.1 (21.9, 28.2)	180.1 (156.7, 203.4)

[1] Results from fasted adults aged 20–79 years, $n = 1621$ (Model 2). Sex, race, diabetes, age, BMI, household income, serum albumin concentration, HbA_{1c}, serum glucose concentration, serum insulin concentration and serum triglyceride concentration were tested in the model. Statistically significant ($p < 0.05$) variables were selected by backwards elimination and retained in the final model. IV, independent variables; Mg, magnesium; [2] Changes in serum Mg concentrations associated with diabetes, a 10 years increment in age, a $10 K increment in yearly household income, a 1 mmol·L^{-1} increment in serum glucose concentration and a 1 pmol·L^{-1} increment in serum insulin concentration; [3] Estimates are adjusted for all IV in the model; [4] Continuous variables were transformed using the 5th and 95th percentiles prior to analysis; [5] Diabetics, $n = 99$.

Table 4. Association of serum Mg with demographic factors, diabetes and HOMA-IR [1].

IV	Estimate (95% CI) [2,3]	Estimate (95% CI) [3,4]	p	Distribution of Continuous IV	
	mmol·L^{-1}			5th (95% CI)	95th (95% CI)
Diabetes [5]	−0.07 (−0.08, −0.06)	-	<0.001	-	-
Age, year	0.01 (0.01, 0.01)	0.04 (0.03, 0.05)	<0.001	20.6 (18.0, 23.3)	70.8 (69.1, 72.5)
Household income, K	0.0008 (0.0004, 0.0012)	0.02 (0.01, 0.02)	<0.001	14.5 (10.3, 18.7)	199.0 (162.0, 236.0)
HOMA-IR	−0.003 (−0.004, −0.002)	−0.02 (−0.02, −0.01)	<0.001	0.80 (0.67, 0.93)	6.99 (6.34, 7.65)

[1] Results from fasted adults aged 20–79 years, $n = 1621$ (Model 3). Sex, race, diabetes, age, BMI, household income, serum albumin concentration, HbA_{1c}, serum triglyceride concentration and HOMA-IR were tested in the model. Statistically significant ($p < 0.05$) variables were selected by backwards elimination and retained in the final model. HOMA-IR, homeostatic model assessment of insulin resistance; IV, independent variables; Mg, magnesium; [2] Changes in serum Mg concentrations associated with diabetes, a 10 years increment in age, a $10 K increment in yearly household income and an increment of 1 for HOMA-IR; [3] Estimates are adjusted for all IV in the model; [4] Continuous variables were transformed using the 5th and 95th percentiles prior to analysis; [5] Diabetics, $n = 99$.

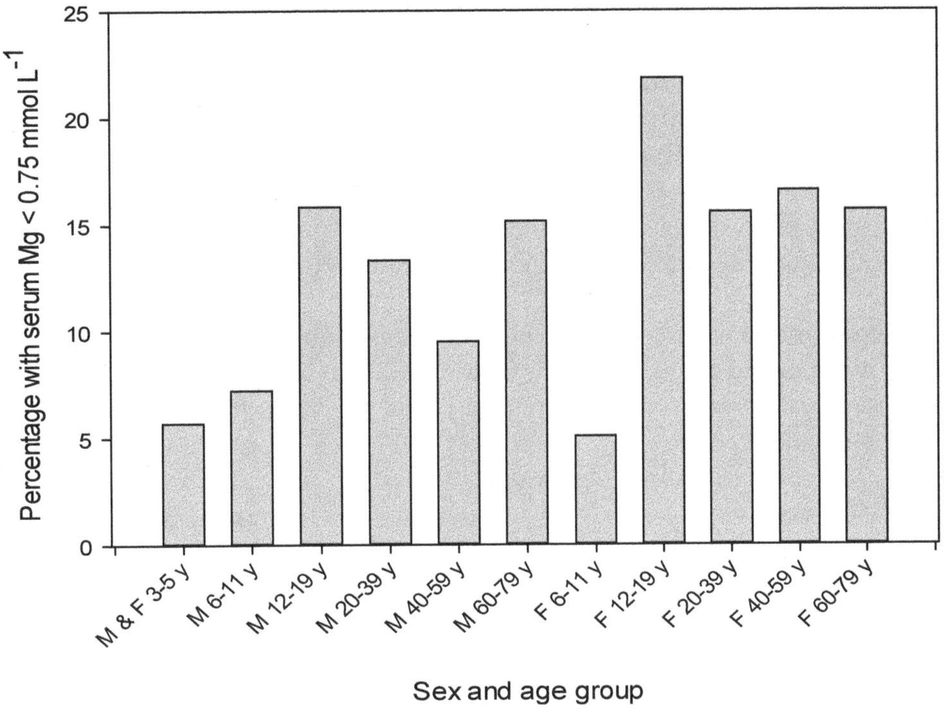

Figure 1. Percentage of each sex and age group with a serum Mg concentration below 0.75 mmol·L^{-1}. The total number of participants (*n*) examined for each sex-age group is shown in Table 1. F, females; M, males; y, years.

4. Discussion

This study describes current (2012–2013) estimates of serum Mg concentrations in a nationally representative sample of the Canadian population for ages 3–79 years. These results are the first national estimates in Canada or the United States since the NHANES I conducted between 1971 and 1973 [14]. Results from that study showed a normal distribution for serum Mg concentration, with 95% of adults aged 18–74 years having a value between 0.75 and 0.955 mmol·L^{-1}. Those estimates were considered as normative for the United States population and were used to establish a population-based reference interval. Serum Mg concentrations in the present study were also normally distributed. Substantial proportions of the adult sex-age groups (9.5%–16.6%) and adolescents aged 12–19 years (15.8%–21.8%) had a serum Mg concentration below 0.75 mmol·L^{-1}, the lower cut-off of the reference interval. All estimates at the 10th percentile for adolescents and adults were also below 0.75 mmol·L^{-1}. In addition, means in this study were lower than means reported in the NHANES I for comparable sex-age groups [14]. Collectively, these results suggest that present-day serum Mg concentrations in Canada are lower compared to concentrations in the United States population in the early 1970s. Since it has been suggested that a serum Mg concentration below 0.75 mmol·L^{-1} represents relatively severe Mg deficiency [11], these results raise suspicions of Mg deficiency in the Canadian population. Estimates at the 95th percentile for all sex-age groups were within the reference interval indicating the rarity of hypermagnesaemia in the population.

Similar to results from the NHANES I, only small differences in serum Mg concentrations were found among sex and age groups. Serum Mg concentrations were highest for children and showed a small increase with age from adolescents 12–19 years to older adults 60–79 years. Among demographic factors, age was the strongest predictor of serum Mg concentration in adults. The magnitudes of associations with sex, race, and household income were considerably smaller. A major finding from the NHANES I was the lower serum Mg in black Americans compared to white Americans [14]. In the present study, being white was associated with a lower serum Mg concentration than being non-white. It should be mentioned that because of the small sample sizes for all racial groups other than whites (including blacks), comparison among races in this study was restricted to the general groups of whites and non-whites.

Boxplot analyses revealed a greater number of older adults with serum Mg values below the lower fence (outliers) indicating that older adults are more prone to marked hypomagnesaemia. Possible explanations include lower dietary Mg intakes, reduced gastrointestinal Mg absorption, and increased renal Mg excretion in the elderly [42]. The higher occurrence of health conditions (e.g., diabetes) and other factors (e.g., use of hypermagnesuric diuretics) that alter Mg metabolism may also contribute [43].

Serum Mg concentrations were compared between fasted and nonfasted participants. Mean serum Mg concentrations were found to be lower for fasted children aged 6–11 years, but higher for fasted females aged 60–79 years. It is presently unclear what accounts for these differences. While the differences could be considered modest, these data offer a caution when interpreting results from a routine serum Mg test for these sex-age groups.

Inverse associations between serum Mg and diabetes and comorbidities such as poor glycemic control and insulin resistance have been well established. However, it is likely that these relationships are affected by factors that can differ among countries or change in populations over time (e.g., dietary Mg intakes, supplement and medication use). Thus, in this study associations of serum Mg concentration with diabetes and measures of glycemic regulation and insulin resistance were investigated in adults to determine the magnitude of these associations in a relatively current nationally-representative dataset. Diabetes was a strong predictor of serum Mg concentration. The estimated lower serum Mg in diabetics (ranging from -0.04 to -0.07 mmol$\cdot$L^{-1} in the various models) accounts for ~20% to 34% of the spread between the lower and upper limits of the normal reference interval. These estimates are substantial and likely have clinical relevance. Serum Mg was also negatively associated with HbA_{1c} and fasting serum glucose concentration. A negative effect of diabetes on Mg status is noteworthy given the high prevalence of diabetes in Canada which is expected to rise to over 10% by the year 2020 [37].

The hyperinsulinemic euglycemic clamp is considered the "gold standard" for assessment of insulin sensitivity, but the complexity of the method limits its use in large studies [44]. In this study, associations between serum Mg and more practical surrogate indices of insulin resistance [45] were examined. Fasting insulin concentration correlates strongly with insulin resistance [46] and HOMA-IR is considered a robust tool for the evaluation of insulin resistance in large epidemiological studies [47,48]. Serum Mg showed a negative association with both fasting insulin and HOMA-IR, indicating a positive relationship between serum Mg and insulin sensitivity. Notably, these relationships were observed in models controlling for diabetes. It should be mentioned that HOMA-IR was determined to be a better predictor of serum Mg concentration compared to other proxy measures of insulin resistance such as QUICKI or McAuley's index that were insignificant ($p \geq 0.05$) in our selection process.

There is evidence indicating that the relationship between Mg deficiency and type 2 diabetes is bidirectional. Mg deficiency is a common manifestation in type 1 and type 2 diabetics [26,27] and may also increase the risk of diabetes and its complications [29–31]. The negative associations between serum Mg and measures of glycemic regulation observed in this study are in agreement with studies indicating that poor glycemic control lowers serum Mg concentrations [33,34]. However, lower serum Mg may also contribute to poorer glycemic regulation and insulin sensitivity. Studies indicate that Mg supplementation improves glucose and insulin sensitivity parameters [49,50]. A meta-analysis of randomized controlled trials showed that Mg supplementation for over four months improved fasting glucose and HOMA-IR in diabetic and non-diabetic subjects [49]. In another meta-analysis, Mg supplementation was shown to reduce fasting plasma glucose in diabetics and improve HOMA-IR and plasma glucose (in a 2 h oral glucose tolerance test) in persons at high risk of diabetes [50]. The mechanisms by which Mg deficiency may increase diabetes risk are poorly understood but may involve increased oxidative stress and inflammation [35,51,52]. It is important to mention that this study does not provide any information on the temporality of the reported associations with serum Mg given the cross-sectional design.

The main strength of this study is the CHMS cycle 3 study design, including the large sample size that is representative of the Canadian population that is ideal for estimating national serum Mg concentrations and population distributions. The use of mixed models and continuous variables (rather than dichotomizing continuous variables) is also a strength. Limitations include the absence of Mg intake data (including supplement use) for comparison with serum Mg concentrations. The different methodologies used to measure serum Mg in this study and the NHANES I (colorimetric vs. atomic absorption spectroscopy) limits, to some extent, the comparison of results between studies; however, serum Mg measurements by the colorimetric method (the most commonly used method) or atomic absorption show excellent agreement ($R > 0.99$) [53]. Also, based on the responses to the household questionnaire, many diabetics in this study could not be categorized as having type 1 or type 2 diabetes. Thus, in our analyses, diabetics included participants with type 1 or type 2 diabetes or both.

The limitations of total serum Mg concentration as a biomarker of Mg status also merit discussion. Only a small fraction (~0.3%) of total body Mg is present in the serum and fluctuations in serum proteins such as albumin can alter Mg concentrations [41]. Furthermore, serum Mg may not always accurately reflect intracellular Mg deficiency. Serum Mg concentration is tightly regulated primarily at the level of renal excretion. Bone also maintains circulating concentrations by acting as a store for Mg and supplementing the serum under conditions of deficiency. This homeostatic regulation is likely a major factor accounting for the poor association observed between serum Mg concentrations and dietary Mg intakes, particularly when intakes meet nutrient requirements [54,55]. Despite these limitations, low serum Mg is usually indicative of Mg deficiency. Serum Mg is decreased in a dose-dependent manner in animal models of dietary Mg deficiency, demonstrating that low Mg intakes (Mg deficiency) reduce serum Mg concentration [56,57]. Human studies have shown that serum Mg is responsive to long-term changes in dietary Mg intakes [58] and increases with Mg supplementation [13,59,60]. A meta-analysis of randomized controlled trials showed that serum Mg concentrations increase in a dose- and time-dependent manner with oral Mg supplementation, and the response is greater when baseline circulating Mg concentrations are lower, suggesting that serum Mg provides useful information about underlying Mg status [13]. It has been suggested that a serum Mg value below 0.75 $mmol{\cdot}L^{-1}$ is a useful measure of relatively severe Mg deficiency, but Mg deficiency cannot be excluded for persons with a value between 0.75 and 0.85 $mmol{\cdot}L^{-1}$ [11,12].

5. Conclusions

This study reports serum Mg concentrations for 11 sex-age groups between 3 and 79 years in the Canadian population. Between 9.5% and 16.6% of the adult sex-age groups were hypomagnesaemic (serum Mg < 0.75 $mmol{\cdot}L^{-1}$) in relation to a population-based reference interval [14]. There is a need to establish an evidence-based reference interval (or at minimum a lower cut-off value) for health that will allow more accurate assessment of the prevalence of Mg deficiency in Canada and related health risk based on results from this study [61]. Among demographic factors, age was the strongest predictor of serum Mg concentration. Serum Mg concentration was negatively associated with diabetes, BMI, serum glucose, serum insulin, HbA_{1c}, and HOMA-IR. These results are consistent with a growing body of evidence indicating a negative effect of diabetes, poor glycemic control, and insulin resistance on Mg status.

Supplementary Materials:

Figure S1: Boxplots of serum Mg concentrations by sex-age group, Table S1: Means and distributions of serum magnesium concentrations by sex and age in fasted and nonfasted Canadians.

Acknowledgments: This research was funded by the Bureau of Nutritional Sciences and the Bureau of Food Surveillance and Science Integration, Health Canada.

Author Contributions: J.B. conceived the study; J.B., K.C.W. and S.H. analyzed the data; J.B. wrote the paper.

References

1. Swaminathan, R. Magnesium metabolism and its disorders. *Clin. Biochem. Rev.* **2003**, *24*, 47–66. [PubMed]
2. Volpe, S.L. Magnesium in disease prevention and overall health. *Adv. Nutr.* **2013**, *4*, 378S–383S. [CrossRef] [PubMed]
3. Elin, R.J. Magnesium: The fifth but forgotten electrolyte. *Am. J. Clin. Pathol.* **1994**, *102*, 616–622. [CrossRef] [PubMed]
4. Wolf, F.I.; Cittadini, A. Magnesium in cell proliferation and differentiation. *Front. Biosci.* **1999**, *4*, D607–D617. [CrossRef] [PubMed]
5. Moshfegh, A.; Goldman, J.D.; Ahuja, J.; Rhodes, D.; LaComb, R. *What We Eat in America, NHANES 2005–2006: Usual Nutrient Intakes from Food and Water Compared to 1997 Dietary Reference Intakes for Vitamin D, Calcium, Phosphorus, and Magnesium*; U.S. Department of Agriculture, Agriculture Research Service: Washington, DC, USA, 2009.
6. Health Canada. Do Canadian Adults Meet Their Nutrient Requirements through Food Intake Alone? Available online: http://www.hc-sc.gc.ca/fn-an/surveill/nutrition/commun/art-nutr-adult-eng.php (accessed on 23 February 2017).
7. Ford, E.S.; Mokdad, A.H. Dietary magnesium intake in a national sample of US adults. *J. Nutr.* **2003**, *133*, 2879–2882. [PubMed]
8. Food and Nutrition Board, Institute of Medicine. *Dietary Reference Intakes for Calcium, Phosphorus, Magnesium, Vitamin D, and Fluoride*; National Academy Press: Washington, DC, USA, 1997; pp. 190–249.
9. EFSA Panel on Dietetic Products, Nutrition and Allergies (NDA). Scientific opinion on dietary reference values for magnesium. *EFSA J.* **2015**, *13*, 4186.
10. Joint FAO/WHO Expert Consultation. *Vitamin and Mineral Requirements in Human Nutrition: Report of a Joint FAO/WHO Expert Consultation*, 2nd ed.; World Health Organization: Geneva, Switzerland, 2004.
11. Arnaud, M.J. Update on the assessment of magnesium status. *Br. J. Nutr.* **2008**, *99*, S24–S36. [CrossRef] [PubMed]
12. Elin, R.J. Assessment of magnesium status for diagnosis and therapy. *Magnes. Res.* **2010**, *23*, S194–S198. [PubMed]
13. Zhang, X.; Del Gobbo, L.C.; Hruby, A.; Rosanoff, A.; He, K.; Dai, Q.; Costello, R.B.; Zhang, W.; Song, Y. The circulating concentration and 24-h urine excretion of magnesium dose- and time-dependently respond to oral magnesium supplementation in a meta-analysis of randomized controlled trials. *J. Nutr.* **2016**, *146*, 595–602. [CrossRef] [PubMed]
14. Lowenstein, F.W.; Stanton, M.F. Serum magnesium levels in the United States, 1971–1974. *J. Am. Coll. Nutr.* **1986**, *5*, 399–414. [CrossRef] [PubMed]
15. Ma, J.; Folsom, A.R.; Melnick, S.L.; Eckfeldt, J.H.; Sharrett, A.R.; Nabulsi, A.A.; Hutchinson, R.G.; Metcalf, P.A. Associations of serum and dietary magnesium with cardiovascular disease, hypertension, diabetes, insulin, and carotid arterial wall thickness: The ARIC study. Atherosclerosis Risk in Communities Study. *J. Clin. Epidemiol.* **1995**, *48*, 927–940. [CrossRef]
16. Zhang, X.; Li, Y.; Del Gobbo, L.C.; Rosanoff, A.; Wang, J.; Zhang, W.; Song, Y. Effects of magnesium supplementation on blood pressure: A meta-analysis of randomized double-blind placebo-controlled trials. *Hypertension* **2016**, *68*, 324–333. [CrossRef] [PubMed]
17. Kieboom, B.C.; Niemeijer, M.N.; Leening, M.J.; van den Berg, M.E.; Franco, O.H.; Deckers, J.W.; Hofman, A.; Zietse, R.; Stricker, B.H.; Hoorn, E.J. Serum magnesium and the risk of death from coronary heart disease and sudden cardiac death. *J. Am. Heart Assoc.* **2016**, *5*, e002707. [CrossRef] [PubMed]
18. Peacock, J.M.; Ohira, T.; Post, W.; Sotoodehnia, N.; Rosamond, W.; Folsom, A.R. Serum magnesium and risk of sudden cardiac death in the Atherosclerosis Risk in Communities (ARIC) Study. *Am. Heart J.* **2010**, *160*, 464–470. [CrossRef] [PubMed]
19. Orchard, T.S.; Larson, J.C.; Alghothani, N.; Bout-Tabaku, S.; Cauley, J.A.; Chen, Z.; LaCroix, A.Z.; Wactawski-Wende, J.; Jackson, R.D. Magnesium intake, bone mineral density, and fractures: Results from the Women's Health Initiative Observational study. *Am. J. Clin. Nutr.* **2014**, *99*, 926–933. [CrossRef] [PubMed]

20. Del Gobbo, L.C.; Imamura, F.; Wu, J.H.; de Oliveira Otto, M.C.; Chiuve, S.E.; Mozaffarian, D. Circulating and dietary magnesium and risk of cardiovascular disease: A systematic review and meta-analysis of prospective studies. *Am. J. Clin. Nutr.* **2013**, *98*, 160–173. [CrossRef] [PubMed]
21. Qu, X.; Jin, F.; Hao, Y.; Li, H.; Tang, T.; Wang, H.; Yan, W.; Dai, K. Magnesium and the risk of cardiovascular events: A meta-analysis of prospective cohort studies. *PLoS ONE* **2013**, *8*, e57720. [CrossRef] [PubMed]
22. Chen, G.C.; Pang, Z.; Liu, Q.F. Magnesium intake and risk of colorectal cancer: A meta-analysis of prospective studies. *Eur. J. Clin. Nutr.* **2012**, *66*, 1182–1186. [CrossRef] [PubMed]
23. Qu, X.; Jin, F.; Hao, Y.; Zhu, Z.; Li, H.; Tang, T.; Dai, K. Nonlinear association between magnesium intake and the risk of colorectal cancer. *Eur. J. Gastroenterol. Hepatol.* **2013**, *25*, 309–318. [CrossRef] [PubMed]
24. Bertinato, J.; Lavergne, C.; Rahimi, S.; Rachid, H.; Vu, N.A.; Plouffe, L.J.; Swist, E. Moderately low magnesium intake impairs growth of lean body mass in obese-prone and obese-resistant rats fed a high-energy diet. *Nutrients* **2016**, *8*, 253. [CrossRef] [PubMed]
25. Veronese, N.; Berton, L.; Carraro, S.; Bolzetta, F.; De Rui, M.; Perissinotto, E.; Toffanello, E.D.; Bano, G.; Pizzato, S.; Miotto, F.; et al. Effect of oral magnesium supplementation on physical performance in healthy elderly women involved in a weekly exercise program: A randomized controlled trial. *Am. J. Clin. Nutr.* **2014**, *100*, 974–981. [CrossRef] [PubMed]
26. De Valk, H.W. Magnesium in diabetes mellitus. *Neth. J. Med.* **1999**, *54*, 139–146. [CrossRef]
27. Pham, P.C.; Pham, P.M.; Pham, S.V.; Miller, J.M.; Pham, P.T. Hypomagnesemia in patients with type 2 diabetes. *Clin. J. Am. Soc. Nephrol.* **2007**, *2*, 366–373. [CrossRef] [PubMed]
28. Kao, W.H.; Folsom, A.R.; Nieto, F.J.; Mo, J.P.; Watson, R.L.; Brancati, F.L. Serum and dietary magnesium and the risk for type 2 diabetes mellitus: The Atherosclerosis Risk in Communities Study. *Arch. Intern. Med.* **1999**, *159*, 2151–2159. [CrossRef] [PubMed]
29. Larsson, S.C.; Wolk, A. Magnesium intake and risk of type 2 diabetes: A meta-analysis. *J. Intern. Med.* **2007**, *262*, 208–214. [CrossRef] [PubMed]
30. Weng, L.C.; Lee, N.J.; Yeh, W.T.; Ho, L.T.; Pan, W.H. Lower intake of magnesium and dietary fiber increases the incidence of type 2 diabetes in Taiwanese. *J. Formos. Med. Assoc.* **2012**, *111*, 651–659. [CrossRef] [PubMed]
31. Gommers, L.M.; Hoenderop, J.G.; Bindels, R.J.; de Baaij, J.H. Hypomagnesemia in type 2 diabetes: A vicious circle? *Diabetes* **2016**, *65*, 3–13. [CrossRef] [PubMed]
32. Bertinato, J.; Xiao, C.W.; Ratnayake, W.M.; Fernandez, L.; Lavergne, C.; Wood, C.; Swist, E. Lower serum magnesium concentration is associated with diabetes, insulin resistance, and obesity in South Asian and white Canadian women but not men. *Food Nutr. Res.* **2015**, *59*, 25974. [CrossRef] [PubMed]
33. Arpaci, D.; Tocoglu, A.G.; Ergenc, H.; Korkmaz, S.; Ucar, A.; Tamer, A. Associations of serum magnesium levels with diabetes mellitus and diabetic complications. *Hippokratia* **2015**, *19*, 153–157. [PubMed]
34. Sinha, S.; Sen, S. Status of zinc and magnesium levels in type 2 diabetes mellitus and its relationship with glycemic status. *Int. J. Diabetes Dev. Ctries.* **2014**, *34*, 220–223. [CrossRef]
35. Kim, D.J.; Xun, P.; Liu, K.; Loria, C.; Yokota, K.; Jacobs, D.R., Jr.; He, K. Magnesium intake in relation to systemic inflammation, insulin resistance, and the incidence of diabetes. *Diabetes Care* **2010**, *33*, 2604–2610. [CrossRef] [PubMed]
36. Shields, M.; Carroll, M.D.; Ogden, C.L. Adult obesity prevalence in Canada and the United States. *NCHS Data Brief* **2011**, *56*, 1–8.
37. Public Health Agency of Canada. Diabetes in Canada: Facts and Figures from a Public Health Perspective. Available online: http://www.phac-aspc.gc.ca/cd-mc/publications/diabetes-diabete/facts-figures-faits-chiffres-2011/index-eng.php (accessed on 23 February 2017).
38. Statistics Canada. Canadian Health Measures Survey (CHMS). Available online: http://www23.statcan.gc.ca/imdb/p2SV.pl?Function=getSurvey&Id=136652 (accessed on 23 February 2017).
39. Giroux, S. Canadian Health Measures Survey: Sampling strategy overview. *Health Rep.* **2007**, *18*, S31–S36.
40. Statistics Canada. Canadian Health Measures Survey (CHMS) Data User Guide: Cycle 1. Available online: http://www23.statcan.gc.ca/imdb-bmdi/document/5071_D2_T1_V1-eng.htm (accessed on 23 February 2017).
41. Kroll, M.H.; Elin, R.J. Relationships between magnesium and protein concentrations in serum. *Clin. Chem.* **1985**, *31*, 244–246. [PubMed]
42. Seelig, M.S.; Preuss, H.G. Magnesium metabolism and perturbations in the elderly. *Geriatr. Nephrol. Urol.* **1994**, *4*, 101–111. [CrossRef]

43. Barbagallo, M.; Belvedere, M.; Dominguez, L.J. Magnesium homeostasis and aging. *Magnes. Res.* **2009**, *22*, 235–246. [PubMed]
44. DeFronzo, R.A.; Tobin, J.D.; Andres, R. Glucose clamp technique: A method for quantifying insulin secretion and resistance. *Am. J. Physiol.* **1979**, *237*, E214–E223. [PubMed]
45. Singh, B.; Saxena, A. Surrogate markers of insulin resistance: A review. *World J. Diabetes* **2010**, *1*, 36–47. [CrossRef] [PubMed]
46. Olefsky, J.; Farquhar, J.W.; Reaven, G. Relationship between fasting plasma insulin level and resistance to insulin-mediated glucose uptake in normal and diabetic subjects. *Diabetes* **1973**, *22*, 507–513. [CrossRef] [PubMed]
47. Matthews, D.R.; Hosker, J.P.; Rudenski, A.S.; Naylor, B.A.; Treacher, D.F.; Turner, R.C. Homeostasis model assessment: Insulin resistance and beta-cell function from fasting plasma glucose and insulin concentrations in man. *Diabetologia* **1985**, *28*, 412–419. [CrossRef] [PubMed]
48. Gutch, M.; Kumar, S.; Razi, S.M.; Gupta, K.K.; Gupta, A. Assessment of insulin sensitivity/resistance. *Indian J. Endocrinol. Metab.* **2015**, *19*, 160–164. [CrossRef] [PubMed]
49. Simental-Mendia, L.E.; Sahebkar, A.; Rodriguez-Moran, M.; Guerrero-Romero, F. A systematic review and meta-analysis of randomized controlled trials on the effects of magnesium supplementation on insulin sensitivity and glucose control. *Pharmacol. Res.* **2016**, *111*, 272–282. [CrossRef] [PubMed]
50. Veronese, N.; Watutantrige-Fernando, S.; Luchini, C.; Solmi, M.; Sartore, G.; Sergi, G.; Manzato, E.; Barbagallo, M.; Maggi, S.; Stubbs, B. Effect of magnesium supplementation on glucose metabolism in people with or at risk of diabetes: A systematic review and meta-analysis of double-blind randomized controlled trials. *Eur. J. Clin. Nutr.* **2016**, *70*, 1354–1359. [CrossRef] [PubMed]
51. Zheltova, A.A.; Kharitonova, M.V.; Iezhitsa, I.N.; Spasov, A.A. Magnesium deficiency and oxidative stress: an update. *BioMedicine* **2016**, *6*, 8–14. [CrossRef] [PubMed]
52. Barbagallo, M.; Dominguez, L.J. Magnesium and type 2 diabetes. *World J. Diabetes* **2015**, *6*, 1152–1157. [CrossRef] [PubMed]
53. Instructions for Use. VITROS Chemistry Products Mg Slides. Available online: https://www.cmmc.org/cmmclab/IFU/Mg_MP2-47_EN_I.pdf (accessed on 23 February 2017).
54. Lakshmanan, F.L.; Rao, R.B.; Kim, W.W.; Kelsay, J.L. Magnesium intakes, balances, and blood levels of adults consuming self-selected diets. *Am. J. Clin. Nutr.* **1984**, *40*, 1380–1389. [PubMed]
55. Misialek, J.R.; Lopez, F.L.; Lutsey, P.L.; Huxley, R.R.; Peacock, J.M.; Chen, L.Y.; Soliman, E.Z.; Agarwal, S.K.; Alonso, A. Serum and dietary magnesium and incidence of atrial fibrillation in whites and in African Americans: Atherosclerosis Risk in Communities (ARIC) Study. *Circ. J.* **2013**, *77*, 323–329. [CrossRef] [PubMed]
56. Bertinato, J.; Lavergne, C.; Plouffe, L.J.; El Niaj, H.A. Small increases in dietary calcium above normal requirements exacerbate magnesium deficiency in rats fed a low magnesium diet. *Magnes. Res.* **2014**, *27*, 35–47. [PubMed]
57. Bertinato, J.; Plouffe, L.J.; Lavergne, C.; Ly, C. Bioavailability of magnesium from inorganic and organic compounds is similar in rats fed a high phytic acid diet. *Magnes. Res.* **2014**, *27*, 175–185. [PubMed]
58. Klevay, L.M.; Milne, D.B. Low dietary magnesium increases supraventricular ectopy. *Am. J. Clin. Nutr.* **2002**, *75*, 550–554. [PubMed]
59. Witkowski, M.; Hubert, J.; Mazur, A. Methods of assessment of magnesium status in humans: A systematic review. *Magnes. Res.* **2011**, *24*, 163–180. [PubMed]
60. Song, Y.; He, K.; Levitan, E.B.; Manson, J.E.; Liu, S. Effects of oral magnesium supplementation on glycaemic control in type 2 diabetes: A meta-analysis of randomized double-blind controlled trials. *Diabet. Med.* **2006**, *23*, 1050–1056. [CrossRef] [PubMed]
61. Costello, R.B.; Elin, R.J.; Rosanoff, A.; Wallace, T.C.; Guerrero-Romero, F.; Hruby, A.; Lutsey, P.L.; Nielsen, F.H.; Rodriguez-Moran, M.; Song, Y.; et al. Perspective: The case for an evidence-based reference interval for serum magnesium: the time has come. *Adv. Nutr.* **2016**, *7*, 977–993. [CrossRef] [PubMed]

11

Effect of Oral Nutritional Supplements with Sucromalt and Isomaltulose versus Standard Formula on Glycaemic Index, Entero-Insular Axis Peptides and Subjective Appetite in Patients with Type 2 Diabetes

Lisse Angarita Dávila [1,*], Valmore Bermúdez [2], Daniel Aparicio [3], Virginia Céspedes [4], Ma. Cristina Escobar [1], Samuel Durán-Agüero [5], Silvana Cisternas [6], Jorge de Assis Costa [7,8], Diana Rojas-Gómez [9], Nadia Reyna [3] and Jose López-Miranda [10,11]

1 Escuela de Nutrición y Dietética, Facultad de Medicina, Universidad Andres Bello, Sede Concepción 4260000, Chile
2 Facultad de Ciencias de la Salud, Universidad Simón Bolívar, Barranquilla 080003, Colombia
3 Centro de Investigaciones Endocrino-Metabólicas "Dr. Félix Gómez", Escuela de Medicina. Facultad de Medicina, Universidad del Zulia, Maracaibo 4001, Venezuela
4 Departamento de Medicina Física y Rehabilitación, Hospital "12 de Octubre", Madrid 28041, Spain
5 Escuela de Nutrición y Dietética, Facultad de Ciencias para el Cuidado de la Salud, Universidad San Sebastián, Santiago 7500000, Chile
6 Escuela de Salud, Universidad Tecnológica de Chile, INACAP, Sede Concepción, Talcahuano 4260000, Chile
7 Faculty of Medicine/UniFAGOC, Ubá 36506-022, Minas Gerais, Brazil
8 Universidade do Estado de Minas Gerais (UEMG), Barbacena 36202-284, Minas Gerais, Brazil
9 Escuela de Nutrición y Dietética, Facultad de Medicina, Universidad Andres Bello, Santiago 8370321, Chile
10 Lipids and Atherosclerosis Unit, Maimonides Institute for Biomedical Research in Cordoba, Reina Sofia University Hospital, University of Córdoba, 14004 Córdoba, Spain
11 CIBER Physiopathology of Obesity and Nutrition (CIBEROBN), Institute of Health Carlos III, 28029 Madrid, Spain
* Correspondence: lisse.angarita@unab.cl

Abstract: Oral diabetes-specific nutritional supplements (ONS-D) induce favourable postprandial responses in subjects with type 2 diabetes (DM2), but they have not been correlated yet with incretin release and subjective appetite (SA). This randomised, double-blind, cross-over study compared postprandial effects of ONS-D with isomaltulose and sucromalt versus standard formula (ET) on glycaemic index (GI), insulin, glucose-dependent insulinotropic polypeptide (GIP), glucagon-like peptide 1 (GLP-1) and SA in 16 individuals with DM2. After overnight fasting, subjects consumed a portion of supplements containing 25 g of carbohydrates or reference food. Blood samples were collected at baseline and at 30, 60, 90, 120, 150 and 180 min; and SA sensations were assessed by a visual analogue scale on separate days. Glycaemic index values were low for ONS-D and intermediate for ET ($p < 0.001$). The insulin area under the curve ($AUC_{0–180\ min}$) ($p < 0.02$) and GIP AUC ($p < 0.02$) were lower after ONS-D and higher GLP-1 AUC when compared with ET ($p < 0.05$). Subjective appetite AUC was greater after ET than ONS-D ($p < 0.05$). Interactions between hormones, hunger, fullness and GI were found, but not within the ratings of SA; isomaltulose and sucromalt may have influenced these factors.

Keywords: glycaemic index; incretins; subjective appetite; isomaltulose; sucromalt; nutritional supplement

1. Introduction

Diabetes mellitus (DM) is a complex metabolic disorder associated with long-term complications as a result of the interplay of genetic, epigenetic, environmental and lifestyle factors [1]. Nowadays, DM is considered a pandemic health problem and one of the top 10 killers, responsible for 1.6 million deaths in 2016 [2]. According to International Diabetes Federation projections, by 2045, 629 million people will be afflicted by DM, exhibiting the fastest rising prevalence of this phenomenon in the history of humanity, which the highest prevalence rates in North America and the Caribbean [3]. Thus, the epidemiological impact of this disease is translated into higher public health expenditures worldwide [4,5].

One of the most important strategies for the prevention and treatment of DM has been correct management of carbohydrate consumption, having been reviewed in dietary guidelines and recommendations stated by many scientific organisations worldwide [6]. The American Diabetes Association (ADA) has highlighted this need, considering nutritional therapy as the fundamental basis of glycaemic control in DM patients [7]. Besides that, the European Association for the Study of Diabetes (EASD) has also focused its recommendations on the amount and type of carbohydrates consumed [8], generating considerable interest in low glycaemic index (LGI) food prescription for management of DM2 [9]. Indeed, a recent international expert consensus debated about the clinical role of GI and glycaemic load (GL) in DM management [10], concluding that low GI and low GL diets have been associated with a reduction in the glycaemic response variability [11], and better appetite control [12,13]. This phenomenon leads us to hypothesise that lower insulin responses exhibited by these supplements could promote satiety and fullness [10,12–14].

Nutritional approaches to type 2 diabetes usually include novel strategies in dietary advice, especially in oral nutritional supplements (ONS) prescription as part of the management of some DM comorbidities or as a complement for daily diet [15,16]. Any ONS designed for people with diabetes (ONS-D) provides better control in postprandial glucose and glycated haemoglobin (HbA_1c) when compared with standard supplements [17], since they are lower in total carbohydrate content (with a variety of sugar substitutes) and enriched with fibre and monounsaturated fatty acids [16,18,19]. Dietary fat and carbohydrate modifications modulate postprandial glycaemic responses by a reduction in glucose absorption rate [20].

The increase in peripheral glucose uptake via entero-insular axis peptides (EIAPs) such as the glucose-dependent insulinotropic peptide (GIP), glucagon-like peptide 1 (GLP-1), and insulin are a group of synergistic pathways counteracting undesirable glucose postprandial peaks [21]. Furthermore, a decrease in GIP secretion drives to adipocyte hypertrophy arrest and insulin resistance amelioration [22]. By contrast, GLP-1 has a direct suppression effect on appetite and protects pancreatic β-cells from programmed cell death [22,23]. It is well known that beverages have a faster gastric emptying and intestinal transit speed than solid food, which results in a rapid glycaemic response and lower perception of satiety [13,23]. For these reasons, the strategies of specific oral supplements designed for people with diabetes should include adaptation in the overall nutrients content [18,19]. Therefore, variations in both EIAP action and gastric emptying modulation by diet could play a fundamental role in short-time appetite regulation and energy intake [24,25].

Use of ONS-Ds in malnourished or sarcopenic diabetic patients enhances energy intake and overall nutritional status, improving glycaemic control, and thus, cause indirect economic benefits [19]. A meta-analysis by Elia et al. [15] on a total of 23 studies and 784 patients receiving oral supplements or tube feeding showed that when compared with standard supplements, ONS-D significantly reduced postprandial rise in blood glucose, peak blood glucose concentration and glucose area under the curve (AUCG) with no significant effects on HDL, total cholesterol, or triglyceride levels. Furthermore, this study reported a reduced insulin requirement (26–71% lower) and fewer complications in patients with ONS-D therapy when compared with standard nutritional supplements [15]. Therefore, in order to tighten glycaemic control, starch modification and sugar substitution [16,26] has become a primary strategy in the formulation of these supplements [15,16]. However, there is a compelling need to conduct more studies in special situations such as hospitalised patients, older people with DM2 or end-stage kidney disease and patients with cancer [27,28].

Recent evidence suggests a favourable glycaemic response after nutritional supplement intake with sucromalt (a natural analogue of sucrose with a lower glycaemic response) in diabetic patients [18,29,30]. Isomaltulose, another sucrose replacer, is a disaccharide composed of glucose and fructose linked by an alpha-1,6-glycosidic bond exhibiting prolonged absorption, LGI (GI = 32), and a 20–25% lower hydrolyzation rate when compared with sucrose [31]. Interestingly, GIP and GLP-1 secretion are affected by this disaccharide [32], resulting in a better insulin secretion profile [33] and a possible reduction in postprandial appetite [34].

Moreover, a study by Pfeiffer et al. [32] gave evidence on the relationship between high-glycaemic index carbohydrates and a faster GIP release pattern in patients with fatty liver disease, subclinical inflammation, DM2 and cardiovascular diseases. On the other hand, LGI carbohydrate consumption would induce a lower GIP release and a higher release of GLP-1 [32], promoting a better metabolic markers profile in both healthy and type DM2 individuals [18]. Therefore, these authors propose the GIP release rate as a determining factor in the "metabolic quality" and in consequence, relevant criteria for the selection of dietary carbohydrates [32].

Several studies in DM-2 subjects have explored incretin release after consumption of oral nutritional supplements with sucromalt or isomaltulose [18,35]; however, GI and GL have only been studied in healthy subjects [35,36] and not in diabetic patients. Likewise, the correlation between the glycaemic response (GI/GL) and SA as well as EIAP behaviour is not sufficiently well described to date, especially during ONS-D intake, digestion and absorption time.

Based on available literature, we hypothesised that an ONS-D that contains slow-digesting carbohydrates (isomaltulose or sucromalt) resulting in a significant release of GLP-1 and lower secretion of both GIP and insulin. As consequence, a reduction in GI/GL index and subjective postprandial appetite ratings would be found when compared with standard nutritional supplements. Thus, the aim of this study was to assess sucromalt/isomaltulose ONS-D effects on the glycaemic response (GI/GL), EIAP release and postprandial SA in type 2 diabetic individuals.

2. Materials and Methods

2.1. Study Design

2.1.1. Design and Ethics Issues

A randomised, double-blind, cross-over study was conducted according to Good Clinical Practice Guidelines, applicable Food and Drug privacy regulations and ethical principles based on the World Medical Association-Helsinki Declaration [37]. This research was approved by the Human Research Ethics Committee of the Endocrine and Metabolic Diseases Research Centre (EMDRC), "Dr. Félix Gómez", School of Medicine at the University of Zulia, Venezuela, and then registered in Clinical Trials.gov (https://clinicaltrials.gov/ct2/show/NCT03829800).

2.1.2. Inclusion and Exclusion Criteria

This study included both male and female DM2 subjects over 50 years old who attended the outpatient diabetes medical clinic at EMDRC [37]. The only antidiabetic therapies allowed were diet/physical activity and/or metformin monotherapy. Body mass index (BMI) between 18.5 kg/m^2–35 kg/m^2 was the only compelling anthropometric marker in order to be included in this trial. Patients with diabetes mellitus type 1 (DM1), diabetic ketoacidosis, hypothyroidism/thyrotoxicosis congestive heart failure, gastric, kidney or hepatic diseases, myocardial infarction, stroke and subjects with insulin therapy or sulfonylureas, antibiotic therapy or corticosteroids, end-stage organ failure, or individuals with organ transplantation, coagulation disorder, bleeding disorders, chronic infectious disease (such as tuberculosis, hepatitis B or C or HIV) were excluded.

2.1.3. Population, Sample Size, and Patient's Selection

Taking into account the criteria mentioned above, the whole EMDRC electronic medical record database was filtered obtaining a population of 57 eligible patients. Literature regarding GI and GL suggests 8 to 10 subjects for a proper meal/supplement assessment [10,36,38]. Thus, a random selection of 23 DM2 patients was made with the purpose of obtaining a sample size with a reasonable accuracy in determining the ONS-D glycaemic impact, GI and GL [36,38]. Since postprandial glycaemia and glycaemic index was our primary outcome, this study was powered to detect the difference among the AUCGs after consuming three oral nutritional supplements (effect size = 0.79) [20,24,35,36,38]. Based on our calculation, at least 15 participants were needed to detect this effect size at 80% statistical power using a cross-over study design [24]. Assuming an attrition rate of 30%, 23 participants were recruited in this study. Eligible subjects were contacted by phone and invited to attend a medical screening visit in order to: (1) be invited to participate in the study, (2) verify if the participant met the inclusion criteria and, (3) asked to give their written consent before beginning the study.

2.1.4. Anthropometric Assessment

Anthropometric data were obtained in fasting state, using light clothing and no shoes. For weight determination and electric bioimpedance study, an UM-018 Digital Scale (Tanita, Tokyo, Japan) was used. Height was measured using a SECA 216 stadiometer (Hamburg, Germany). Body mass index was calculated using the equation: BMI (kg/m^2) = mass (Kg)/height (m^2).

2.2. Study Protocol

2.2.1. Oral Nutritional Supplements Composition

In this study, three oral nutritional supplements were examined: (1) non-diabetes-specific standard oral nutritional supplements (ET; Ensure® Abbott Nutrition, Columbus, OH, USA); (2) oral supplements with a blend of slow-digesting carbohydrates including resistant maltodextrin and sucromalt (GS; Glucerna SR® Abbott Nutrition, Columbus, OH, USA); and (3) oral supplements composed of lactose, isomaltulose, and resistant starch (DI; Diasip® Nutricia Advanced, Medical Nutrition, Dublin, Ireland).

The macronutrient composition of these formulas per 100 mL is shown in Table 1. Considering that two of the supplements contained a relatively low amount of total carbohydrates, a standardised portion with 25 g of this nutrient was administered in each patient for all tests. This criterion is recommended when the carbohydrate load in the food is low, in order not to overestimate portion size [35,38]. Therefore, all supplements were compared with a glucose load of 25 g (GB), as a reference food (anhydrous glucose dissolved in 250 mL plain water) (100 Kcal) [35,38]. It is important to mention that there was no significant difference in the volume of formulations supplied in this study (Table 2).

Table 1. Macronutrient composition of the oral nutritional supplements per 100 mL.

Composition	ET	DI	GS
Calories (kcal)	105	104	93
Protein (g)	3.8	4.9	4.3
Fat (g)	2.5	3.8	3.5
Saturates (g)	0.4	0.5	0.3
Monounsaturates (g)	0.8	2.2	2.1
Polyunsaturates (g)	1.3	1.1	0.9
Total carbohydrate (g)	17.3	11.7	10.9
Sugar (g)	10.0	8.3	1.7
Dietary Fibre (g)	1.0	2.0	1.8

Table 1. *Cont.*

Composition	ET	DI	GS
Soluble (g)	0.0	1.6	1.8
Non-soluble (g)	0.0	0.4	0.0
Chromium (μg)	12.7	12.0	5.0
Portion size (mL)	100	100	100

Ensure® (ET): A standard oral nutritional supplement which is non-specific for diabetic patients. Diasip® (DI): Isomaltulose and resistant starch oral nutritional supplement. Glucerna® (GS): Resistant maltodextrin and sucromalt oral nutritional supplement.

Table 2. Nutrient composition of oral nutritional supplements based on 25 g available carbohydrate.

Composition	ET	DI	GS
Calories (kcal)	149	223	214
Protein (g)	5.3	10.5	9.9
Fat (g)	3.5	8.1	8.1
Saturates (g)	0.5	1.0	0.6
Monounsaturated (g)	1.1	4.7	4.9
Polyunsaturated (g)	1.8	2.3	2.0
Total carbohydrate (g)	25.0	25.0	25.0
Sugar (g)	14.1	8.3	0.0
Dietary Fibre (g)	0.9	4.3	4.1
Soluble (g)	0.0	3.4	4.1
Non-soluble (g)	0.0	0.8	0.0
Chromium (μg)	12.4	25.8	11.5
Portion size (mL)	141	214	230

Ensure® (ET): A standard oral nutritional supplement not specific for diabetic patients. Diasip® (DI): Isomaltulose and resistant starch oral nutritional supplement. Glucerna® (GS): Resistant maltodextrin and sucromalt oral nutritional supplement.

The three oral nutritional supplements delivered energy ranging from 149 to 223 kcal (Table 2). Both DI and GS contained 208 kcal per 200 mL versus 205 Kcal per 220 mL, respectively (recommended daily serving size). Supplement DI had a lower percentage of carbohydrate (47 energy%) and protein (19%) but higher percentage of fat (32 energy%, of which 18.5% was monounsaturated fatty acids (MUFAs). On the other hand, the composition of GS was more comparable with DI; a lower percentage of carbohydrate 47.7% and protein 18.42%, and higher percentage of fat 33.81% (MUFA: 20.5%), while the composition of ET had a higher percentage of carbohydrate: 55.68%; lower percentage of fat: 29.45%; and protein: 14.87%; with 250 Kcal per 237 mL. The GI values were calculated according to the information reported in the nutritional labelling of each supplement.

2.2.2. Experimental Protocol

Background Diet, Physical Activities and Other Measurements

Subjects were informed about diet and physical activity restrictions to be followed before each session, which included: (1) 10–12 h fasting, (2) abstinence from alcohol, caffeine or smoking and not exercising excessively 24 h before each session; (3) avoiding the metformin morning dose or other medications allowed on trial days until instructed, and to do so at the health centre. Participants were evaluated before each treatment by a licenced nutritionist. In this evaluation, patients had to submit a 3 day food record in order to confirm adherence to the meal plan. The day before the administration of supplements, the nutritionist recommended a standardised dinner before 21:00 and were asked not to consume anything before arriving at the laboratory except water, which was allowed until midnight [14,39]. In order to ensure that participants complied with established protocols, they had to complete a compliance survey. In case they did not comply with the previous test protocols, the test sessions were rescheduled.

During the appetite test sessions, patients engaged in 60 min of sedentary activities (word puzzles, reading, board games, etc.) [14,39]. The activities were performed in a friendly, non-competitive manner to avoid emotional excitement or stress. Any food-related topics were avoided for the duration of the sessions [14]. Research team members evaluated the compliance of the experimental protocol verifying the correct administration to all patients in each visit. Participants had access to water during the day of the trial. The leading investigator reviewed these records before performing the food tolerance test. During each test day subjects were allowed to drink water each hour (maximum 150 mL each hour) immediately after filling in the appetite questionnaires. Water consumed during the test session on the first day was recorded and repeated on the other test days [14,39].

Randomisation

All participants were randomly assigned to eight consumption tests: two for the standard glucose solutions and two for each of the three nutritional supplements. This scheme was carried out with an interval of 1 week between tests in random sequences. The test supplement selection was randomised using a computerized randomisation matrix. The order of supplement was further randomised for each subject. The number of tests in each patient was done according to methodological considerations for glycaemic index protocols [38]. Appetite was assessed twice for the same subject before and after supplement intake on two different occasions [14,39].

Previous-evening lunch standardisation: the dinner consumed by all participants the night before each session day consisted of meat with boiled rice and a fruit cake for dessert ~505 kcal [14]. The energy content of this meal was 35% of the daily estimated energy needs of each participant [40]. The distribution of energy in the evening meal was 50% from carbohydrate, 37% from fat and 13% from protein [14,39].

2.3. Measurement of EIAP/GI and Subjective Appetite Evaluation

2.3.1. EIAP and Glycaemic Index

Participants attended the EMDRC following 10–12 h fasting at 07:00. Both duplicated blood capillary samples (0.5 mL) and venous samples were taken in basal state, and then each patient was randomly assigned to drink one of both the ONS (ET DI or GS) supplement or the reference food (glucose 25 g in plain water) during a period not exceeding 15 min [35,36,38]. The reference food (GB) (glucose solution) was used for glucose and insulin AUC determination only. Subsequently, samples of capillary and venous blood were obtained at 30, 60, 90, 120 and 180 min for serum glucose, insulin, GIP and GLP-1 measurement. During this phase, subjects were comfortably seated in a room with a quiet environment [38]. This process was repeated seven more times, on different days, with one week interval until all consumption tests were done [36,38].

2.3.2. Subjective Appetite Assessment

The appetite sensations measured in this study were: hunger, desire to eat, prospective food consumption and fullness assessed on different days from those in which the GI was determined. The visual analogue scale (VAS) chart was supplied in every session [39] and the subjects were asked to fill this instrument at baseline (0 min), 30, 60, 90, 120, 150 and 180 min after the ingestion of each supplement. This instrument contemplates four questions: What is your feeling of fullness? How hungry are you? How intense is your desire to eat? And how much food do you think you could eat? [14,39].

The VAS structure consisted of 100 mm lines anchored at each end with opposite statements with a scale of 0 to 100 mm, in which 0 means absence of perception and 100 maximum perception. The distance between 0 and the marked point (an "x" placed by the participants on the line to indicate their assessment at that time) was measured to quantify the perceived sensations. The score was calculated by measuring the distance in millimetres from the beginning of the line to the "x" position (from left to right) [39].

The following equation was used to calculate the ratings of subjective appetite [41]: "Subjective appetite = (desire to eat + hunger + (100 − fullness) + prospective food consumption)/4".

2.3.3. Laboratory Determinations

Capillary glycaemia was determined by the glucose oxidase method using a portable glucometer (Optium Xceed, Abbott Laboratories, Dallas, TX, USA) Both intra-assay and inter-assay coefficients of variation were 3.2 and 10.8%, respectively. Plasma Insulin (mU/L) was measured by an enzyme-linked immunosorbent assay (10-1113; Mercodia, Uppsala, Sweden) with a minimum detectable limit of 1.0 mU/L, and an intra- and inter-assay variation coefficients of 3.0% and 8.7%. Glycated haemoglobin HbA1c was determined using a cationic exchange resin separation method (SIGMA, St. Louis, MO, USA). Plasma total GIP (pg/mL) and GLP-1 (pmol/L) were measured by radioimmunoassay (RIA) (SIGMA, St. Louis, MO, USA). The minimum detectable limits were 2 pmol/L and 3 pmol/L with an intra- and inter-assay coefficient of variation for GIP of 3.9% and 9%, and for GLP-1 6.3% and 10.3%, respectively. Total cholesterol, triacylglycerides, and HDL-C were determined by commercial enzymatic-colorimetric kits (Human Gesellschaft für Biochemica und Diagnostica MBH, Wiesbaden, HE, Germany). Serum LDL-C levels were calculated according to Friedewald's equation.

2.4. Data Processing and Statistical Analyses

Statistical analyses were performed using IBM SPSS Statistics for Windows, version 23.0 (IBM Corp., 2015, Armonk, NY, USA). Shapiro–Wilk test was used for the normality distribution assessment of quantitative variables.

Incremental areas under the curves (IAUCs) were determined according to the trapezoidal method for all variables using NCSS statistical software version 12.0 (NCSS, LLC, 2018, Kaysville, UT, USA). A 2 h glycaemic response curve was generated for each subject for test foods. Any area below the baseline fasting value was ignored. The calculated median of AUCG for three test foods from 16 participants was compared with the response to reference food or glucose solution (median of two measurements), and the GI value of the glucose solution was set as 100.

The GI was calculated using the following equation [36,38]: GI = (AUCG value for the test food/AUCG value for the reference food) × 100.

Data obtained was classified in low GI (≤55), intermediate (55–69) and high (≥70) [41]. Glycaemic load (GL) was represented by a derivative measure of the GI of the nutritional supplement tested and calculated by the following formula: GL = (GI × grams of carbohydrate per food portion)/100 [36,38].

All quantitative variables were presented as mean ± standard error of the mean (SEM). Plasma glucose, insulin, GIP, GLP-1, perceptions of hunger, desire to eat, prospective food consumption, fullness and SA had a normal distribution and its arithmetic means were analysed using ANOVA for repeated measures with the Tukey's HSD (honestly significant difference) test. Significant statistical differences between ONS were evaluated through one-way ANOVA. The bivariate relation between variables such as the AUC, blood glucose, EIAP and SA was analysed by correlation coefficients for each oral test. Statistical significance was accepted at $p < 0.05$.

3. Results

At the beginning of the study, the initial sample was 23 individuals (12 women, 11 men), but seven subjects did not complete the trial for different reasons: (1) two subjects needed both corticosteroid and antibiotic therapy; (2) two subjects initiated a vigorous physical activity program by medical prescription; and (3) three voluntarily withdrew from the study. At the end of the study, only 16 subjects (seven women and nine men) completed all the test protocols. Table 3 shows the general characteristics of the sample.

Table 3. General characteristics of the enrolled patients.

	Sex					
	Female		Male		Total	
	Mean	SEM *	Mean	SEM	Mean	SEM
Age (years)	54.75	1. 65	57.83	1.35	56.0	1.11
Weight (cm)	87.75	3.73	90.17	1.22	89.0	1.58
Height (m)	1.68	0.04	1.69	0.01	1.68	0.01
BMC (kg/m^2)	30.90	0.44	31.04	0.36	30.8	0.26
Waist circumference (cm)	106.00	1.58	111.00	0.89	106	0.77
Base glycaemia (mmol/L)	7.51	0.40	6.75	0.30	7.05	0.26
Total cholesterol (mg/dL)	209.60	5.71	213.77	8.84	212.10	5.56
High-density lipoprotein (mg/dL)	44.70	4.63	44.30	2.32	44.46	2.16
Low-density lipoprotein (mg/dL)	130.95	4.37	133.28	1.54	132.35	1.87
Triglycerides (mg/dL)	161.70	2.56	158.06	4.45	159.52	2.80
Glycated haemoglobin HbA1c (%)	6.95	0.30	6.98	0.30	6.97	0.20

* Standard error of the mean. There were no significant differences between sexes.

The protocol was well tolerated by all subjects. No individual reported nausea, dizziness or vomiting after taking the nutritional supplements or the reference product. Basal concentrations of serum glucose, insulin, GLP-1 and GIP (Table 4 and Figure 1) did not show significant differences according to sex or among weekly visits. Similarly, hunger perception, fullness, desire to eat, prospective food consumption in fasting state and SA ratings (Table 5 and Figure 2) did not show significant differences among gender or study session ($p > 0.05$).

Table 4. Serum glucose concentration and EIAP according to each treatment.

Supplement	Time (min)	Serum Glucose (mmol/L)	Insulin (mU/L)	GLP-1 (pmol/L)	GIP (pg/mL)
ET	0	6.52 ± 0.07	6.44 ± 0.32	6.26 ± 0.28	29.64 ± 0.50
	30	10.14 ± 0.07 ^{bc}	22.84 ± 1.00 ^{bc}	12.93 ± 0.21 ^{bc}	55.44 ± 0.58 ^{bc}
	60	10.80 ± 0.12 ^{bd}	33.91 ± 0.97 ^{bc}	8.35 ± 0.22 ^{bc}	62.27 ± 0.89 ^{bc}
	90	9.39 ± 0.16 ^{b}	36.20 ± 0.64 ^{bc}	7.78 ± 0.15 ^{b}	74.68 ± 0.72 ^{bc}
	120	8.76 ± 0.17 ^{b}	25.90 ± 0.70 ^{bc}	7.16 ± 0.27 ^{b}	71.23 ± 0.36 ^{bc}
	150	8.14 ± 0.21 ^{bc}	16.80 ± 0.56 ^{bc}	6.55 ± 0.12 ^{b}	67.77 ± 0.50 ^{bc}
	180	7.13 ± 0.21 ^{b}	9.91 ± 0.81	5.99 ± 0.21 ^{b}	62.86 ± 1.26 ^{bc}
GS	0	6.64 ± 0.08	6.49 ± 0.11	6.95 ± 0.36 ^{c}	29.97 ± 0.40
	30	6.68 ± 0.13 ^{ac}	17.24 ± 0.31 ^{a}	18.16 ± 0.26 ^{ac}	45.57 ± 0.42 ^{a}
	60	9.10 ± 0.06 ^{ac}	18.16 ± 0.24 ^{ac}	14.75 ± 0.24 ^{ac}	50.85 ± 0.15 ^{ac}
	90	8.53 ± 0.07 ^{ac}	19.09 ± 0.20 ^{a}	12.73 ± 0.24 ^{ac}	54.23 ± 0.21 ^{ac}
	120	7.92 ± 0.05 ^{ac}	14.38 ± 0.16 ^{ac}	11.63 ± 0.14 ^{ac}	55.99 ± 1.09 ^{ac}
	150	6.98 ± 0.12 ^{a}	12.93 ± 0.19 ^{a}	10.86 ± 0.19 ^{ac}	57.87 ± 0.31 ^{a}
	180	6.16±0.10 ^{a}	10.87 ± 0.18	8.91 ± 0.21 ^{ac}	52.85 ± 1.69 ^{ac}
DI	0	6.66 ± 0.10	6.50 ± 0.40	6.20 ± 0.53	28.70 ± 1.07
	30	7.47 ± 0.12 ^{ab}	19.04 ± 0.27 ^{a}	14.51 ± 0.22 ^{ab}	46.00 ± 0.71 ^{a}
	60	10.17 ± 0.05 ^{ab}	24.86 ± 0.35 ^{ab}	10.26 ± 0.11 ^{ab}	56.51 ± 1.12 ^{ab}
	90	9.10 ± 0.05 ^{b}	21.14 ± 0.36 ^{a}	8.09 ± 0.17 ^{b}	63.78 ± 0.63 ^{ab}
	120	8.56 ± 0.07 ^{b}	17.98 ± 0.30 ^{ab}	7.35 ± 0.14 ^{b}	61.10 ± 0.51 ^{ab}
	150	7.33 ± 0.07 ^{a}	13.24 ± 0.25 ^{a}	6.95 ± 0.09 ^{b}	57.52 ± 0.50 ^{a}
	180	6.61 ± 0.12	11.13 ± 0.21	6.56 ± 0.20 ^{b}	45.19 ± 0.96 ^{ab}

Treatment groups were defined as a standard nutritional supplement not specific for people with diabetes (ET); resistant maltodextrin and sucromalt supplement (GS); isomaltulose and resistant starch supplement (DI). GIP: glucose-dependent insulinotropic polypeptide; GLP-1: glucagon-like peptide 1; SEM: standard error of the mean. ^{a} $p < 0.05$ versus ET. ^{b} $p < 0.05$ versus GS. ^{c} $p < 0.05$ versus DI.

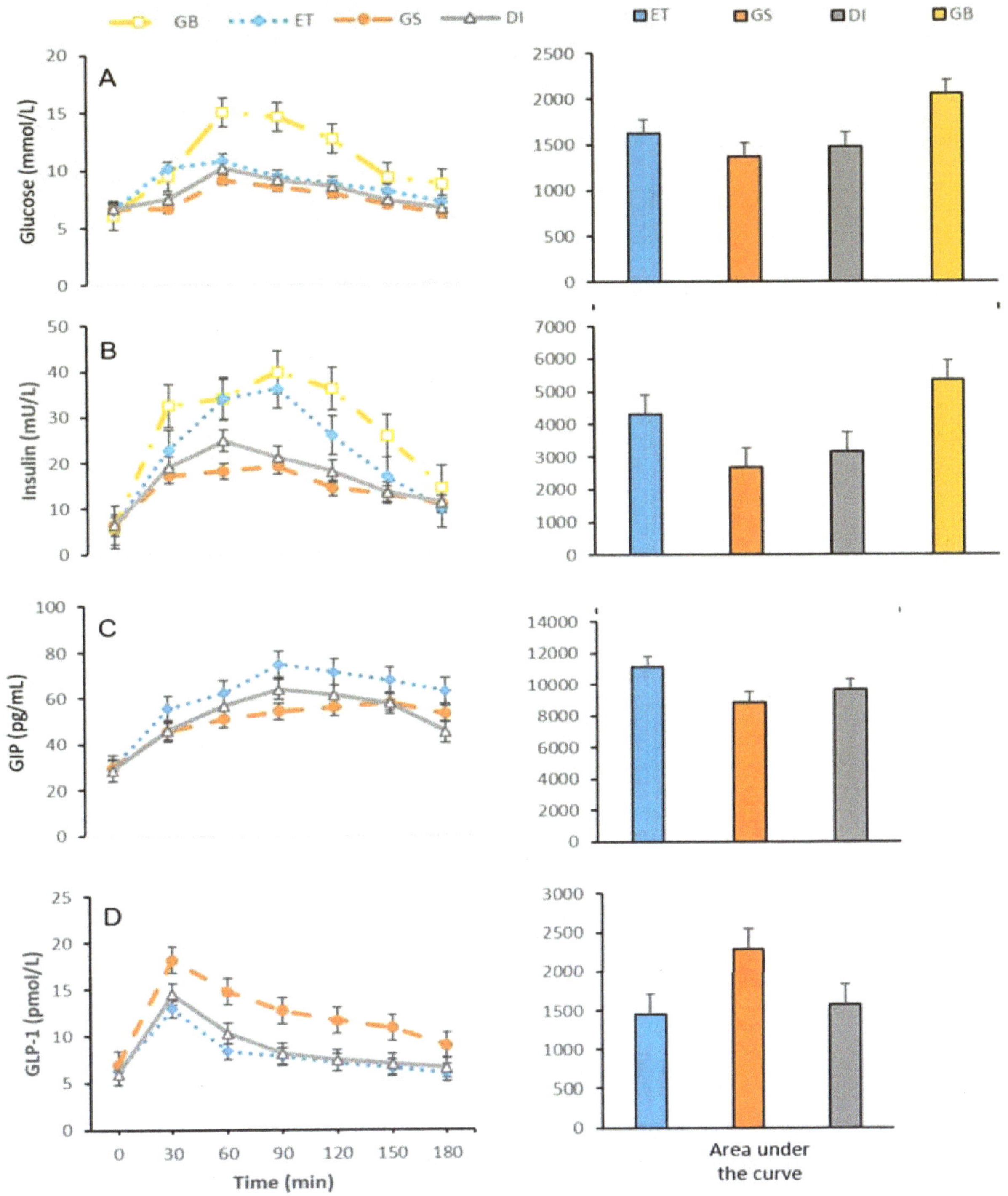

Figure 1. Time course and $AUC_{0-180\ min}$ of serum glucose, insulin GIP and GPL-1 concentrations following ingestions of GB, ET, GS and DI. (**A**) Glucose in relation with time and $AUC_{0-180\ min}$, (**B**) insulin in relation with time and $AUC_{0-180\ min}$, (**C**) GIP in relation with time and $AUC_{0-180\ min}$, and (**D**) GLP-1 in relation with time and $AUC_{0-180\ min}$ for all the different types of treatments. Data are expressed as means ± SEM; $n = 16$. The same colour scheme was used for all the graphs. All $AUC_{0-180\ min}$ means significant differences ($p < 0.02$) in each group. Treatment groups: (GB) Glucose solution or reference product; (ET) standard nutritional supplement not specific for diabetics; (GS) resistant maltodextrin and sucromalt supplement; (DI) isomaltulose and resistant starch supplement. GIP: glucose-dependent insulinotropic polypeptide; GLP-1: glucagon-like peptide 1.

Table 5. Subjective appetite measurements according to each treatment.

Supplement	Time (min)	Hunger(mm)	Fullness(mm)	Desire to Eat(mm)	Prospective Food Consumption (mm)	SA (mm)
ET	0	63.80 ± 1.70	34.30 ± 0.88	61.80 ± 1.14	21.40 ± 1.88	53.18 ± 0.40
	30	33.60 ± 2.45	62.50 ± 1.60 [b]	32.10 ± 1.19	28.90 ± 2.04 [b]	33.03 ± 0.91 [bc]
	60	37.10 ± 1.10 [bc]	55.70 ± 2.32 [b]	42.60 ± 1.11 [bc]	35.50 ± 0.91 [bc]	40.08 ± 0.56 [bc]
	90	46.00 ± 1.00 [bc]	38.40 ± 3.14 [bc]	43.40 ± 0.82 [bc]	38.00 ± 1.97 [b]	47.05 ± 1.08 [bc]
	120	47.20 ± 1.58 [bc]	32.60 ± 2.02 [bc]	46.00 ± 1.00 [bc]	41.80 ± 0.95 [bc]	50.60 ± 0.53 [bc]
	150	56.60 ± 1.41 [bc]	30.40 ± 2.10 [bc]	54.30 ± 1.39 [bc]	46.80 ± 1.44 [b]	56.83 ± 0.74 [bc]
	180	70.60 ± 1.92 [bc]	20.50 ± 1.71 [bc]	73.60 ± 1.06 [bc]	55.90 ± 1.27 [b]	69.90 ± 0.91 [bc]
GS	0	66.40 ± 1.42	32.50 ± 1.76	63.50 ± 0.93	19.20 ± 0.80	54.15 ± 0.62
	30	30.80 ± 1.78	70.10 ± 2.12 [a]	30.80 ± 1.65	20.60 ± 0.69 [a]	28.03 ± 0.85 [a]
	60	28.50 ± 1.66 [a]	65.90 ± 1.57 [a]	27.80 ± 1.80 [ac]	22.00 ± 1.09 [ac]	28.10 ± 0.58 [ac]
	90	27.30 ± 1.95 [ac]	63.70 ± 1.92 [ac]	31.00 ± 1.69 [a]	24.40 ± 1.75 [ac]	29.75 ± 0.93 [ac]
	120	29.80 ± 1.70 [ac]	58.60 ± 1.99 [ac]	35.60 ± 0.83 [a]	33.30 ± 1.12 [a]	35.03 ± 0.77 [ac]
	150	34.30 ± 1.16 [ac]	46.00 ± 1.74 [ac]	43.90 ± 1.16 [a]	36.60 ± 0.90 [ac]	40.20 ± 0.42 [ac]
	180	62.30 ± 1.51 [a]	34.90 ± 1.47 [ac]	58.80 ± 1.90 [a]	45.00 ± 1.32 [ac]	57.80 ± 0.64 [ac]
DI	0	63.20 ± 1.30	32.80 ± 1.18	65.20 ± 1.24	21.40 ± 1.27	54.25 ± 0.59
	30	32.30 ± 1.50 [a]	68.40 ± 1.38	29.60 ± 1.97	23.90 ± 1.30	29.35 ± 0.85 [a]
	60	28.60 ± 2.03 [ab]	60.60 ± 1.35	34.60 ± 1.48 [ab]	25.50 ± 0.91 [ab]	32.03 ± 0.68 [ab]
	90	33.90 ± 1.38 [ab]	54.80 ± 1.17 [ab]	35.00 ± 1.22 [a]	35.00 ± 1.02 [b]	37.28 ± 0.64 [ab]
	120	39.00 ± 1.13 [ab]	45.90 ± 1.49 [ab]	36.90 ± 1.17 [a]	36.70 ± 1.27 [a]	40.93 ± 0.58 [ab]
	150	44.90 ± 0.99 [ab]	38.30 ± 2.39 [ab]	47.40 ± 1.97 [a]	44.90 ± 1.50 [b]	49.73 ± 0.63 [ab]
	180	60.60 ± 2.02 [a]	27.00 ± 1.71 [ab]	61.90 ± 2.36 [a]	52.00 ± 1.21 [b]	61.88 ± 076 [ab]

Treatment groups were defined as a standard nutritional supplement not specifically for people with diabetes (ET); resistant maltodextrin and sucromalt supplement (GS); isomaltulose and resistant starch supplement (DI). GIP: glucose-dependent insulinotropic polypeptide; GLP-1: glucagon-like peptide 1; SEM: standard error of the mean. [a] $p < 0.05$ versus ET. [b] $p < 0.05$ versus GS. [c] $p < 0.05$ versus DI. SA: Subjective appetite.

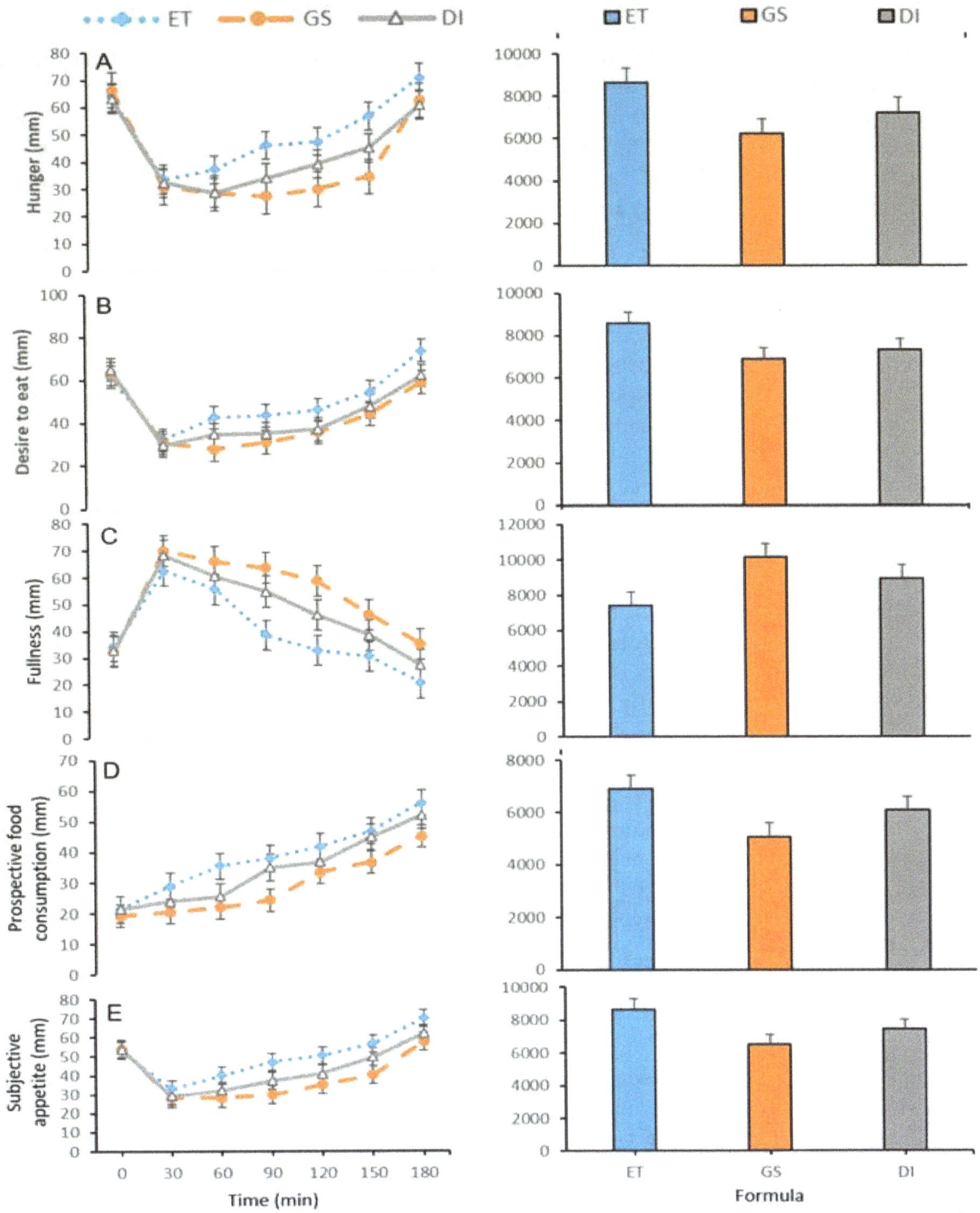

Figure 2. Time course and formula of postprandial perception of hunger, desire to eat, fullness, prospective food consumption, subjective appetite and $AUC_{0-180\ min}$ values following ingestions of GB, ET, GS and DI. (**A**) hunger in relation with time and formula; (**B**) desire to eat in relation with time and formula, (**C**) fullness in relation to time and formula, (**D**) prospective food consumption in relation with time and formula and (**E**) subjective appetite in relation with time and formula. Data are expressed as means ± SEM, ($n = 16$). Data comparisons about differences in subjective measurements of appetite according to consumption tests are described in Table 5. The same colour scheme was used for all graphs. All means of $AUC_{0-180\ min}$ showed significant differences ($p < 0.02$) in each group. Treatment groups: (ET) standard nutritional supplement not specifically for people with diabetes. (GS) Resistant maltodextrin and sucromalt supplement. (DI) Isomaltulose and resistant starch supplement.

3.1. Glycaemic Response and EIAP Concentrations

Glycaemic curves, as well as the mean and SEM of the glucose $AUC_{0-180\ min}$ after ingestion of both the reference product (glucose) and the nutritional supplements, are shown in Figure 1. Glucose maximum peak was observed at 60 min (Table 4) for all products but significantly higher for GB 15.03 ± 0.20 when compared with ET 10.80 ± 0.12mmol/L ($p < 0.001$), DI 10.17 ± 0.05 ($p < 0.001$) and GS 9.10 ± 0.06 mmol/L ($p < 0.001$). Glucose at 180 min was significantly higher in comparison with both, fasting level for GB ($p < 0.001$) and for ET ($p < 0.024$). The $AUC_{0-180\ min}$ of ET ($p < 0.001$) was significantly higher than DI ($p < 0.001$) and GS ($p < 0.01$) (Figure 1).

3.1.1. Insulin

Plasma insulin concentrations increased after the consumption of all supplements and the reference product, reaching significant differences at 90 min for GB (serum peak) in comparison to ET ($p < 0.05$), GS ($p < 0.001$) and DI ($p < 0.001$), respectively (Figure 1). At 150 min, ET presented a higher glucose concentration than DSF ($p < 0.001$), but no significant differences were found in insulin concentration between DI and GS ($p = 0.976$), see Table 4. The $AUC_{0-180\ min}$ in insulin response was significantly lower in GS when compared with the other supplements ($p < 0.001$) (Figure 1).

3.1.2. GLP-1

Maximum GLP-1 concentration was observed at 30 min after the intake of the three supplements, significantly higher for GS in comparison to ET ($p < 0.05$) and DI ($p < 0.05$). At 150 min, concentrations of GLP-1 in ET and DI supplements were similar ($p = 0.841$), but the value of this incretin was significantly higher for GS when compared with both, ET ($p < 0.001$) and DI ($p < 0.001$), (Table 4). The $AUC_{0-180\ min}$ of the GLP-1 response was significantly higher in GS in contrast to the ET ($p < 0.001$) and DI ($p < 0.001$), (Figure 1).

3.1.3. GIP

The GIP plasma concentration increased after consumption of all supplements. The maximum peak of this incretin was observed at 90 min with ET and DI, which was higher when compared to GS levels ($p < 0.05$). At 150 min, ET presented higher GIP concentrations when compared to GS ($p < 0.001$) and DI ($p < 0.001$), however, DSF levels did not show significant differences ($p = 0.844$), Table 4. The $AUC_{0-180\ min}$ of the GIP response for GS was lower when compared to DI ($p < 0.001$) and ET ($p < 0.001$, (Figure 1).

3.2. Subjective Appetite Measurements

Hunger sensation, fullness, desire to eat, prospective food consumption and SA from baseline to 180 min are shown in Figure 2. Consumption of the different treatments promoted an immediate decrease in hunger and desire to eat accompanied by an increase in the perception of fullness, reversing these sensations over the curve as time passed.

The arithmetic mean of hunger perception decreased after the consumption of all supplements, registering the lowest level at 30 min for E, while the minimum value for GS was evidenced at 90 min, significantly lower when compared to ET ($p < 0.05$) and DI ($p < 0.05$), (Table 5). The $AUC_{0-180\ min}$ of hunger sensation for GS was significantly lower when compared to ET ($p < 0.001$) and DI ($p < 0.001$), (Figure 2).

Regarding fullness sensation, the maximum level was found at 30 min in the three groups, without significant differences between DI and GS, while the peak of fullness sensation was significantly lower with ET ($p < 0.05$), (Table 5). The $AUC_{0-180\ min}$ of this sensation was significantly higher in GS when compared to DI ($p < 0.001$) and ET ($p < 0.05$), (Figure 2). On the other hand, the desire to eat $AUC_{0-180\ min}$ was significantly lower for GS when compared to DI ($p = 0.035$) and ET ($p < 0.001$), (Figure 2).

This same pattern was evidenced in the prospective food consumption, in which the $AUC_{0\text{–}180\ min}$ was significantly lower in GS when compared with ET ($p < 0.001$) and DI ($p < 0.001$), (Figure 2). Subjective appetite SA decreased to a minimum value at 30 min and then increased 60 min after the three treatments for all subjects; this score was higher with ET when compared to GS ($p < 0.01$) and DI ($p < 0.01$), (Table 5). The $AUC_{0\text{–}180\ min}$ of SA was significantly lower with GS than with DI ($p < 0.01$) and ET ($p < 0.001$), (Figure 2).

3.3. Correlation Analysis Between EIAP, Serum Glucose and Subjective Appetite

After ET intake, insulin concentration $AUC_{0\text{–}180\ min}$ and subjective sensation of fullness were directly related ($r = 0.713$, $p = 0.021$), while an inverse relationship between fullness perception and GLP-1 concentration $AUC_{0\text{–}180\ min}$ ($r = -0.756$, $p = 0.011$) and serum glucose ($r = -0.687$; $p = 0.028$) was observed. The value SA was directly correlated with serum glucose ($r = 0.659$, $p = 0.038$), see Table 6. No statistically significant correlations were found for $AUC_{0\text{–}180\ min}$ concentrations of these peptides with DI and GS.

Table 6. Coefficient correlations between AUC values of glycaemia, EIAP and subjective measurements of appetite according to consumption tests.

	Hunger		**Fullness**		**Desire to Eat**		**Prospective Food Consumption**		**Subjective Appetite**	
ET	*r*	*p*	*r*	*p*	*r*	*p*	*r*	*p*	*r*	*p*
Glycaemia	0.060	0.868	−0.687	0.028	0.217	0.547	−0.025	0.945	0.659	0.038
Insulin	−0.215	0.552	0.713	0.021	−0.046	0.900	0.362	0.304	−0.437	0.321
GLP-1	−0.133	0.714	−0.756	0.011	0.392	0.262	−0.543	0.105	0.321	0.540
GIP	0.219	0.544	−0.082	0.821	0.486	0.155	0.399	0.253	0.540	0.107
DI	*r*	*p*	*r*	*p*	*r*	*p*	*r*	*p*	*r*	*p*
Glycaemia	0.004	0.992	−0.226	0.530	−0.069	0.849	0.173	0.633	0.357	0.311
Insulin	0.190	0.599	−0.163	0.652	−0.455	0.187	−0.196	0.587	−0.254	0.479
GLP-1	0.483	0.158	0.140	0.700	0.158	0.662	−0.407	0.243	0.098	0.787
GIP	0.294	0.410	0.099	0.785	−0.615	0.058	0.069	0.850	−0.540	0.107
GS	*r*	*p*	*r*	*p*	*r*	*p*	*r*	*p*	*r*	*p*
Glycaemia	−0.192	0.595	0.019	0.958	−0.152	0.674	0.128	0.726	−0.154	0.672
Insulin	0.466	0.175	−0.020	0.957	0.217	0.548	−0.175	0.628	0.344	0.330
GLP-1	0.308	0.386	0.072	0.843	0.436	0.208	−0.421	0.226	0.191	0.596
GIP	0.231	0.521	−0.046	0.900	−0.135	0.710	−0.076	0.834	0.086	0.813

Treatment groups: (ET) standard nutritional supplement not specifically for diabetes patients; (DI) isomaltulose and resistant starch supplement; (GS) resistant maltodextrin and sucromalt supplement. GIP: glucose-dependent insulinotropic polypeptide; GLP-1: glucagon-like peptide 1; SEM: standard error of the mean. The values presented correspond to *r* coefficients and *p*-value for all subject correlations between subjective perceptions of appetite and concentrations hormones according to the treatment group. *p*-values were significant when $p < 0.05$.

Correlations between baseline and postprandial concentrations at 30, 90 and 120 min of glucose, EIAP and SA measures were accomplished in all treatments. Insulin at 30 min for ET was inversely related to hunger sensation ($r = -0.745$, $p = 0.012$) and SA ($r = -0.849$, $p = 0.002$) (Supplementary Materials Table S1). DI intake was correlated with glycaemia and prospective food consumption at 30 min ($r = 0.775$, $p = 0.008$) and, GLP-1 with the desire to eat at 120 min ($r = 0.667$ $p = 0.035$); whereas, SA was inversely correlated at 30 min with GIP ($r = -0.688$, $p = 0.028$) (Supplementary Materials Table S2).

GS evidenced a direct relationship between glycaemia at 90 min with sensation of fullness ($r = 0.698$, $p = 0.025$) and levels of GIP with sensation of hunger ($r = 0.825$, $p = 0.003$). GLP-1 at 30 min and prospective food consumption were inversely related ($r = -0.722$, $p = 0.018$). SA was directly correlated with blood glucose levels at 30 min ($r = 0.711$, $p = 0.021$) (Supplementary Materials Table S3).

3.4. Glycaemic Index and Glycaemic Load

ET presented a GI mean higher than that calculated for DI ($p < 0.001$) and GS ($p < 0.001$), respectively. Comparing both specific supplements for diabetics, the lowest value for this indicator was evidenced in GS ($p < 0.001$). Concerning GL, ET showed the highest mean compared to the rest of treatments ($p < 0.001$), and the lowest mean value for DI (11.28 ± 0.14, $p < 0.001$), (Table 7).

Table 7. Glycaemic index and glycaemic load according to consumption tests.

Treatment Groups	Mean ± SEM
Glycaemic Index (GI)	
ET	56.40 ± 0.43 [bc]
DI	51.44 ± 0.60 [ab]
GS	47.59 ± 0.49 [ac]
Glycaemic Load (GL)	
ET	23.69 ± 0.18 [bc]
DI	12.04 ± 0.14 [ac]
GS	11.42 ± 0.12 [ab]

Treatment groups: (ET) standard nutritional supplement not specifically for people with diabetes; (DI) isomaltulose and resistant starch supplement; (GS) resistant maltodextrin and sucromalt supplement. SEM: Standard error of the mean. There were no significant differences between sexes. ANOVA and post-hoc Tukey HSD for intragroup comparisons; p-value was significant when $p < 0.05$. [a] $p < 0.001$ versus ET. [b] $p < 0.001$ versus GS. [c] $p < 0.001$ versus DI.

3.5. EIAP and SA Relation with GI and GL

In relation to each supplement, it was found that hunger sensation $AUC_{0-180\ min}$ was directly correlated with GI ($r = 0.777$, $p = 0.008$) and GL ($r = 0.777$, $p = 0.008$) for ET; while DI, both GI and GL were inversely related to GIP ($r = -0.867$, $p = 0.001$). GS, GI and GL were inversely related with fullness sensation ($r = -0.698$, $p = 0.025$). SA ratings did not correlate significantly with any of these indexes ($p > 0.05$), (Supplementary Materials Table S4).

4. Discussion

This study assessed ONS-D with isomaltulose and sucromalt versus a standard oral supplement on GI/GL, insulin response, incretin release and SA in DM2 patients. In this regard, the main finding of this study confirmed that ONS-D intake in diabetic subjects stimulated GLP-1 release, reducing GIP levels with a subsequent decrease in insulin secretion. This particular EIAP pattern promotes a lower IG/CG index when compared with a standard supplement. In spite of the former, there was a reduction of SA and $AUC_{0-180\ min}$ after ONS-D intake; only correlation between hunger perception, fullness and some metabolic variables were found after GS intake.

These findings confirm that ONS-D consumption promotes a better metabolic profile in diabetic subjects than standard supplements, allowing greater control in postprandial appetite. Specifically, this investigation demonstrates that plasma glucose levels and glucose $AUC_{0-180\ min}$ were significantly lower after the ingestion of ONS-D than ET. Our observations are consistent with previous research carried out with slow-digesting carbohydrates supplements [18,29,42,43]. In this study, after the consumption of GS, the mean glycaemic peak was consistent with ADA recommendations for glucose level < 180 mg/dL (9.99 mmol/L), with elevated HbA1c in DM patients [7] and IDF of 160 mg/dL goal, both in the postprandial period [6]. Similar to observations by Mottalib et al. [42] this study shows that serum glucose level after ONS-D ingestion returned to baseline in a shorter period (150 min) when compared with ET (180 min) [42], see Figure 1 and Table 4 [18,29,42]. These differences in glycaemic profile can be attributed, at least in part, to the low GI of ONS-D [18,29,35,42], a point of paramount importance to avoid cardiovascular complications [44] because of pro-inflammatory cytokines and oxygen free radical overproduction [44,45]. In this trial, the consumption of GS produced lower values of GI/GL, a lower increment of GIP/insulin and more significant release of GLP-1.

Among the different factors that influence the GI of a food, the source and carbohydrate type are very relevant aspects. High GI carbohydrates differ from those with LGI, not only in postprandial glycaemic and insulinemic response but also in GIP release [45–47]. In this regard, Pfeiffer et al. [32], suggest a novel concept that encompasses the intake of LGI CHO with a lower release of GIP and a greater GLP-1 secretion results in improvements of metabolic markers in healthy [45], type 2 and insulin-resistant individuals [46].

This concept relates to GI of each food to different secretory responses of GIP and GLP -1, which are released in different segments of the small intestine [21,45–47]. These authors propose that both a fast and pronounced GIP release in the proximal small intestine by high GI carbohydrates programming the intermediary metabolism towards useful energy storage but adversely promoting fatty liver disease [46], insulin resistance [48], obesity [49], subclinical inflammation and hypertriglyceridemia [46]. This program could represent an evolutionary advantage in times that rapid energy storage was required [32,46]. Complete understanding of the pathophysiological mechanisms of foods with a high GI provides a basis for the development of nutritional and therapeutic solutions [10,11,41,46].

Nonetheless, it is essential to differentiate the digestion (di, oligo and polysaccharides) and absorption rate (monosaccharide), from the particular metabolism of each monosaccharide. This is because certain simple sugars, such as fructose, with a relatively low GI (=23) [36], could induce insulin-independent additional metabolic effects [50] on uric acid levels, blood pressure, liver cell triacylglycerides content and hepatic insulin sensitivity when consumed in high amounts [51]. On the other hand, tagatose is a low GI (=3) monosaccharide [36], that promoting a GLP-1 release in a similar extent to fructose without any significant GIP secretion response [52] and exhibiting an interesting glucose-lowering effect [53]. In this study, we assessed two of the most employed slow-digesting carbohydrates in ONS-D: isomaltulose and sucromalt.

Beneficial metabolic effects have been reported when low GI disaccharides = 32, such as isomaltulose [31,36], are added to oral supplements in people with DM2 [29]. This disaccharide has an α-1,6-glycosidic bond replacing the original sucrose´s 1,2-glycosidic linkage by enzymatic isomerisation rearrangement obtained from beet sugar [33]. This molecular reorganisation leads to slower digestion and, in consequence, delayed intestinal uptake of glucose and fructose [33,54]. Unlike sucrose, isomaltulose administration prevents proximal K cells stimulation, secreting less GIP and promoting a smaller insulin release [32,33]. For its part, the low glycaemic response to sucromalt showed a sustained increase in GLP-1 secretion at 4 h post intake, suggesting an almost complete uptake by the small intestine [30]. Thus, it is important to distinguish the effects in GI from those caused by changes in gut microbiota that occur when sugar reaches the colon and alter microbiome composition, affecting long-term carbohydrate metabolism and insulin response [55–57].

In this study, ONS-D insulinemic behaviour interestingly showed a lower $AUC_{0–180\ min}$ level in ET, especially after GS at 90 min, the time when the maximum peak of this hormone occurs. Meanwhile, the maximum insulin concentration after DI intake occurred at the 60 min (Figure 1). The maximum increase in GIP levels after GS occurred after the rest of the treatments (150 min), but it was only statistically different from ET (Table 4). Likewise, the $AUC_{0–180\ min}$ for GIP was lower for ONS-D compared with the ET, and lowest for GS versus DI, (Figure 1). This finding could confirm the theory mentioned above about the effect of slow digestion carbohydrates on the release of insulin and GIP, although insulinemic peak after ET also occurred in 90 min, but with a much higher incretin concentration than that produced by ONS ($p < 0.05$ for both).

It has been proposed that slow-digestion carbohydrates can reach the more distal segments of the small intestine before being absorbed, hence, stimulating a late-plasma increase of GLP-1 [30,52]. In this trial, the $AUC_{0–180\ min}$ of GLP-1 was higher after ONS-D consumption when compared to ET, and higher for GS when compared with DI, (Figure 1). Our results were similar to those reported by Devitt et al. [29] regarding metabolic differences after specific supplement ingestion composed of a variety of carbohydrates like tapioca dextrins, isomaltulose, tapioca starch/fructose and sucromalt in DM2 patients. In this study, patients showed an increase in $AUC_{0–240\ min}$ for GLP-1 after sucromalt-based supplement intake, but it was only significantly higher after supplements made with tapioca dextrin in comparison with the standard ET [29].

Some benefits of increased GLP-1 secretion in DM2 patients are an improvement in insulin–glucagon ratio, suppression of endogenous glucose production and the increase in first-pass splanchnic glucose uptake [47,58]. It is currently unclear whether inhibition of L-cell secretion or GLP-1 enhanced degradation entails to the characteristic blunted-effect of this incretin in DM2. Also, the exact mechanism of GLP-1 effects on glucose control has not yet been elucidated [18,21]. Although there are studies about this incretin for isomaltulose and sucromalt in healthy subjects [46], other studies have reported benefits in individuals with metabolic syndrome, obesity and DM2 after isomaltulose versus sucrose consumption [31,58–60], but few have compared the effects of cross-consumption of pre-loads elaborated with these types of carbohydrates in DM2. To date, only one study has determined a higher release of GLP-1 after the consumption of isomaltulose in individuals with diabetes [58]. Our results showed an $AUC_{0-180\ min}$ of GLP-1 higher after the consumption of GS versus DI, (Figure 1) exhibiting a synergistic effect of these carbohydrates.

In this sense, it is well-known that GLP-1 secretion is directly related to macronutrients composition, in particular to both carbohydrates and monounsaturated fatty acids (MUFAs) [61,62] without any significant effect on insulin levels [61,63,64]. This is consistent with our results and with the Mottalib et al. work regarding GLP-1 secretion and MUFA content in ONS-D when compared to ET [42]. In a study by Printz [65], adequate glycaemic and insulinemic responses were found after the intake of three enteral supplements for diabetics in subjects with DM2, but no significant differences in the release of GIP and GLP-1 were found [65]. In fact, carbohydrates used in Printz's [65] study, such as glucose, fructose, lactose and maltose [65], probably resulted in both changes in the final place of the intraluminal digestion and the speed of absorption, which could explain these results, especially when comparing the forenamed carbohydrates with those administered in our study. Even though DI also contains disaccharides such as lactose, its metabolic profile could be sufficient to produce a more significant GLP-1 release of and less GIP than ET, but not enough to produce a better effect on incretins and insulin than GS. This observation confirms previous findings that both the amount and type of carbohydrates and fats influence incretin release 18,24,29,45], as well as in the GI and GL.

Our study could be one of the first demonstrating ONS-D effects on GI in DM2 subjects. In fact, when compared with glucose solution, the evaluated supplements turned out to have an intermediate GI value in people with diabetes for ET = 56. Meanwhile for GS = 47 and DI = 51, the result was a low GI. Whereas, GL was high for ET = 23 and intermediate for GS = 11 and DI = 12, (Table 7). The mean of these values is higher than the reported in the international GI and GL tables for healthy subjects [36]: GI for ET = 48, GS = 23, DI = 12; with an intermediate GL: ET = 16, GS = 6 DI = 3. In a randomised cross-over study conducted by Hofman et al. [35], in which the GI of 12 supplements was evaluated in healthy subjects, the mean GI value in the ONS-D was 19.4 ± 1.8, and from 42.1 ± 5.9 in standard supplements [35].

Significant differences have been reported in the GI value of different foods and/or typical foods between healthy subjects and DM2 [66]. It is well known that the subject's characteristics does not have a significant effect on mean IG values [38], but the variation of the values can differ in different groups, being higher in people suffering from type 1 diabetes (29%) than in healthy subjects (22%) or in DM2 patients (15%) [38]. Our results are comparable with a previous study in which the GI for a DM oral specific supplement was assessed in healthy subjects (IG = 27) and DM2 (IG = 54), finding a significant difference between groups [67].

This situation can be explained by a greater relative increase in the glycaemic response after consumption of the reference food (GB) in people with diabetes compared to healthy subjects [38,68]. One possible explanation in that a defective insulin secretion is unable to counteract greater glycaemic excursions in DM2 patients. At the same time [68], healthy people preserve their insulin secretory machinery, preventing a greater glycaemic increase especially for the lowest digestion rates [38,68].

As mentioned above, we found a higher GI for DI, even though a lower GI value has been reported in healthy subjects when compared to the rest of the treatments [35,36]. However, in the study conducted by Hofman et al. [35], both supplements GS and DI contained fructose 1.9 g/100 mL, and a higher amount of MUFAs, DI = 3.6 g/100 mL versus GS = 3.8 g/100 mL than the supplements evaluated in this study, therefore, it is not possible to make an exact comparison [35].

The GI value for DI in DM2 patients could be explained in part by the quantitative sugar content (which has an 8.3 g versus 0.0 g to GS per portion given in this study) (Table 2). The rest of the components like both the amount and type of fibre can also influence these results. Moreover, soluble fibre can decrease the GI by many factors such as postprandial glucose fluctuation cushioning, and, by its action on intestinal motility, on peptide action and gastrointestinal enzymes [29,69,70].

In this study, total fibre concentration in DI was 2 g/100 mL, whose proportion corresponds to the 80:20 ratio of soluble/insoluble fibre compared to GS, whose total amount corresponds to 1.8 g/100 mL soluble (Table 1). In this regard, identical fibre concentrations generated different GI, such is the case of supplements with 1.5 g/100 mL of fibre and with GI = 26 and 17, respectively, in healthy subjects [35,36], constituted by different fibre mixtures based on fructooligosaccharides, inulin, oligofructose, Arabic gum, soybean polysaccharides and cellulose. Furthermore, it has been reported that soluble fibre can stimulate appetite-regulating peptides such as GLP-1 and pancreatic peptide YY (PYY) in rodents as well as in human [69–71]. It is important to note that DI has resistant starch, whereas GS contains a modified and resistant maltodextrin linked to soluble fibre [69]. In a study in healthy subjects, an increase in peptide YY concentrations and GLP-1 was observed alongside a corresponding decrease in the sensation of hunger and an increased satiety perception after the consumption of tea with 10 g of this component [69].

Few investigations about OSF-D intake have correlated SA with incretin concentrations as it has been evaluated in this study. This indicator was quantified through a score that included variables such as perception of hunger, desire to eat, prospective consumption of food and fullness [14]. It was observed in this investigation that plasma insulin, GIP and GLP-1 were related to some of these parameters but observing a lower SA ratings $AUC_{0\text{–}180\text{ min}}$ in the ET (Supplementary Materials Table S4). It is known that appetite regulation is a complex process stimulated by several central and peripheral signals in response to energy and, mainly, to food composition, where emotional, sensory and environmental factors can influence the overall response [71,72].

There is a lack of consensus regarding GI/GL usefulness in predicting appetite and food intake [12,73,74]. Although GI is not synonymous with glycaemic response, the debate is anchored to the controversy toward the effect of postprandial glycaemic level and its effects on SA reduction [14,75]. Some authors state that the evidence about these affirmations are not conclusive [73,76], postulating that postprandial glycaemic and appetite are not related and considering that insulin response [74], but not the glycaemic response is the real mediator of the short-term appetite reduction, as shown by Flint et al. [14,76]. Specifically, Flint et al. has reported that the maximum insulinemic peak after meal ingestion was related to a decrease in hunger sensation and a satiety increase.

Likewise, in our study, precisely at 30 min and not at the maximum peak, insulin values were inversely related to the sensation of hunger and the overall of SA rating after ET intake, but not the perception of fullness (Supplementary Materials Table S1). However, the same behaviour for these variables was not evident after the consumption of ONS-D. Possibly, this was due to the higher and faster insulin increase produced by ET at this point of the curve, based on the type and amount of non-extended release carbohydrates of this ONS, and more than half corresponded to free sugars (14.1 g/per portion given in this study) (Table 2). Despite this premise, a relationship between glycaemia concentration and prospective food consumption 30 min after DI intake was found, (Supplementary Materials Table S2) and a direct relationship between glycaemic levels in 90 min with the sensation of fullness after the consumption of GS (Supplementary Materials Table S3). The observed feeling of fullness could be related to another mechanism produced via carbohydrate type and fibre content in GS, a supplement that besides sucromalt also has amylase-resistant maltodextrin, in which fibre-viscosity addition could increase the fullness sensation [69].

It is important to note there was an inverse correlation between GLP-1 levels and prospective consumption of food 30 min after GS ingestion (Supplementary Materials Table S3). In other studies [24,77], a relationship between GLP-1 and delayed gastric emptying has been evidenced. This gastrointestinal response would influence the feeling of fullness after GS intake at this curve time. Niwano [12] showed that high GI foods consumption are associated with increased hunger and short-term satiety reduction in humans, but not over the long-term [74].

It is relevant to highlight the inverse correlation between GIP and GI/GL after ONS-D ingestion (Supplementary Materials Table S4). This finding could confirm the theory proposed by Pfeiffer et al. [32] regarding the role of this incretin as an indicator of "carbohydrate metabolic quality" [32]. On the other hand, we confirmed our hypothesis that ONS-D with slow-digesting carbohydrates strongly stimulates GLP-1 release with a subsequent decrease in GIP and insulin secretion, promoting a lower IG/CG index in DM2 subjects when compared with a standard supplement. Although ONS-D reduced the $AUC_{0\text{–}180\ min}$ of subjective appetite, only GS exhibited both a hunger sensation decreasing effect and an increased fullness perception in some points of the postprandial response. Finally, these results were also consistent with Peters et al. [78], who evaluated the digestibility of three carbohydrates on appetite and its relation to blood glucose levels and postprandial insulin, reporting that glycaemic response had minimal effects on appetite when the products only differed in the rate and extension of carbohydrate digestibility [78].

The limitations of our research comprised the lack of evaluation of some variables such as gastric emptying. Although the number of subjects who completed this study was sufficient to assess GI/GL accurately, a higher number of patients is recommended for SA evaluation. On the other hand, one of the strengths of this study is that the results of these indicators, especially GI/GL, could be the first of their kind in the literature done in diabetic individuals from Latin America. It is also one of the first to combine these variables with subjective appetite and incretin levels. It would be a matter of interest to extend the curve's time after consumption in order to evaluate the intake suppression force to the following meal, along with intervention protocols regarding intestinal microbiota in this type of individual.

5. Conclusions

The results of this study showed lower values in postprandial subjective appetite ratings and better metabolic profile after ONS-D intake when compared to standard supplements. A more attenuated glycaemic and insulinemic response along with a lower GIP release and higher levels of GLP-1 confirmed the synergistic effect of slow-digesting carbohydrates along MUFA addition. Isomaltulose and sucromalt may have influenced these factors. In this study, GI/GL in subjects with DM2 after ONS-D consumption were lower than the reference food (glucose solution) and the standard supplement, and lower for GS than DI.

Strategies in food technology, such as intestinal amylase-resistant dextrins along with new functional fibres, need to be considered in low GI product development in order to obtain adequately managed metabolic responses of fullness perception after ONS-D consumption. Our study qualifies two of these supplements as optimal for prescription in people with diabetes when compared with a standard supplement. However, it is necessary to conduct more investigations allowing to correlate long-term appetite suppression with the EG/CG of these supplements.

Supplementary Materials:

Table S1: Correlation coefficients between biochemical variables and subjective measurements of appetite in 0, 30, 90 and 120 min at standard oral nutritional supplements not specific for diabetic patients (ET). Table S2: Correlations coefficients between biochemical variables and subjective measurements of appetite in 0, 30, 90 and 120 min at isomaltulose and resistant starch supplement (DI). Table S3: Correlations coefficients between biochemical variables and subjective measurements of appetite in 0, 30, 90 and 120 min at resistant maltodextrin and sucromalt supplement (GS). Table S4: Correlations coefficients between glycaemic index and glycaemia load with AUC values of hormones and subjective measurements of appetite.

Author Contributions: Conceptualization, L.A.D., V.B. and J.L.-M.; methodology, L.A.D., V.B., N.R., J.d.A.C. and J.L.-M.; software, D.A.; validation, V.C. and N.R.; formal analysis, D.A. and V.C.; investigation, J.d.A.C., S.D.-A. and D.R.-G.; resources, V.B., S.D.-A. and S.C.; data handling, D.A. and V.C.; writing—original draft preparation, L.A.D., V.B. and J.L.-M.; writing—review and editing, L.A.D., V.B., J.L.-M. and M.C.E.; visualization, M.C.E., D.R.-G., J.d.A.C. and S.C.; supervision, L.A.D.; project administration, L.A.D. and N.R.; funding acquisition, L.A.D., N.R. and V.B. All authors conducted the drafting of the manuscript and agreed on the final approval of the version to be published.

Acknowledgments: The authors thank Valmore Bermúdez and Nadia Reina Villasmil for their laboratory assistance and the Endocrine and Metabolic Diseases Research Centre (EMDRC) and Andres Bello University for this publication.

Abbreviations

ADA	American Diabetes Association
BMI	Body mass index
DI	Isomaltulose and resistant starch supplement
DM2	Diabetes mellitus type 2
ET	Standard nutritional supplement not specific for diabetics
GB	Glucose solution or reference food
GI	Glycaemic index
GIP	Glucose-dependent insulinotropic polypeptide
GL	Glycaemic load
GLP-1	Glucagon-like peptide 1
GS	Resistant maltodextrin and sucromalt supplement
HbA1c	Glycated haemoglobin (HbA1c)
IDF	International Diabetes Federation
ONS-D	Oral nutritional supplements specific for diabetics
SEM	Standard error of the mean
VAS	Visual analogue scale
LGL	Low glycaemic load
AUCG	Area under the curve glucose

References

1. Rosen, E.D.; Kaestner, K.H.; Natarajan, R.; Patti, M.-E.; Sallari, R.; Sander, M.; Susztak, K. Epigenetics and Epigenomics: Implications for Diabetes and Obesity. *Diabetes* **2018**, *67*, 1923–1931. [CrossRef]
2. World Health Organization. The Top 10 Causes of Death. 2018. Available online: https://www.who.int/news-room/fact-sheets/detail/the-top-10-causes-of-death (accessed on 31 March 2019).
3. World Health Organization. Diabetes. 2018. Available online: https://www.who.int/en/news-room/fact-sheets/detail/diabetes (accessed on 31 March 2019).
4. Unnikrishnan, R.; Pradeepa, R.; Joshi, S.R.; Mohan, V. Type 2 Diabetes: Demystifying the Global Epidemic. *Diabetes* **2017**, *66*, 1432–1442. [CrossRef] [PubMed]
5. International Diabetes Federation (IDF). The 8th Edition of the Diabetes Atlas. 2017. Available online: http://diabetesatlas.org/resources/2017-atlas.html (accessed on 31 March 2019).
6. International Diabetes Federation Guideline Development Group. Guideline for management of postmeal glucose in diabetes. *Diabetes Res. Clin. Pract.* **2014**, *103*, 256–268. [CrossRef]
7. American Diabetes Association. 15. Diabetes Advocacy: Standards of Medical Care in Diabetes—2018. *Diabetes Care* **2018**, *41*, S152–S153. [CrossRef] [PubMed]
8. Diabetes and Nutrition Study Group of the European Association for the Study of Diabetes Recommendations for the nutritional management of patients with diabetes mellitus. *Eur. J. Clin. Nutr.* **2000**, *54*, 353–355. [CrossRef]

9. Willett, W.; Manson, J.; Liu, S. Glycemic index, glycemic load, and risk of type 2 diabetes. *Am. J. Clin. Nutr.* **2002**, *76*, 274S–280S. [CrossRef]
10. Augustin, L.S.A.; Kendall, C.W.C.; Jenkins, D.J.A.; Willett, W.C.; Astrup, A.; Barclay, A.W.; Björck, I.; Brand-Miller, J.C.; Brighenti, F.; Buyken, A.E.; et al. Glycemic index, glycemic load and glycemic response: An International Scientific Consensus Summit from the International Carbohydrate Quality Consortium (ICQC). *Nutr. Metab. Cardiovasc. Dis.* **2015**, *25*, 795–815. [CrossRef] [PubMed]
11. Ojo, O.; Ojo, O.O.; Adebowale, F.; Wang, X.-H. The Effect of Dietary Glycaemic Index on Glycaemia in Patients with Type 2 Diabetes: A Systematic Review and Meta-Analysis of Randomized Controlled Trials. *Nutrients* **2018**, *10*, 373. [CrossRef] [PubMed]
12. Niwano, Y.; Adachi, T.; Kashimura, J.; Sakata, T.; Sasaki, H.; Sekine, K.; Yamamoto, S.; Yonekubo, A.; Kimura, S. Is glycemic index of food a feasible predictor of appetite, hunger, and satiety? *J. Nutr. Sci. Vitaminol. (Tokyo)* **2009**, *55*, 201–207. [CrossRef]
13. Sun, F.-H.; Li, C.; Zhang, Y.-J.; Wong, S.; Wang, L. Effect of Glycemic Index of Breakfast on Energy Intake at Subsequent Meal among Healthy People: A Meta-Analysis. *Nutrients* **2016**, *8*, 37. [CrossRef] [PubMed]
14. Flint, A.; Møller, B.K.; Raben, A.; Sloth, B.; Pedersen, D.; Tetens, I.; Holst, J.J.; Astrup, A. Glycemic and insulinemic responses as determinants of appetite in humans. *Am. J. Clin. Nutr.* **2006**, *84*, 1365–1373. [CrossRef]
15. Elia, M.; Ceriello, A.; Laube, H.; Sinclair, A.J.; Engfer, M.; Stratton, R.J. Enteral nutritional support and use of diabetes-specific formulas for patients with diabetes: A systematic review and meta-analysis. *Diabetes Care* **2005**, *28*, 2267–2279. [CrossRef]
16. Ojo, O.; Brooke, J. Evaluation of the Role of Enteral Nutrition in Managing Patients with Diabetes: A Systematic Review. *Nutrients* **2014**, *6*, 5142–5152. [CrossRef] [PubMed]
17. De Luis DA, D.M. A randomized clinical trial with two enteral diabetes-specific supplements in patients with diabetes mellitus type 2: Metabolic effects. *Eur. Rev. Med. Pharmacol. Sci.* **2008**, *12*, 261–266.
18. Voss, A.C.; Maki, K.C.; Garvey, W.T.; Hustead, D.S.; Alish, C.; Fix, B.; Mustad, V.A. Effect of two carbohydrate-modified tube-feeding formulas on metabolic responses in patients with type 2 diabetes. *Nutrition* **2008**, *24*, 990–997. [CrossRef]
19. Sanz-Paris, A.; Boj-Carceller, D.; Lardies-Sanchez, B.; Perez-Fernandez, L.; Cruz-Jentoft, A. Health-Care Costs, Glycemic Control and Nutritional Status in Malnourished Older Diabetics Treated with a Hypercaloric Diabetes-Specific Enteral Nutritional Formula. *Nutrients* **2016**, *8*, 153. [CrossRef] [PubMed]
20. Tan, S.Y.; Siow, P.C.; Peh, E.; Henry, C.J. Influence of rice, pea and oat proteins in attenuating glycemic response of sugar sweetened beverages. *Eur. J. Nutr.* **2018**, *57*, 2795–2803. [CrossRef] [PubMed]
21. Yabe, D.; Seino, Y.; Seino, Y. Incretin concept revised: The origin of the insulinotropic function of glucagon-like peptide-1 -the gut, the islets or both? *J. Diabetes Investig.* **2018**, *9*, 21–24. [CrossRef]
22. Rojas, J.; Bermudez, V.; Palmar, J.; Martínez, M.S.; Olivar, L.C.; Nava, M.; Tomey, D.; Rojas, M.; Salazar, J.; Garicano, C.; et al. Pancreatic Beta Cell Death: Novel Potential Mechanisms in Diabetes Therapy. *J. Diabetes Res.* **2018**, *2018*, 1–19. [CrossRef]
23. Prinz, P. The role of dietary sugars in health: Molecular composition or just calories? *Eur. J. Clin. Nutr.* **2019**. [CrossRef]
24. Giezenaar, C.; Trahair, L.G.; Luscombe-Marsh, N.D.; Hausken, T.; Standfield, S.; Jones, K.L.; Lange, K.; Horowitz, M.; Chapman, I.; Soenen, S. Effects of randomized whey-protein loads on energy intake, appetite, gastric emptying, and plasma gut-hormone concentrations in older men and women. *Am. J. Clin. Nutr.* **2017**, *106*, 865–877. [CrossRef] [PubMed]
25. Steinert, R.E.; Feinle-Bisset, C.; Asarian, L.; Horowitz, M.; Beglinger, C.; Geary, N. Ghrelin, CCK, GLP-1, and PYY(3-36): Secretory controls and physiological roles in eating and glycemia in health, obesity, and after RYGB. *Physiol. Rev.* **2017**, *97*, 411–463. [CrossRef] [PubMed]
26. Behall, K.M.; Scholfield, D.J.; Canary, J. Effect of starch structure on glucose and insulin responses in adults. *Am. J. Clin. Nutr.* **1988**, *47*, 428–432. [CrossRef] [PubMed]
27. McMahon, M.M.; Nystrom, E.; Braunschweig, C.; Miles, J.; Compher, C.; the American Society for Parenteral and Enteral Nutrition (A.S.P.E.N.) Board of Directors. A.S.P.E.N. Clinical Guidelines: Nutrition Support of Adult Patients with Hyperglycemia. *J. Parenter. Enter. Nutr.* **2013**, *37*, 23–36. [CrossRef] [PubMed]

28. Doola, R.; Todd, A.S.; Forbes, J.M.; Deane, A.M.; Presneill, J.J.; Sturgess, D.J. Diabetes-Specific Formulae Versus Standard Formulae as Enteral Nutrition to Treat Hyperglycemia in Critically Ill Patients: Protocol for a Randomized Controlled Feasibility Trial. *JMIR Res. Protoc.* **2018**, *7*, e90. [CrossRef]
29. Devitt, A.A.; Williams, J.A.; Choe, Y.S.; Hustead, D.S.; Mustad, V.A. Glycemic responses to glycemia-targeted specialized-nutrition beverages with varying carbohydrates compared to a standard nutritional beverage in adults with type 2 diabetes. *Adv. Biosci. Biotechnol.* **2013**, *4*, 1–10. [CrossRef]
30. Grysman, A.; Carlson, T.; Wolever, T.M.S. Effects of sucromalt on postprandial responses in human subjects. *Eur. J. Clin. Nutr.* **2008**, *62*, 1364–1371. [CrossRef]
31. Maresch, C.C.; Petry, S.F.; Theis, S.; Bosy-Westphal, A.; Linn, T. Low Glycemic Index Prototype Isomaltulose-Update of Clinical Trials. *Nutrients* **2017**, *9*, 381. [CrossRef]
32. Pfeiffer, A.F.H.; Keyhani-Nejad, F. High Glycemic Index Metabolic Damage—A Pivotal Role of GIP and GLP-1. *Trends Endocrinol. Metab.* **2018**, *29*, 289–299. [CrossRef]
33. Holub, I.; Gostner, A.; Theis, S.; Nosek, L.; Kudlich, T.; Melcher, R.; Scheppach, W. Novel findings on the metabolic effects of the low glycaemic carbohydrate isomaltulose (Palatinose). *Br. J. Nutr.* **2010**, *103*, 1730–1737. [CrossRef]
34. Kendall, F.E.; Marchand, O.; Haszard, J.J.; Venn, B.J. The Comparative Effect on Satiety and Subsequent Energy Intake of Ingesting Sucrose or Isomaltulose Sweetened Trifle: A Randomized Crossover Trial. *Nutrients* **2018**, *10*, 1504. [CrossRef] [PubMed]
35. Hofman, Z.; De Van Drunen, J.; Kuipers, H. The Glycemic Index of standard and diabetes-specific enteral formulas. *Asia Pac. J. Clin. Nutr.* **2006**, *15*, 412–417. [PubMed]
36. Atkinson, F.S.; Foster-Powell, K.; Brand-Miller, J.C. International Tables of Glycemic Index and Glycemic Load Values: 2008. *Diabetes Care* **2008**, *31*, 2281–2283. [CrossRef] [PubMed]
37. World Medical Association. Ethical Principles for Medical Research Involving Human Subjects. 64ª General Assembly. 2013. Available online: https://www.wma.net/policies-post/wma-declaration-of-helsinki-ethical-principles-for-medical-research-involving-human-subjects/ (accessed on 24 March 2019).
38. Brouns, F.; Bjorck, I.; Frayn, K.N.; Gibbs, A.L.; Lang, V.; Slama, G.; Wolever, T.M. Glycaemic index methodology. *Nutr. Res. Rev.* **2005**, *18*, 145–171. [CrossRef] [PubMed]
39. Parker, B.A.; Sturm, K.; Macintosh, C.G.; Feinle, C.; Horowitz, M.; Chapman, I.M. Relation between food intake and visual analogue scale ratings of appetite and other sensations in healthy older and young subjects. *Eur. J. Clin. Nutr.* **2004**, *58*, 212–218. [CrossRef] [PubMed]
40. World Health Organization. Energy and Protein Requirements: Report of a Joint FAO/WHO/UNU Expert Consultation. 1981. Available online: https://apps.who.int/iris/handle/10665/39527 (accessed on 24 March 2019).
41. Akilen, R.; Deljoomanesh, N.; Hunschede, S.; Smith, C.E.; Arshad, M.U.; Kubant, R.; Anderson, G.H. The effects of potatoes and other carbohydrate side dishes consumed with meat on food intake, glycemia and satiety response in children. *Nutr. Diabetes* **2016**, *6*, e195. [CrossRef]
42. Mottalib, A.; Mohd-Yusof, B.-N.; Shehabeldin, M.; Pober, D.; Mitri, J.; Hamdy, O. Impact of Diabetes-Specific Nutritional Formulas versus Oatmeal on Postprandial Glucose, Insulin, GLP-1 and Postprandial Lipidemia. *Nutrients* **2016**, *8*, 443. [CrossRef]
43. Alish, C.J.; Garvey, W.T.; Maki, K.C.; Sacks, G.S.; Hustead, D.S.; Hegazi, R.A.; Mustad, V.A. A Diabetes-Specific Enteral Formula Improves Glycemic Variability in Patients with Type 2 Diabetes. *Diabetes Technol. Ther.* **2010**, *12*, 419–425. [CrossRef]
44. Ceriello, A.; Davidson, J.; Hanefeld, M.; Leiter, L.; Monnier, L.; Owens, D.; Tajima, N.; Tuomilehto, J. Postprandial hyperglycaemia and cardiovascular complications of diabetes: An update. *Nutr. Metab. Cardiovasc. Dis.* **2006**, *16*, 453–456. [CrossRef]
45. Yoshizane, C.; Mizote, A.; Yamada, M.; Arai, N.; Arai, S.; Maruta, K.; Mitsuzumi, H.; Ariyasu, T.; Ushio, S.; Fukuda, S. Glycemic, insulinemic and incretin responses after oral trehalose ingestion in healthy subjects. *Nutr. J.* **2017**, *16*. [CrossRef]
46. Kawaguchi, T.; Nakano, D.; Oriishi, T.; Torimura, T. Effects of isomaltulose on insulin resistance and metabolites in patients with non-alcoholic fatty liver disease: A metabolomic analysis. *Mol. Med. Rep.* **2018**. [CrossRef] [PubMed]

47. Nauck, M.A.; Meier, J.J. The incretin effect in healthy individuals and those with type 2 diabetes: Physiology, pathophysiology, and response to therapeutic interventions. *Lancet Diabetes Endocrinol.* **2016**, *4*, 525–536. [CrossRef]
48. Holst, J.J. On the Physiology of GIP and GLP-1. *Horm. Metab. Res.* **2004**, *36*, 747–754. [CrossRef] [PubMed]
49. Nasteska, D.; Harada, N.; Suzuki, K.; Yamane, S.; Hamasaki, A.; Joo, E.; Iwasaki, K.; Shibue, K.; Harada, T.; Inagaki, N. Chronic Reduction of GIP Secretion Alleviates Obesity and Insulin Resistance Under High-Fat Diet Conditions. *Diabetes* **2014**, *63*, 2332. [CrossRef] [PubMed]
50. Bray, G.A. Potential health risks from beverages containing fructose found in sugar or high-fructose corn syrup. *Diabetes Care* **2013**, *36*, 11–12. [CrossRef] [PubMed]
51. Herman, M.A.; Samuel, V.T. The Sweet Path to Metabolic Demise: Fructose and Lipid Synthesis. *Trends Endocrinol. Metab.* **2016**, *27*, 719–730. [CrossRef] [PubMed]
52. Donner, T.W.; Wilber, J.F.; Ostrowski, D. D-tagatose, a novel hexose: Acute effects on carbohydrate tolerance in subjects with and without type 2 diabetes. *Diabetes Obes. Metab.* **1999**, *1*, 285–291. [CrossRef]
53. Guerrero-Wyss, M.; Durán Agüero, S.; Angarita Dávila, L. D-Tagatose Is a Promising Sweetener to Control Glycaemia: A New Functional Food. *BioMed Res. Int.* **2018**, *2018*, 8718053. [CrossRef]
54. Maeda, A.; Miyagawa, J.-I.; Miuchi, M.; Nagai, E.; Konishi, K.; Matsuo, T.; Tokuda, M.; Kusunoki, Y.; Ochi, H.; Murai, K.; et al. Effects of the naturally-occurring disaccharides, palatinose and sucrose, on incretin secretion in healthy non-obese subjects. *J. Diabetes Investig.* **2013**, *4*, 281–286. [CrossRef]
55. Ruiz-Ojeda, F.J.; Plaza-Díaz, J.; Sáez-Lara, M.J.; Gil, A. Effects of Sweeteners on the Gut Microbiota: A Review of Experimental Studies and Clinical Trials. *Adv. Nutr. (Bethesda Md.)* **2019**, *10*, S31–S48. [CrossRef]
56. Zeevi, D.; Korem, T.; Zmora, N.; Israeli, D.; Rothschild, D.; Weinberger, A.; Ben-Yacov, O.; Lador, D.; Avnit-Sagi, T.; Lotan-Pompan, M.; et al. Personalized Nutrition by Prediction of Glycemic Responses. *Cell* **2015**, *163*, 1079–1094. [CrossRef] [PubMed]
57. Angarita, L.; Bermudez, V.; Reina, N.; Cisternas, S.; Díaz, W.; Escobar, M.C.; Carrasco, P.; Durán, S.; Buhring, K.; Buhring, R.; et al. New Insights into Alleviating Diabetes Mellitus: Role of Gut Microbiota and a Nutrigenomic Approach. In *Diabetes Food Plan*; Waisundara, V., Ed.; InTech: London, UK, 2018; ISBN 978-1-78923-274-5.
58. Ang, M.; Linn, T. Comparison of the effects of slowly and rapidly absorbed carbohydrates on postprandial glucose metabolism in type 2 diabetes mellitus patients: A randomized trial. *Am. J. Clin. Nutr.* **2014**, *100*, 1059–1068. [CrossRef] [PubMed]
59. König, D.; Theis, S.; Kozianowski, G.; Berg, A. Postprandial substrate use in overweight subjects with the metabolic syndrome after isomaltulose (Palatinose TM) ingestion. *Nutrition* **2012**, *28*, 651–656. [CrossRef] [PubMed]
60. Van Can, J.G.P.; van Loon, L.J.C.; Brouns, F.; Blaak, E.E. Reduced glycaemic and insulinaemic responses following trehalose and isomaltulose ingestion: Implications for postprandial substrate use in impaired glucose-tolerant subjects. *Br. J. Nutr.* **2012**, *108*, 1210–1217. [CrossRef]
61. Sloth, B.; Due, A.; Larsen, T.M.; Holst, J.J.; Heding, A.; Astrup, A. The effect of a high-MUFA, low-glycaemic index diet and a low-fat diet on appetite and glucose metabolism during a 6-month weight maintenance period. *Br. J. Nutr.* **2008**, *101*, 1846–1858. [CrossRef] [PubMed]
62. Drucker, D.J. The biology of incretin hormones. *Cell Metab.* **2006**, *3*, 153–165. [CrossRef]
63. Rocca, A.S.; LaGreca, J.; Kalitsky, J.; Brubaker, P.L. Monounsaturated Fatty Acid Diets Improve Glycemic Tolerance through Increased Secretion of Glucagon-Like Peptide-1*. *Endocrinology* **2001**, *142*, 1148–1155. [CrossRef]
64. Storm, H.; Holst, J.J.; Hermansen, K.; Thomsen, C. Differential effects of saturated and monounsaturated fats on postprandial lipemia and glucagon-like peptide 1 responses in patients with type 2 diabetes. *Am. J. Clin. Nutr.* **2003**, *77*, 605–611. [CrossRef]
65. Printz, H.; Recke, B.; Fehmann, H.C.; Göke, B. No apparent benefit of liquid formula diet in NIDDM. *Exp. Clin. Endocrinol. Diabetes* **2009**, *105*, 134–139. [CrossRef]
66. Noreberg, C.; Indar-Brown, K.; Madar, Z. Glycemic and insulinemic responses after ingestion of ethnic foods by NIDDM and healthy subjects. *Am. J. Clin. Nutr.* **1992**, *55*, 89–95. [CrossRef]
67. Aguirre, P.C.; Galgani, F.J.; Díaz, B.E. Determinación del índice glicémico del alimento nutridiabetic® destinado a diabéticos tipo 2. *Rev. Chil. Nutr.* **2006**, *33*, 14–21. [CrossRef]

68. Rizkalla, S.W.; Laromiguiere, M.; Champ, M.; Bruzzo, F.; Boillot, J.; Slama, G. Effect of baking process on postprandial metabolic consequences: Randomized trials in normal and type 2 diabetic subjects. *Eur. J. Clin. Nutr.* **2006**, *61*, 175. [CrossRef] [PubMed]
69. Ye, Z.; Arumugam, V.; Haugabrooks, E.; Williamson, P.; Hendrich, S. Soluble dietary fibre (Fibersol-2) decreased hunger and increased satiety hormones in humans when ingested with a meal. *Nutr. Res.* **2015**, *35*, 393–400. [CrossRef] [PubMed]
70. Delzenne, N.M.; Cani, P.D.; Daubioul, C.; Neyrinck, A.M. Impact of inulin and oligofructose on gastrointestinal peptides. *Br. J. Nutr.* **2005**, *93*, S157–S161. [CrossRef] [PubMed]
71. Kirkmeyer, S.V.; Mattes, R.D. Effects of food attributes on hunger and food intake. *Int. J. Obes.* **2000**, *24*, 1167–1175. [CrossRef]
72. Stafleu, A.; Hendriks, H.F.; Smeets, P.A.; Blom, W.A.; de Graaf, C. Biomarkers of satiation and satiety. *Am. J. Clin. Nutr.* **2004**, *79*, 946–961.
73. Thomas, D.; Elliott, E.; Baur, L. Low glycaemic index or low glycaemic load diets for overweight and obesity. *Cochrane Database Syst. Rev.* **2007**. [CrossRef]
74. Bornet, F.R.J.; Jardy-Gennetier, A.-E.; Jacquet, N.; Stowell, J. Glycaemic response to foods: Impact on satiety and long-term weight regulation. *Appetite* **2007**, *49*, 535–553. [CrossRef]
75. Van Dam, R.M.; Seidell, J.C. Carbohydrate intake and obesity. *Eur. J. Clin. Nutr.* **2007**, *61*, S75. [CrossRef]
76. Flint, A.; Gregersen, N.T.; Gluud, L.L.; Møller, B.K.; Raben, A.; Tetens, I.; Verdich, C.; Astrup, A. Associations between postprandial insulin and blood glucose responses, appetite sensations and energy intake in normal weight and overweight individuals: A meta-analysis of test meal studies. *Br. J. Nutr.* **2007**, *98*, 17–25. [CrossRef]
77. Giezenaar, C.; van der Burgh, Y.; Lange, K.; Hatzinikolas, S.; Hausken, T.; Jones, K.; Horowitz, M.; Chapman, I.; Soenen, S. Effects of Substitution, and Adding of Carbohydrate and Fat to Whey-Protein on Energy Intake, Appetite, Gastric Emptying, Glucose, Insulin, Ghrelin, CCK and GLP-1 in Healthy Older Men—A Randomized Controlled Trial. *Nutrients* **2018**, *10*, 113. [CrossRef] [PubMed]
78. Peters, H.P.F.; Ravestein, P.; van der Hijden, H.T.W.M.; Boers, H.M.; Mela, D.J. Effect of carbohydrate digestibility on appetite and its relationship to postprandial blood glucose and insulin levels. *Eur. J. Clin. Nutr.* **2010**, *65*, 47. [CrossRef] [PubMed]

12

The Effect of Selenium Supplementation on Glucose Homeostasis and the Expression of Genes Related to Glucose Metabolism

Ewa Jablonska [1,*], Edyta Reszka [1], Jolanta Gromadzinska [2], Edyta Wieczorek [1], Magdalena B. Krol [2], Sara Raimondi [3], Katarzyna Socha [4], Maria H. Borawska [4] and Wojciech Wasowicz [2]

1 Nofer Institute of Occupational Medicine, Department of Toxicology and Carcinogenesis, Sw. Teresy 8 Street, 91-348 Lodz, Poland; edyta.reszka@imp.lodz.pl (E.R.); edyta.wieczorek@imp.lodz.pl (E.W.)
2 Nofer Institute of Occupational Medicine, Department of Biological and Environmental Monitoring, Sw. Teresy 8 Street, 91-348 Lodz, Poland; jolanta.gromadzinska@imp.lodz.pl (J.G.); magdalena.krol@imp.lodz.pl (M.B.K.); wojciech.wasowicz@imp.lodz.pl (W.W.)
3 European Institute of Oncology, Division of Epidemiology and Biostatistics, via Ripamonti 435, Milan 20139, Italy; sara.raimondi@ieo.it
4 The Medical University of Bialystok, Department of Bromatoloy, A. Mickiewicza 2D Street, 15-222 Bialystok, Poland; sara.raimondi@ieo.it (K.S.); borawska@umb.edu.pl (M.H.B.)
* Correspondence: ewa.jablonska@imp.lodz.pl

Abstract: The aim of the study was to evaluate the effect of selenium supplementation on the expression of genes associated with glucose metabolism in humans, in order to explain the unclear relationship between selenium and the risk of diabetes. For gene expression analysis we used archival samples of cDNA from 76 non-diabetic subjects supplemented with selenium in the previous study. The supplementation period was six weeks and the daily dose of selenium was 200 μg (as selenium yeast). Blood for mRNA isolation was collected at four time points: before supplementation, after two and four weeks of supplementation, and after four weeks of washout. The analysis included 15 genes encoding selected proteins involved in insulin signaling and glucose metabolism. In addition, HbA1c and fasting plasma glucose were measured at three and four time points, respectively. Selenium supplementation was associated with a significantly decreased level of HbA1c but not fasting plasma glucose (FPG) and significant down-regulation of seven genes: *INSR, ADIPOR1, LDHA, PDHA, PDHB, MYC,* and *HIF1AN*. These results suggest that selenium may affect glycemic control at different levels of regulation, linked to insulin signaling, glycolysis, and pyruvate metabolism. Further research is needed to investigate mechanisms of such transcriptional regulation and its potential implication in direct metabolic effects.

Keywords: selenium; gene expression; insulin signaling; glucose metabolism; glycolysis; pyruvate metabolism; energy metabolism; glycated hemoglobin; fasting plasma glucose

1. Introduction

Selenium (Se) is a trace element with multiple biological functions. The majority of studies related to this nutrient and human health were devoted to its potential anticancer activity and chemoprevention based on Se supplementation [1–3]. However recent scientific focus has been switched towards possible harmful effects of Se supplementation, especially in terms of its unclear link with glucose metabolism and diabetes [4–6]. The increased risk of diabetes type II (T2DM) in humans associated with elevated Se status has been suggested for the first time on the basis of reanalysis of a placebo-controlled randomized trial (NPC, Nutritional Prevention of Cancer) conducted in the USA in the years 1983–1991 in a group of 1312 subjects. In that study, there was a significant increase in the risk of diabetes among Se-supplemented subjects who had the highest Se status (plasma concentration >121.6 ng/mL) before supplementation (Risk Ratio (RR) = 2.40; $p = 0.01$) [7]. In another American study (SELECT, Selenium and Vitamin E Cancer Prevention Trial) conducted in 35,533 individuals, there was a non-significant increase in the risk of diabetes among Se- supplemented arm (RR = 1.07%, $p = 0.16$) [8]. Results of this large and well-designed, randomized, placebo-controlled trial generated much controversy and up to now, no clear conclusion have been made with respect to the potentially diabetogenic properties of Se. Several observational studies, as well as Se supplementation trials, in which the association between Se status/Se intake and the risk of diabetes or markers of glucose metabolism has been investigated, generated inconsistent results [4,9–12]. On the other hand, animal studies indicated that Se supplementation may lead to hyperinsulinemia, insulin resistance, and glucose intolerance [13]. To complicate this, previous in vivo studies indicated protective role of Se in diabetes [14,15]. The link between Se and glucose seems very complex and is supposed to be reflected by a non-linear U-shaped dose-response relationship [16].

The insights from experimental studies in animals indicate that Se is involved in glucose metabolism via Se-dependent proteins (selenoproteins), which possess redox properties. It is assumed that they may influence the insulin-dependent metabolic pathways, because both insulin release and insulin signaling are regulated by the cellular redox potential [17]. In particular, the essential role in the regulation of both processes is attributed to hydrogen peroxide, which is one of the reactive oxygen species produced inter alia by dismutation of superoxide anion radical (catalyzed by superoxide dismutase, SOD). Hydrogen peroxide is reduced to water with the participation of enzymes, such as Se-dependent glutathione peroxidase (GPx) and catalase (CAT). The role of GPx in the metabolism of insulin appears to be significant and complex, which is reflected by a relatively low expression of mRNA for GPx1 and its low enzymatic activity in the pancreas (1%–5% of the value observed in the liver; the study in mice) [18]. Moreover, it was shown that global overexpression of GPx1 mRNA in mice fed with a normal Se diet (0.4 mg/kg) was associated with hyperglycemia, hyperinsulinemia, and an increase in plasma leptin concentrations [19]. Another selenoprotein potentially important in the etiology of diabetes is selenoprotein P (Sepp1) which is produced mainly in the liver and secreted into plasma, acting as a Se transporter, and having also antioxidant properties. Misu et al. observed a positive correlation between the level of Sepp1 mRNA and insulin resistance in humans [20]. The same authors also demonstrated in vitro that cells stimulated exogenously with purified Sepp1 were characterized by impaired insulin signaling and impaired glucose metabolism [20]. Recently it has been also observed that serum concentration of Sepp1 was positively correlated with fasting plasma glucose (FPG) concentration ($r = 0.35$, $p = 0.037$) and negatively correlated with serum adiponectin levels ($r = -0.355$, $p = 0.034$; $r = -0.367$, $p = 0.028$) in patients with T2DM [21].

Altogether, mechanisms of action of Se in humans at the level of glucose metabolism and its potential role in the etiology of diabetes are unknown and point to the need for more studies relevant to human metabolism. The aim of this study was to assess the effect of Se supplementation on the expression of genes related to glucose metabolism, including genes encoding hormones responsible for glycemic control (insulin, glucagon, leptin, and adiponectin), receptors for these hormones, enzymes involved in glycolysis, as well as key transcription factors involved in the regulation of glycolysis. To our knowledge this is the first study conducted in humans, which aimed to investigate more in-depth molecular effects of Se with respect to glucose homeostasis.

2. Materials and Methods

2.1. Study Design

For the purpose of this study we used archival samples of cDNA obtained from subjects who were supplemented with Se during the trial conducted by us previously. Details of the trial, as well as subjects' exclusion criteria, were described elsewhere [22]. The exclusion criteria for subjects' recruitment included inter alia current smoking and self-reported prevalence of diabetes. Briefly, the 95 non-smoking and non-diabetic individuals were supplemented with 200 μg of Se/day (in the form of Se yeast) for six weeks and fasting blood was collected at four time points: at baseline, after two weeks of supplementation, after six weeks of supplementation, and after four weeks of washout. In the present study, gene expression analysis was performed with the use of cDNA obtained from 76 subjects, randomly selected out of the entire study group, including 36 males and 40 females. Table 1 presents basic characteristics of the subjects. Plasma Se concentration was measured previously (as described in [22]) and mean plasma Se levels calculated for 76 subjects at each time points are presented also in Table 1.

Written informed consent was obtained from all the study participants and the study was approved by the Local Ethics Committee (Ethical Institutional Review Board at the Nofer Institute of Occupational Medicine, Lodz, Poland, Resolution No. 3/2010).

Table 1. Basic characteristics of the study group (76 subjects supplemented with selenium).

Variable	All (n = 76)	Males (n = 36)	Females (n = 40)	p (Males vs. Females)
Age (years)	34.8 ± 10.4	35 ± 18	36 ± 18	0.7549 [a]
BMI (kg/m^2)	24.0 ± 2.9	25.0 ± 2.7	23.0 ± 2.9	**0.0009** [a]
Smoking, n (%)				
Current	0 (0)	0 (0)	0 (0)	
Ever	18 (24)	8 (23)	10 (24)	
Never	58 (76)	27 (77)	31 (76)	ns
Use of Se-containing supplements in the past 6 months, n (%)				
Yes	5 (7)	3 (9)	2 (5)	
No	71 (93)	32 (91)	39 (95)	ns
Mean plasma Se ± SD (μg/L)				
Baseline	65.2 ± 16.5	65.2 ± 16.6	65.3 ± 16.5	0.9729 [b]
After two weeks	101.1 ± 24.5	98.7 ± 22.8	103.3 ± 26.1	0.3907 [a]
After six weeks	99.1 ± 20.3	95.0 ± 16.9	102.7 ± 22.4	0.0928 [b]
After four weeks of washout	76.5 ± 15.6	75.3 ± 15.3	77.6 ± 16.1	0.7777 [b]
p (ANOVA)	**<0.0001**	**<0.0001**	**<0.0001**	

[a]—Mann-Whitney U test; [b]—Student's t-test. Significant p values are in bold.

2.2. Gene Expression Experiment

mRNA for gene expression analysis was isolated from white blood cells (WBC). The description of material preservation, mRNA isolation, quantification, and quality assessment were described previously [22]. For reverse transcription we used a QuantiTect Kit (Qiagen, Hilden, Germany). Gene expression was analyzed by means of qPCR and conducted on a QuantStudioTM 12K Flex Real-Time PCR System (Thermo Fisher Scienific, Waltham, MA, USA), using Custom Taqman® array cards and TaqMan® Universal Master Mix (Thermo Fisher Scienific, Waltham, MA, USA). For each array card 6 μg of cDNA was taken. Reaction conditions were as follows: 95 °C of initial denaturation for 10 min followed by 50 cycles of 95 °C for 15 s and 60 °C for 60 s. The analysis included 15 genes encoding selected proteins involved in insulin signaling and glucose metabolism. The expression was normalized against *GAPDH*. The list of all targets is presented in Table 2. The genes were divided into four groups according to the type of encoded protein: (1) hormones: insulin (*INS*), glucagon (*GCG*), adiponectin (*ADIPOQ*), and leptin (*LEP*); (2) hormone receptors: insulin receptor (*INSR*), glucagon receptor (*GCGR*), adiponectin receptors (*ADIPOR1*, *ADIPOR2*), and leptin receptor (*LEPR*); (3) enzymes involved in pyruvate metabolism: lactic acid dehydrogenase (*LDHA*), pyruvate dehydrogenase, alpha subunit (*PDHA1*) and beta subunit (*PDHB*); (4) transcription factors or their inhibitors driving glycolysis: transcription factor HIF1 (*HIF1A*), HIF1A inhibitor (*HIF1AN*), and nuclear transcription factor MYC (*MYC*).

Table 2. Genes of interest selected for the study.

Gene	Locus	Gene Product	Protein Group
INS	11p15.5	insulin	hormones
GCG	2q36-q37	glucagon	
ADIPOQ	3q27	adiponectin	
LEP	1p31	leptin	
INSR	19p13.3-p13.2	insulin receptor	hormone receptors
GCGR	17q25	glucagon receptor	
ADIPOR1	1q32.1	adiponectin receptor 1	
ADIPOR2	12p13.31	adiponectin receptor 2	
LEPR	7q31.3	leptin receptor	
LDHA	11p15.4	lactate dehydrogenase	enzymes involved in pyruvate metabolism
PDHA1	Xp22.1	pyruvate dehydrogenase (lipoamide) alpha 1 subunit	
PDHB	3p21.1-p14.2	pyruvate dehydrogenase (lipoamide) beta subunit	
HIF1A	14q23.2	hypoxia inducible factor 1, alpha subunit	transcription factors and their inhibitors, involved in the regulation of glycolysis
HIF1AN	10q24	hypoxia inducible factor 1, alpha subunit inhibitor	
MYC	8q24.21	v-myc avian myelocytomatosis viral oncogene homolog	

2.3. HbA1c, Fasting Plasma Glucose

Levels of HbA1c (glycated hemoglobin) were determined in 10 μL of whole blood (heparinized tube) immediately after the blood was collected. The analysis was performed commercially in the certified laboratory of clinical diagnostics, using immunoturbidimetric assay on an INTEGRA 400 system (Roche Diagnostics, Rotkreuz, Switzerland). The enzymic colorimetric method was based on an oxidase/peroxidase method and the respective commercial kit (Alpha Diagnostics, Warsaw, Poland) was used to analyze FPG. All absorbance values were measured on a UV4 Unicam UV-VIS spectrophotometer (Cambridge, UK). Intra- and inter-assay coefficients of variation for FPG analyses were 2.52% ($n = 10$) and 4.57% ($n = 32$), respectively.

2.4. Statistical Analysis

The analysis on gene expression data was performed on the log-transformed values in order to have a normal distribution. Repeated measures analysis of variance (MANCOVA) with an unstructured covariance matrix was carried out to test the effects of time on FPG, HbA1c, and gene expression. With this analysis, markers (FPG, HbA1c, gene expression) at different time points were considered as dependent variables, while covariates (age, sex, BMI, and baseline Se) were included in the models as independent variables. The possible correlation between variation of Se and of gene expression values at different time points was investigated by a linear regression model with the difference of gene expression at two time points as the dependent variable, and the difference of Se, age, sex, BMI, baseline Se, and baseline gene expression as independent variables. All of the analyses were carried out in the whole group of subjects and separately in women and men. Post-hoc comparisons between pairwise time points were performed by contrast tests, using Bonferroni correction. All of the other statistical tests were performed at a significance level of $\alpha = 0.05$. To adjust the results for multiple comparisons, we performed a false discovery rate (FDR) analysis. Statistical analyses were conducted using SAS software, version 9.2 (SAS Institute, Cary, NC, USA).

3. Results

3.1. The Effect of Se Supplementation on HbA1c and Fasting Plasma Glucose

Significant changes in HbA1c levels were observed upon Se supplementation ($p < 0.0001$), with post hoc tests indicating a significant decrease both after six weeks of supplementation and after four weeks of washout ($p < 0.0001$ and $p = 0.02$ vs. baseline, respectively) (Table 3). On the contrary, FPG concentration remained unaffected upon supplementation trial ($p = 0.553$).

Table 3. The effect of Se supplementation on fasting plasma glucose concentration, HbA1c levels and gene expression. Data for all study subjects ($n = 76$).

Marker	Time Points				p (MANCOVA *)
	Baseline	Two Weeks	Six Weeks	Washout	
FPG (mg/dL)	91.96 ± 13.94	90.55 ± 14.07	91.00 ± 14.15	91.56 ± 13.79	0.55
HbA1c (%)	4.74 ± 0.80	na	**4.44 ± 0.63** [c]	**4.57± 0.65** [a]	**<0.05**
INSR	1.23 ± 0.67	**0.98 ± 0.25** [b]	**1.02 ± 0.27** [b]	**0.95 ± 0.25** [c]	**0.005**
ADIPOR1	2.05 ± 0.23	**2.00 ± 0.18** [a]	2.07 ± 0.21	2.04 ± 0.23	**0.002**
ADIPOR2	1.88 ± 0.23	1.84 ± 0.18	1.84 ± 0.19	1.80 ± 0.19	0.08
LEPR	0.87 ± 0.35	0.80 ± 0.34	0.80 ± 0.29	0.82 ± 0.38	0.26
LDHA	2.74 ± 0.30	**2.59 ± 0.26** [c]	**2.49 ± 0.21** [c]	**2.51 ± 0.27** [c]	**<0.0001**
PDHA	2.03 ± 0.29	**1.93 ± 0.24** [a]	**1.90 ± 0.20** [c]	**1.90 ± 0.26** [b]	**0.0002**
PDHB	1.92 ± 0.25	1.86 ± 0.20	**1.81 ± 0.18** [c]	**1.81 ± 0.21** [b]	**0.0008**
HIF1A	2.37 ± 0.26	2.29 ± 0.23	2.29 ± 0.24	2.30 ± 0.27	0.16
HIF1AN	1.71 ± 0.32	**1.61 ± 0.19** [b]	1.70 ± 0.20	1.67 ± 0.21	**0.0001**
MYC	2.31 ± 0.29	**2.22 ± 0.26** [a]	**2.14 ± 0.22** [c]	**2.18 ± 0.25** [a]	**<0.0001**

Values significantly different as compared to baseline are in bold, [a]—$p < 0.05$, [b]—$p < 0.01$, [c]—$p < 0.001$; *—Multivariate analysis of covariance, model included age, sex, BMI and baseline selenium; na—not analyzed (HbA1c was not analyzed after two weeks of supplementation).

3.2. The Effect on Gene Expression

In the first step of analysis, we excluded genes which were not expressed or which had very low expression. These were five genes: *INS, GCG, GCGR, ADIPOQ,* and *LEP*. Further analysis of the remaining 10 genes indicated a significant reduction in mRNA expression of seven targets, including *INSR, ADIPOR1, LDHA, PDHA, PDHB, MYC,* and *HIF1AN*. In the case of *INSR, LDHA, PDHA,* and *MYC*, a significant decrease was observed at all measurement points as indicated by contrast tests (during supplementation and the washout period). For genes *ADIPOR2, LEPR,* and *HIF1A* there was no statistically significant changes over time (Table 3).

Further analysis aimed to test whether the variation of gene expression depended on the variation of Se. We conducted this analysis for all 10 genes and all time points regardless of the fact whether the overall effect was significant or not. Significant correlations between Se status and gene expression were found in the case of *ADIPOR1* after six weeks of supplementation ($p = 0.012$) and in the case of *HIF1AN* after two weeks ($p = 0.045$) and six weeks ($p = 0.002$) of supplementation. All data are shown in Table S3.

3.3. Sex Differences

At baseline, males had significantly higher levels of FPG ($p = 0.01$) as compared to females, however, both sexes did not differ significantly in the level of HbA1c ($p = 0.175$). No modifying effect of sex was observed at the level of both markers upon time (during supplementation and after washout period, as assessed in the MANCOVA model; $p = 0.55$ and $p = 0.09$ for time interaction with sex for FPG and HbA1c, respectively). Data on FPG, HbA1c, and on gene expression analyzed separately for males and females are presented in the supplementary materials (Tables S1 and S2). The results of analysis stratified by sex were less powered and some p-values were no more significant. However, general trends were similar. Analogically to the analyses conducted in the whole group, we tested the correlation between variations in plasma Se levels and in gene expression. In males significant correlation was found for *HIF1AN* after six weeks of supplementation ($p = 0.038$). In females significant correlations were observed for four genes after six weeks of supplementation: *ADIPOR1* ($p = 0.047$), *PDHB* ($p = 0.034$), *HIF1AN* ($p = 0.035$), and *MYC* ($p = 0.048$). Regression analysis data are shown in Tables S4 (for males) and S5 (for females).

3.4. False Discovery Rate Analysis

P-values for the effect on gene expression (Table 3, Tables S1 and S2) were still statistically significant after FDR adjustment for multiple comparisons, except for two genes in women: *ADIPOR1* and *HIF1AN* (in both cases the FDR-adjusted *p*-value was 0.06).

4. Discussion

In this study we observed that six weeks of supplementation with 200 μg of Se in the form of Se yeast had significantly decreased the level of HbA1c in the subjects with relatively low baseline Se status. On the other hand we did not observe any changes at the level of FPG. However, FPG reflects the glycemic status at the time of measurement. HbA1c is regarded as a more reliable marker since it indicates long-term changes in the glycemic control. Thus, the impact of Se supplementation on HbA1c levels observed in this study confirms that Se is involved in the metabolism of glucose. Moreover, significant decrease in HbA1c levels was maintained four weeks after supplementation discontinuation, which clearly shows that the effect of Se on the glycemic control was relatively strong. There are only a few other studies reporting the effect of Se supplementation on glucose homeostasis in humans. Three of them, being all randomized, placebo-controlled trials (RCTs), have shown beneficial effect of short-term Se supplementation in specific groups of women. In the first study, 70 women with gestational diabetes were supplemented with Se at a dose of 200 μg per day for six weeks. Improved glucose homeostasis was observed as reflected by decreased levels of FPG and serum insulin as well as decreased HOMA-IR values (homeostasis model of assessment of insulin resistance) [23]. The second study was conducted in 70 women with polycystic ovary syndrome. After eight weeks of supplementation with Se at 200 μg per day, there was a significant decrease in serum insulin levels, HOMA-IR, HOMA-B (homeostatic model of assessment of beta-cell function) values, and an increase in QUICKI (quantitative insulin sensitivity check index), whereas FPG remained unchanged [24]. The last study investigated the effect of Se supplementation in women with central obesity. After six weeks of Se supplementation (200 μg/day), significant decrease in serum insulin levels and HOMA-IR values was observed [25]. Another study which was conducted in 60 subjects of both sexes (20 males and 40 females) diagnosed with T2DM and coronary heart disease also showed beneficial effects of Se supplementation (200 μg/day for eight weeks) in terms of decreased insulin, HOMA-IR, HOMA-B parameters, and increased QUICKI [26]. On the contrary, only one RCT, conducted in patients with T2DM ($n = 60$, including 34 males and 26 females), indicated that three months of Se supplementation (200 μg/day) led to the increased FPG levels [27]. To compare with short term supplementation, long-term RCTs did not indicate any effects on glucose homeostasis upon Se supplementation, as shown at the level of serum glucose concentration in 140 men with prostate cancer (supplemented with Se at dose 200 μg/day for five years) or at the level of FPG in 3146 participants of the SU.VI.MAX trial (supplemented with 100 μg of Se in combination with zinc (Zn) and vitamins C, E, and beta-carotene, for 7.5 years) [28,29]. Overall, the inconsistent results of the above RCTs coincide with a lack of compliance in the observational studies investigating the link between Se and diabetes. These studies also suggest that Se-induced effects may largely depend on specific health conditions (notably none of them has been conducted in the general population). A similar conclusion has been drawn from recent studies in mice, which were fed with a high-fat diet in order to induce insulin resistance [30]. It was observed that pre-treatment with Se protected animals against developing insulin resistance, whereas post-treatment with Se exacerbated this metabolic disorder. The effects of pre-treatment and post-treatment with Se were different in the context of adipogenesis and lipolysis, showing increased adipocyte differentiation and fat accumulation in adipose tissue in pre-treated mice, whereas post-treated mice were characterized by increased lipolysis and ectopic lipid deposition [30]. The above study clearly shows that Se exerts differential effects under different health conditions.

Along with HbA1c decrease upon Se supplementation, we have observed in this study a significant decrease of leukocyte mRNA levels for seven genes involved in different steps of glucose metabolism regulation. The first group of mRNA targets (*INSR* and *ADIPOR1*) concerned receptors for endocrine hormones: insulin and adiponectin, which are key players in insulin signaling responsible for cellular glucose uptake. Suppressive effects of Se on insulin receptors was observed previously in a study of gestating rats and their offspring [31]. In that experiment, decreased mRNA expression for *Insr*, as well as other insulin signaling genes, including *Irs-1* (insulin receptor substrate 1), *Irs-2* (insulin receptor substrate 2), and *Akt2* (serine/threonine protean kinase 2), was observed in the liver of dams supplemented with 3 mg Se/kg diet (as compared to dams fed basal diet). Importantly, similar changes in the liver, additionally accompanied by decreased protein levels of insulin receptors, were observed in the offspring of dams also receiving a high Se diet. At the same time, high Se diet was associated in both dams and the offspring with hyperinsulinemia, insulin resistance and glucose intolerance [31]. The impact of a high Se diet on protein levels for insulin receptors was also investigated in pigs, showing tissue-specific changes, with up-regulation in the liver and down-regulation in the muscle. However, no changes in both tissues were observed for insulin receptors at the level of mRNA [32]. Similarly, another study conducted in pigs also failed to show any effect of supranutritional intake of Se on insulin receptor mRNA levels, analyzed in liver, muscle, and visceral adipose tissue [33]. Significant reduction of mRNA expression for the adiponectin receptor, *ADIPOR1*, observed in our study after two weeks of supplementation, was accompanied by a borderline significant decrease in *ADIPOR2* ($p = 0.08$). AdipoR2 is expressed mainly in the liver; thus, in blood leukocytes it was more probable to observe a significant effect in the case of AdipoR1, which is expressed ubiquitously [34]. Both receptors bind adiponectin, a hormone produced by adipocytes and involved in glucose metabolism via modulating insulin sensitivity [34]. Though our study may suggest some effect of Se on adiponectin signaling, two supplementation trials failed to show any effect of Se administration on plasma adiponectin levels in humans [35,36]. Nevertheless, the suppressive effect on *INSR* and *ADIPOR1* indicated in this study deserves further research, as decreased expression of mRNA levels for these receptors has been linked to insulin resistance and diabetes in humans and animals [37–39]. Decreased expression of essential genes involved in glucose metabolism, such as those encoding receptors for insulin and adiponectin, may indicate rather detrimental effects of Se supplementation in the study group. On the other hand, the effect at the level of HbA1c was somewhat positive. The hypothetical explanation for these contradictory observations may be that the potentially beneficial decrease in HbA1c level reflects an adaptive response which counteracts the adverse effects of the metalloid on glucose homeostasis and that this response is rather short-term. This adaptive mechanism when induced in a constant manner (by introducing the factor day by day for several weeks) may be strong enough to influence the level of HbA1c, however, not in the long-term. The hypothesis about short-term adaptive response is in line with overall observations from Se supplementation trials, indicating mainly beneficial effects of Se on glucose metabolism in the case of short-term administration and, on the other hand, null or negative effects upon long-term supplementation with this nutrient. Alternative explanation for decreased levels of HbA1c upon Se is the possibility that Se may prevent the process of hemoglobin glycation. This may be suggested on the basis of a recent study by Yu and colleagues, showing Se nanoparticles prevent protein glycation in vitro [40]. Nevertheless, it is not clear whether changes observed in our study at the level of leukocyte gene expression reflect changes in insulin-sensitive tissues. If they do, down-regulation of *INSR* and *ADIPOR1* in blood leukocytes could serve as an early biomarker of adverse health effects of Se supranutrition in humans, leading to impaired glucose homeostasis.

The second group of down-regulated genes in this study included *LDH*, *PDHA*, and *PDHB*, all three encoding enzymes involved in pyruvate metabolism. Pyruvate is the end product of glycolysis and its further metabolism depends on cellular oxygen concentration. Under anaerobic conditions, it is transformed by lactate dehydrogenase (LDH) to lactic acid whereas, under normal aerobic conditions, it is metabolized by pyruvate dehydrogenase complex (PDC) to acetyl coenzyme A (acetyl CoA). The latter reaction links glycolysis to the Krebs cycle. Importantly, pyruvate recycling (occurring across mitochondrial membranes) is an important regulator of insulin secretion due to the generation of NADPH (the reduced form of nicotinamide adenine dinucleotide phosphate), the pivotal molecule required for insulin granule exocytosis in beta cells [41]. Pyruvate metabolism was shown to be implicated in diabetes, as reflected by increased activity of pyruvate dehydrogenase kinase (PDK) in diabetic subjects (PDK plays significant role in glucose disposal as it decreases the activity of PDC) [42]. In general, glycolytic pathway was shown to be dysregulated in diabetes [43]. A study in rats showed, for example, that an alloxan-induced diabetic state significantly altered the activities of glycolytic enzymes in lymphocytes [44]. Importantly, recent animal studies suggest that Se interferes with glycolytic targets and pyruvate metabolism, supporting our observation. Pigs fed with a supranutritional dose of Se exhibited decreased expression of mRNA for pyruvate kinase (enzyme responsible for pyruvate synthesis in the last step of glycolysis) [33]. Interestingly, increased pyruvate levels in the liver and increased expression of pyruvate metabolizing enzymes (pyruvate carboxylase (Pcx) and pyruvate dehydrogenase (Pdh)) were shown in mice with a knocked out gene for selenocysteine lyase (SCLY, the enzyme catalyzing conversion of selenocysteine into alanine and selenide, an important step in Se metabolism, as selenide is a substrate for selenoprotein biosynthesis) [45]. Recently it has been also shown that Se affects glycolysis in cancer cells, suggesting that down-regulation of glycolytic enzymes is a novel mechanism of Se toxicity in cancer and that this mechanism targets the well-known metabolic hallmark of cancer cells associated with enhanced glycolysis, which is called the Warburg effect [46]. In our study we have observed, additionally that Se may affect also transcriptional regulation of glycolysis, leading to significantly decreased expression of *MYC*. c-MYC protein, encoded by *MYC* gene, is responsible for transcriptional regulation of all glycolytic targets, including pyruvate kinase, pyruvate kinase dehydrogenase and lactate dehydrogenase [47]. Importantly, it was also shown to regulate the expression of glucose transporter 2 (GLUT2) and 4 (GLUT4) [47]. mRNA expression of the second major transcriptional regulator of glycolytic targets, HIF1 [47] was not affected upon Se supplementation in our study, whereas a significant decrease was observed for its inhibitor (but only after two weeks of supplementation). Altogether, these results suggest the need for a more in-depth investigation of the link between Se and glycolysis in humans.

We were not able to detect the expression of genes encoding: insulin (*INS*), glucagon (*GCG*), adiponectin (*ADIPOQ*), and leptin (*LEP*) in leukocytes. This was not surprising as all of these hormones are produced either by pancreas (insulin, glucagon) or by adipocytes (adiponectin, leptin). Similarly, *GCGR* levels were not detectable in leukocytes, which was also expected, as the glucagon receptor is expressed mainly in the liver, in which it mediates glucagon effects: glycogen breakdown and glucose release into the bloodstream.

The last analysis in this study concerned the correlation between the variation in gene expression and variation in plasma Se concentrations at a particular time point. There were only a few significant correlations and those that were significant were very small, indicating that changes in gene expression were not high enough to correlate with changes in Se.

Since this report presents secondary outcomes of the supplementation trial, it has several weaknesses. First of all, due to the short-term supplementation (six weeks) we were not able to assess changes in HbA1c levels after the whole life span of erythrocytes (which is about 120 days). HbA1c levels reflect the cumulative history of glycemic control in the past two to three months [48]. After this period the measurement of HbA1c levels is most indicative. However it is possible to observe changes earlier, as shown by studies investigating the effects of glucose-lowering drugs [49]. Since erythrocytes are produced constantly (meaning that the whole pool of erythrocytes contains cells of different ages) the effect observed in our study resulted from HbA1c reduction in the youngest erythrocytes. Nevertheless, one could speculate that these changes might have occurred due to some potential confounders present in the study during several weeks before the beginning of the trial, such as pharmacological or dietary factors. However, none of the supplemented subjects declared to be taking any drugs or supplements that could affect glucose metabolism (we asked all subjects about their use of glucose-lowering drugs or supplements before and during the trial). As for the influence of diet, none of the individuals reported a change to his/her dietary habits during the trial.

The second major weakness of this study is attributable to the fact that the trial was not randomized (subjects were selected for the study according to genotype) and not placebo controlled (for details see [22]). Since no separate control group was investigated, we compared all data with respect to baseline values, measured on the first day of the trial, before taking the first pill with the supplement. Finally, gene expression was analyzed in this study in blood leukocytes and it is not clear whether these changes reflect general reactions to Se at the molecular level in humans or if they are tissue specific. In addition we did not analyze the protein levels for genes of interest; thus, we were unable to show any correspondence between transcriptomic and proteomic expression and elucidate whether observed subtle changes in mRNA have any further consequences.

To conclude, results of this study suggest that Se may affect glycemic control at different levels of regulation, linked not only to insulin signaling, but also to glycolytic pathway and pyruvate metabolism. Further research is needed to investigate mechanisms of negative transcriptional regulation in blood leukocytes upon Se treatment, its relevance to other tissues, correspondence to protein levels and, finally, potential implications in direct metabolic and cellular effects. Overall, findings of this study added more insight into the controversial topic of possible diabetogenic effects of Se supplementation in humans. What is the exact impact of Se supplementation on glucose homeostasis and the risk of diabetes remains still an open question. The answer will not be obtained without studies unraveling the underlying mechanisms, as well as factors which may modify Se effects with respect to glucose homeostasis, in addition to these already suggested, such as sex and genotype [50,51], as well as Se speciation [52,53]. Explaining the link between Se, glucose metabolism, and diabetes is currently one of the priority goals in Se research because it will determine the further direction of studies focusing on Se as a potential chemopreventive agent.

Supplementary Materials:
Table S1: The effect of Se supplementation on fasting plasma glucose concentration, HbA1c levels and gene expression. Data for male subjects (n = 36); Table S2: The effect of Se supplementation on fasting plasma glucose concentration, HbA1c levels and gene expression. Data for female subjects (n = 40); Table S3: Correlation between changes in Se and changes in gene expression measured between two different time points. Data for all subjects (n = 76); Table S4: Correlation between changes in Se and changes in gene expression measured between two different time points in male subjects (calculated only for genes which were shown to be significantly changed upon Se supplementation). Data for male subjects (n = 36); Table S5: Correlation between changes in Se and changes in gene expression measured between two different time points in all subjects (calculated only for genes which were shown to be significantly changed upon Se supplementation). Data for female subjects (n = 40).

Acknowledgments: This study was supported by The Polish Ministry of Science and Higher Education (grant 1666/B/P01/2011/40) and NIOM Internal Grant IMP 1.36/2015-2016).

Author Contributions: E.J. designed the study, performed data analysis and wrote the manuscript, E.R. and E.W. performed gene expression experiments, S.R. performed statistical analysis, M.B.K. collected blood and questionnaire data from the subjects and performed biochemical analyses, K.S. analyzed plasma for selenium concentration, J.G., M.H.B. and W.W. supplied materials and reagents, E.R. revised the manuscript. All authors have read and accepted the final version of the manuscript.

References

1. Labunskyy, V.M.; Hatfield, D.L.; Gladyshev, V.N. Selenoproteins: Molecular pathways and physiological roles. *Physiol. Rev.* **2014**, *94*, 739–777. [CrossRef] [PubMed]
2. Hatfield, D.L.; Tsuji, P.A.; Carlson, B.A.; Gladyshev, V.N. Selenium and selenocysteine: Roles in cancer, health, and development. *Trends Biochem. Sci.* **2014**, *39*, 112–120. [CrossRef] [PubMed]
3. Vinceti, M.; Dennert, G.; Crespi, C.M.; Zwahlen, M.; Brinkman, M.; Zeegers, M.P.A.; Horneber, M.; D'Amico, R.; Del Giovane, C. Selenium for preventing cancer. *Cochrane Database Syst. Rev.* **2014**, *3*, CD005195.
4. Rayman, M.P.; Stranges, S. Epidemiology of selenium and type2 diabetes: Can we make sense of it? *Free Radic. Biol. Med.* **2013**, *65*, 1557–1564. [CrossRef] [PubMed]
5. Mueller, A.S.; Mueller, K.; Wolf, N.M.; Pallauf, J. Selenium and diabetes: An enigma? *Free Radic. Res.* **2009**, *43*, 1029–1059. [CrossRef] [PubMed]
6. Rocourt, C.R.; Cheng, W.H. Selenium supranutrition: Are the potential benefits of chemoprevention outweighed by the promotion of diabetes and insulin resistance? *Nutrients* **2013**, *5*, 1349–1365. [CrossRef] [PubMed]

7. Stranges, S.; Marshall, J.R.; Natarajan, R.; Donahue, R.P.; Trevisan, M.; Combs, G.F.; Cappuccio, F.P.; Ceriello, A.; Reid, M.E. Effects of long-term selenium supplementation on the incidence of type 2 diabetes: A randomized trial. *Ann. Intern. Med.* **2007**, *147*, 217–223. [CrossRef] [PubMed]
8. Lippman, S.M.; Klein, E.A.; Goodman, P.J.; Lucia, M.S.; Thompson, I.M.; Ford, L.G.; Parnes, H.L.; Minasian, L.M.; Gaziano, J.M.; Hartline, J.A.; et al. Effect of selenium and vitamin e on risk of prostate cancer and other cancers: The selenium and vitamin e cancer prevention trial (select). *JAMA* **2009**, *301*, 39–51. [CrossRef] [PubMed]
9. Gao, H.; Hagg, S.; Sjogren, P.; Lambert, P.C.; Ingelsson, E.; van Dam, R.M. Serum selenium in relation to measures of glucose metabolism and incidence of type 2 diabetes in an older swedish population. *Diabet. Med. A J. Br. Diabet. Assoc.* **2014**, *31*, 787–793. [CrossRef] [PubMed]
10. Wei, J.; Zeng, C.; Gong, Q.Y.; Yang, H.B.; Li, X.X.; Lei, G.H.; Yang, T.B. The association between dietary selenium intake and diabetes: A cross-sectional study among middle-aged and older adults. *Nutr. J.* **2015**, *14*, 18. [CrossRef] [PubMed]
11. Yuan, Z.; Xu, X.; Ye, H.; Jin, L.; Zhang, X.; Zhu, Y. High levels of plasma selenium are associated with metabolic syndrome and elevated fasting plasma glucose in a chinese population: A case-control study. *J. Trace Elem. Med. Biol.* **2015**, *32*, 189–194. [CrossRef] [PubMed]
12. Thompson, P.A.; Ashbeck, E.L.; Roe, D.J.; Fales, L.; Buckmeier, J.; Wang, F.; Bhattacharyya, A.; Hsu, C.H.; Chow, H.H.; Ahnen, D.J.; et al. Selenium supplementation for prevention of colorectal adenomas and risk of associated type 2 diabetes. *J. Natl. Cancer Inst.* **2016**, *108*. [CrossRef] [PubMed]
13. Zhou, J.; Huang, K.; Lei, X.G. Selenium and diabetes-evidence from animal studies. *Free Radic. Biol. Med.* **2013**, *65*, 1548–1556. [CrossRef] [PubMed]
14. Ezaki, O. The insulin-like effects of selenate in rat adipocytes. *J. Biol. Chem.* **1990**, *265*, 1124–1128. [PubMed]
15. Müller, A.S.; Most, E.; Pallauf, J. Effects of a supranutritional dose of selenate compared with selenite on insulin sensitivity in type II diabetic dbdb mice. *J. Anim. Physiol. Anim. Nutr.* **2005**, *89*, 94–104. [CrossRef] [PubMed]
16. Wang, X.L.; Yang, T.B.; Wei, J.; Lei, G.H.; Zeng, C. Association between serum selenium level and type 2 diabetes mellitus: A non-linear dose-response meta-analysis of observational studies. *Nutr. J.* **2016**, *15*, 48. [CrossRef] [PubMed]
17. Steinbrenner, H. Interference of selenium and selenoproteins with the insulin-regulated carbohydrate and lipid metabolism. *Free Radic. Biol. Med.* **2013**, *65*, 1538–1547. [CrossRef] [PubMed]
18. Lenzen, S.; Drinkgern, J.; Tiedge, M. Low antioxidant enzyme gene expression in pancreatic islets compared with various other mouse tissues. *Free Radic. Biol. Med.* **1996**, *20*, 463–466. [CrossRef]
19. McClung, J.P.; Roneker, C.A.; Mu, W.; Lisk, D.J.; Langlais, P.; Liu, F.; Lei, X.G. Development of insulin resistance and obesity in mice overexpressing cellular glutathione peroxidase. *Proc. Natl. Acad. Sci. USA* **2004**, *101*, 8852–8857. [CrossRef] [PubMed]
20. Misu, H.; Takamura, T.; Takayama, H.; Hayashi, H.; Matsuzawa-Nagata, N.; Kurita, S.; Ishikura, K.; Ando, H.; Takeshita, Y.; Ota, T.; et al. A liver-derived secretory protein, selenoprotein p, causes insulin resistance. *Cell Metab.* **2010**, *12*, 483–495. [CrossRef] [PubMed]
21. Misu, H.; Ishikura, K.; Kurita, S.; Takeshita, Y.; Ota, T.; Saito, Y.; Takahashi, K.; Kaneko, S.; Takamura, T. Inverse correlation between serum levels of selenoprotein p and adiponectin in patients with type 2 diabetes. *PLoS ONE* **2012**, *7*, e34952. [CrossRef] [PubMed]
22. Jablonska, E.; Raimondi, S.; Gromadzinska, J.; Reszka, E.; Wieczorek, E.; Krol, M.B.; Smok-Pieniazek, A.; Nocun, M.; Stepnik, M.; Socha, K.; et al. DNA damage and oxidative stress response to selenium yeast in the non-smoking individuals: A short-term supplementation trial with respect to gpx1 and sepp1 polymorphism. *Eur. J. Nutr.* **2015**, *55*, 2469–2484. [CrossRef] [PubMed]
23. Asemi, Z.; Jamilian, M.; Mesdaghinia, E.; Esmaillzadeh, A. Effects of selenium supplementation on glucose homeostasis, inflammation, and oxidative stress in gestational diabetes: Randomized, double-blind, placebo-controlled trial. *Nutrition* **2015**, *31*, 1235–1242. [CrossRef] [PubMed]
24. Jamilian, M.; Razavi, M.; Fakhrie Kashan, Z.; Ghandi, Y.; Bagherian, T.; Asemi, Z. Metabolic response to selenium supplementation in women with polycystic ovary syndrome: A randomized, double-blind, placebo-controlled trial. *Clin. Endocrinol. (Oxf.)* **2015**, *82*, 885–891. [CrossRef] [PubMed]

25. Alizadeh, M.; Safaeiyan, A.; Ostadrahimi, A.; Estakhri, R.; Daneghian, S.; Ghaffari, A.; Gargari, B.P. Effect of L-arginine and selenium added to a hypocaloric diet enriched with legumes on cardiovascular disease risk factors in women with central obesity: A randomized, double-blind, placebo-controlled trial. *Ann. Nutr. Metab.* **2012**, *60*, 157–168. [CrossRef] [PubMed]
26. Farrokhian, A.; Bahmani, F.; Taghizadeh, M.; Mirhashemi, S.M.; Aarabi, M.H.; Raygan, F.; Aghadavod, E.; Asemi, Z. Selenium supplementation affects insulin resistance and serum hs-crp in patients with type 2 diabetes and coronary heart disease. *Horm. Metab. Res.* **2016**, *48*, 263–268. [CrossRef] [PubMed]
27. Faghihi, T.; Radfar, M.; Barmal, M.; Amini, P.; Qorbani, M.; Abdollahi, M.; Larijani, B. A randomized, placebo-controlled trial of selenium supplementation in patients with type 2 diabetes: Effects on glucose homeostasis, oxidative stress, and lipid profile. *Am. J. Ther.* **2014**, *21*, 491–495. [CrossRef] [PubMed]
28. Algotar, A.M.; Stratton, M.S.; Stratton, S.P.; Hsu, C.H.; Ahmann, F.R. No effect of selenium supplementation on serum glucose levels in men with prostate cancer. *Am. J. Med.* **2010**, *123*, 765–768. [CrossRef] [PubMed]
29. Czernichow, S.; Couthouis, A.; Bertrais, S.; Vergnaud, A.C.; Dauchet, L.; Galan, P.; Hercberg, S. Antioxidant supplementation does not affect fasting plasma glucose in the supplementation with antioxidant vitamins and minerals (Su.Vi.Max) study in France: Association with dietary intake and plasma concentrations. *Am. J. Clin. Nutr.* **2006**, *84*, 395–399. [PubMed]
30. Wang, X.; Wu, H.; Long, Z.; Sun, Q.; Liu, J.; Liu, Y.; Hai, C. Differential effect of Se on insulin resistance: Regulation of adipogenesis and lipolysis. *Mol. Cell Biochem.* **2016**, *415*, 89–102. [CrossRef] [PubMed]
31. Zeng, M.-S.; Li, X.; Liu, Y.; Zhao, H.; Zhou, J.-C.; Li, K.; Huang, J.-Q.; Sun, L.-H.; Tang, J.-Y.; Xia, X.-J.; et al. A high-selenium diet induces insulin resistance in gestating rats and their offspring. *Free Radic. Biol. Med.* **2012**, *52*, 1335–1342. [CrossRef] [PubMed]
32. Zhao, Z.; Barcus, M.; Kim, J.; Lum, K.L.; Mills, C.; Lei, X.G. High dietary selenium intake alters lipid metabolism and protein synthesis in liver and muscle of pigs. *J. Nutr.* **2016**, *146*, 1625–1633. [CrossRef] [PubMed]
33. Pinto, A.; Juniper, D.T.; Sanil, M.; Morgan, L.; Clark, L.; Sies, H.; Rayman, M.P.; Steinbrenner, H. Supranutritional selenium induces alterations in molecular targets related to energy metabolism in skeletal muscle and visceral adipose tissue of pigs. *J. Inorg. Biochem.* **2012**, *114*, 47–54. [CrossRef] [PubMed]
34. Freitas Lima, L.C.; Braga, V.A.; do Socorro de Franca Silva, M.; Cruz, J.C.; Sousa Santos, S.H.; de Oliveira Monteiro, M.M.; Balarini, C.M. Adipokines, diabetes and atherosclerosis: An inflammatory association. *Front. Physiol.* **2015**, *6*, 304. [CrossRef] [PubMed]
35. Rayman, M.P.; Blundell-Pound, G.; Pastor-Barriuso, R.; Guallar, E.; Steinbrenner, H.; Stranges, S. A randomized trial of selenium supplementation and risk of type-2 diabetes, as assessed by plasma adiponectin. *PLoS ONE* **2012**, *7*, e45269. [CrossRef] [PubMed]
36. Mao, J.; Bath, S.C.; Vanderlelie, J.J.; Perkins, A.V.; Redman, C.W.; Rayman, M.P. No effect of modest selenium supplementation on insulin resistance in UK pregnant women, as assessed by plasma adiponectin concentration. *Br. J. Nutr.* **2016**, *115*, 32–38. [CrossRef] [PubMed]
37. Kadowaki, T.; Yamauchi, T.; Kubota, N.; Hara, K.; Ueki, K.; Tobe, K. Adiponectin and adiponectin receptors in insulin resistance, diabetes, and the metabolic syndrome. *J. Clin. Investig.* **2006**, *116*, 1784–1792. [CrossRef] [PubMed]
38. Foti, D.; Chiefari, E.; Fedele, M.; Iuliano, R.; Brunetti, L.; Paonessa, F.; Manfioletti, G.; Barbetti, F.; Brunetti, A.; Croce, C.M.; et al. Lack of the architectural factor hmga1 causes insulin resistance and diabetes in humans and mice. *Nat. Med.* **2005**, *11*, 765–773. [CrossRef] [PubMed]
39. Boucher, J.; Kleinridders, A.; Kahn, C.R. Insulin receptor signaling in normal and insulin-resistant states. *Cold Spring Harb. Perspect. Biol.* **2014**, *6*, a009191. [CrossRef] [PubMed]
40. Yu, S.X.; Zhang, W.T.; Liu, W.; Zhu, W.X.; Guo, R.C.; Wang, Y.S.; Zhang, D.H.; Wang, J.L. The inhibitory effect of selenium nanoparticles on protein glycation in vitro. *Nanotechnology* **2015**, *26*, 145703. [CrossRef] [PubMed]
41. Luo, X.; Li, R.; Yan, L.J. Roles of pyruvate, NADH, and mitochondrial complex I in redox balance and imbalance in beta cell function and dysfunction. *J. Diabetes Res.* **2015**, *2015*, 512618. [CrossRef] [PubMed]
42. Jeoung, N.H. Pyruvate dehydrogenase kinases: Therapeutic targets for diabetes and cancers. *Diabetes Metab. J.* **2015**, *39*, 188–197. [CrossRef] [PubMed]
43. Guo, X.; Li, H.; Xu, H.; Woo, S.; Dong, H.; Lu, F.; Lange, A.J.; Wu, C. Glycolysis in the control of blood glucose homeostasis. *Acta Pharm. Sin. B* **2012**, *2*, 358–367. [CrossRef]

44. Otton, R.; Mendonca, J.R.; Curi, R. Diabetes causes marked changes in lymphocyte metabolism. *J. Endocrinol.* **2002**, *174*, 55–61. [CrossRef] [PubMed]
45. Seale, L.A.; Gilman, C.L.; Hashimoto, A.C.; Ogawa-Wong, A.N.; Berry, M.J. Diet-induced obesity in the selenocysteine lyase knockout mouse. *Antioxid. Redox Signal.* **2015**, *23*, 761–774. [CrossRef] [PubMed]
46. Bao, P.; Chen, Z.; Tai, R.Z.; Shen, H.M.; Martin, F.L.; Zhu, Y.G. Selenite-induced toxicity in cancer cells is mediated by metabolic generation of endogenous selenium nanoparticles. *J. Proteome Res.* **2015**, *14*, 1127–1136. [CrossRef] [PubMed]
47. Yeung, S.J.; Pan, J.; Lee, M.H. Roles of p53, myc and hif-1 in regulating glycolysis—The seventh hallmark of cancer. *Cell Mol. Life Sci.* **2008**, *65*, 3981–3999. [CrossRef] [PubMed]
48. Sherwani, S.I.; Khan, H.A.; Ekhzaimy, A.; Masood, A.; Sakharkar, M.K. Significance of hba1c test in diagnosis and prognosis of diabetic patients. *Biomark. Insights* **2016**, *11*, 95–104. [PubMed]
49. Hirst, J.A.; Stevens, R.J.; Farmer, A.J. Changes in hba1c level over a 12-week follow-up in patients with type 2 diabetes following a medication change. *PLoS ONE* **2014**, *9*, e92458. [CrossRef] [PubMed]
50. Ogawa-Wong, A.N.; Berry, M.J.; Seale, L.A. Selenium and metabolic disorders: An emphasis on type 2 diabetes risk. *Nutrients* **2016**, *8*, 80. [CrossRef] [PubMed]
51. Hellwege, J.N.; Palmer, N.D.; Ziegler, J.T.; Langefeld, C.D.; Lorenzo, C.; Norris, J.M.; Takamura, T.; Bowden, D.W. Genetic variants in selenoprotein p plasma 1 gene (sepp1) are associated with fasting insulin and first phase insulin response in hispanics. *Gene* **2014**, *534*, 33–39. [CrossRef] [PubMed]
52. Mueller, A.S.; Pallauf, J.; Rafael, J. The chemical form of selenium affects insulinomimetic properties of the trace element: Investigations in type ii diabetic dbdb mice. *J. Nutr. Biochem.* **2003**, *14*, 637–647. [CrossRef] [PubMed]
53. Kiersztan, A.; Lukasinska, I.; Baranska, A.; Lebiedzinska, M.; Nagalski, A.; Derlacz, R.A.; Bryla, J. Differential effects of selenium compounds on glucose synthesis in rabbit kidney-cortex tubules and hepatocytes. In vitro and in vivo studies. *J. Inorg. Biochem.* **2007**, *101*, 493–505. [CrossRef] [PubMed]

13

Dietary Patterns Related to Triglyceride and High-Density Lipoprotein Cholesterol and the Incidence of Type 2 Diabetes in Korean Men and Women

Sihan Song [1] and Jung Eun Lee [1,2,*]

[1] Department of Food and Nutrition, College of Human Ecology, Seoul National University, 1 Gwanak-ro, Gwanak-gu, Seoul 08826, Korea; songsihan@snu.ac.kr

[2] Research Institute of Human Ecology, Seoul National University, 1 Gwanak-ro, Gwanak-gu, Seoul 08826, Korea

* Correspondence: jungelee@snu.ac.kr

Abstract: We aimed to examine whether dietary patterns that explain the variation of triglyceride (TG) to high-density lipoprotein cholesterol (HDL-C) ratio were associated with the incidence of type 2 diabetes in Korean adults. We included a total of 5097 adults without diabetes at baseline with a mean follow-up of 11.54 years. Usual diet was assessed by a validated food frequency questionnaire, and serum levels of TG and HDL-C were measured at baseline. We derived dietary pattern scores using 41 food groups as predictors and the TG/HDL-C ratio as a response variable in a stepwise linear regression. We calculated the odds ratio (OR) with the 95% confidence interval (CI) of type 2 diabetes according to pattern scores using multivariate logistic regression. A total of 1069 incident cases of type 2 diabetes were identified. A list of foods characterizing the dietary pattern differed by sex. Higher dietary pattern scores were associated with an increased risk of type 2 diabetes; ORs (95% CIs) comparing extreme quintiles were 1.53 (1.12–2.09; p for trend = 0.008) for men and 1.33 (0.95–1.86; p for trend = 0.011) for women. Our study suggests the evidence that dietary patterns associated with low levels of TG/HDL-C ratio may have the potential to reduce the burden of type 2 diabetes.

Keywords: dietary pattern; triglyceride; high-density lipoprotein cholesterol; type 2 diabetes

1. Introduction

The estimated global prevalence of diabetes mellitus has increased about 50% over the last decade, increased from 5.9% in 2007 to 8.8% in 2017 according to the International Diabetes Foundation [1,2] Over 90% of diabetes cases are of type 2 [2], and the rapid increase is largely attributed to changes in lifestyle factors, such as being overweight or obese, physical inactivity, unhealthy diet, and smoking [3,4]. To reduce the burden of diabetes and its complications, the early detection and treatment of diabetes and evidence-based guideline for diabetes prevention or management are important [5]. The World Health Organization (WHO) and the Food and Agriculture Organization (FAO) provide dietary recommendations for type 2 diabetes prevention, which include limiting saturated fat and obtaining an adequate fiber intake [6]. In addition, WHO recommends reducing the free sugar intake to prevent non-communicable diseases (NCDs), including type 2 diabetes [7].

Because nutrients and foods are consumed in combination, dietary pattern analysis can provide more practical evidence than single-nutrient analysis [8,9]. In addition, the consumption of dietary factors associated with the risk of type 2 diabetes may correlate with each other; therefore, dietary pattern analysis that reflects the complexity of diets may provide scientific insight and practical strategies for disease prevention. Approaches to assess the effects of dietary patterns on the risk of diabetes have been implemented in epidemiologic studies [10,11]. Several previous studies have found significant associations between the risk of type 2 diabetes and posteriori-derived dietary patterns that explain the variation in diabetes-related biomarkers, such as blood glucose, lipids, or inflammatory markers [12–21].

Insulin resistance, a phenomenon involving the resistance to insulin-stimulated glucose uptake, is involved in the pathogenesis of type 2 diabetes, hypertension, and coronary heart disease [22,23]. Indices derived from fasting glucose and insulin including homoeostasis model assessment-insulin resistance (HOMA-IR) and quantitative insulin-sensitivity check index (QUICKI) are widely used to quantify insulin resistance [24]. In addition, the triglyceride (TG) to high-density lipoprotein cholesterol (HDL-C) ratio has been suggested as a simple measure of insulin resistance [25–28]. Vega et al. [29] found that a high TG/HDL-C ratio was associated with an increased risk of type 2 diabetes and cardiovascular disease (CVD) mortality among men participating in the Cooper Center Longitudinal Study (CCLS). In the Korean population, the TG/HDL-C ratio was also significantly associated with insulin resistance [30,31], and the risk of type 2 diabetes [32].

The aim of our study was to identify posteriori-dietary patterns that explain variation in the TG/HDL-C ratio and to examine their association with the risk of type 2 diabetes in Korean adults. Given the sex-differences in TG and HDL-C levels [33] and dietary behavior [34], we identified the dietary patterns among men and women separately.

2. Materials and Methods

2.1. Study Population

The Ansan and Ansung study is part of the Korean Genome and Epidemiology Study (KoGES), which was designed to prospectively investigate the genetic and environmental influences on chronic disease in Korean adults [35]. The Ansan and Ansung study included 10,030 adults (4758 men and 5272 women) aged 40–69 years from the general population of urban (Ansan) and rural (Ansung) areas in 2001–2002. Clinical examination and interviewer-administered questionnaires were conducted at baseline and at biennial follow up. The follow-up rate was 62.8% at the 6th follow-up in 2013–2014 from baseline [35]. All participants provided informed consent. This study was approved by the Seoul National University Institutional Review Board (IRB No. E1811/001-009).

Of 10,030 participants at baseline, we excluded participants who had been diagnosed with or treated for diabetes (n = 683), cancer (n = 247), CVD (n = 408) or had missing data on relevant information (n = 7); those who had used insulin treatment (n = 93), an oral hypoglycemic drug (n = 360) or stroke medication (n = 21). We further excluded participants who did not have baseline fasting plasma glucose, 2-h plasma glucose after a 75 g oral glucose tolerance test (OGTT), or hemoglobin A1c (HbA1c) measurements (n = 67) as well as undiagnosed diabetes cases who met the American Diabetes Association (ADA) criteria for the diagnosis of diabetes (n = 692). We also excluded participants who did not have serum TG or HDL measurements (n = 1) or had outlier values for TG or HDL-C levels as determined by a box-plot method (greater than 3*interquartile range; n = 4).

KoGES provided food frequency questionnaires (FFQs) data after excluding individuals who: 1) did not answer any questions on the FFQs, 2) left more than 12 blanks for frequency questions, 3) did not answer any questions about rice intake, or 4) had extremely low (<100 kcal/day) or high (≥10,000 kcal/day) energy intake [36], resulting in exclusion of 255 participants. Furthermore, we excluded individuals who reported implausible energy intake (<500 or >3500 kcal/day for women and <800 or >4200 kcal/day for men; n = 230) or did not have data on alcohol consumption (n = 247). Among those participants who met the inclusion criteria at baseline (n = 7338), we excluded those who were not followed at the 5th (2011–2012) or 6th (2013–2014) follow up (n = 2228) as well as for those whose information on the ascertainment of type 2 diabetes during the follow-up (n = 754) was not available. As a result, a total of 5097 participants (2410 men and 2687 women) were included in the current study. Flow diagram of inclusion for study participants is presented in Figure S1.

2.2. Dietary Assessment

Usual dietary intake was assessed using an interviewer-administered semi-quantitative 103 item FFQ at baseline. The questionnaire was previously validated using 12-day dietary records among 124 participants of KoGES; Pearson's correlation coefficients for energy-adjusted nutrient intakes ranged from 0.23 (vitamin A) to 0.64 (carbohydrate) [37]. Daily energy and nutrient intake were estimated based on the seventh edition of the Food Composition Tables of the Korean Nutrition Society [38]. Participants were asked to report the frequency and portion size of each food item during the previous year. Nine frequency categories ranging from "never or seldom" to "three times or more a day" and three portion sizes (small, medium, or large) were given as options. Alcoholic beverage consumption was assessed separately at baseline and at each biennial follow up. Alcohol drinking status was defined as nondrinker, past drinker, or current drinker. Current alcohol drinkers were asked to report the amount and frequency of alcohol beverage consumption in the previous month, and total alcohol consumption (g/day) was calculated based on the alcohol content of one standard drink.

2.3. Ascertainment of Type 2 Diabetes and Biomarker Assessment

A diagnostic test for diabetes and interviewer-administered questionnaires on diabetes diagnosis or treatment were repeated at biennial follow up. We defined incident type 2 diabetes cases as those who had: 1) a diagnosis of diabetes according to the ADA criteria including HbA1c $\geq$ 6.5% or fasting plasma glucose $\geq$ 126 mg/dl or 2-h plasma glucose $\geq$ 200 mg/dl after a 75 g OGTT [39]; or 2) a diagnosis of type 2 diabetes by physicians or treatment with insulin or oral hypoglycemic medication. Participants who developed type 2 diabetes after baseline were classified as diabetes cases and were otherwise categorized as non-cases.

Blood samples were collected after an overnight fast (at least 8 h) at baseline and at each biennial follow-up examination. Fasting plasma glucose, 1-h and 2-h plasma glucose after a 75 g OGTT were measured enzymatically using an automatic analyzer (ADIVA 1650; Siemens, USA). Whole blood HbA1c level was measured by high-performance liquid chromatography (BIO-RAD Variant II—Turbo; BIORAD, Japan). Serum TG and HDL-C were measured enzymatically using an automatic analyzer (ADIVA 1650; Siemens, USA). The TG/HDL-C ratio was calculated as the ratio of TG to HDL-C.

2.4. Covariate Assessment

Trained interviewers administered a questionnaire regarding sociodemographic factors, lifestyle factors, disease history or current treatment, medication history, family disease history, and reproductive factors. Smoking status was categorized into nonsmoker, past smoker, or current smoker. Pack-years of smoking were calculated using detailed information on smoking history among past or current smokers. When information regarding age at menopause was missing (n = 326), we considered the participant postmenopausal if they had been diagnosed after the age of 50, which was the median age of menopause in Korean postmenopausal women aged 40–69 years in 2001 [40]. Participants were asked to report: 1) the hours per day spent on four-intensity physical activity levels (sedentary, light, moderate, and vigorous activity) and 2) the frequency of leisure time spent on physical activity per week and the hours spent on each activity (aerobic, jogging, walking, swimming, tennis, golf, bowling, health club exercise, and mountain climbing). Physical activity was expressed as metabolic equivalents (METs) hours per week by multiplying the hours per week engaged in that activity by the activity's corresponding MET value [41,42]. Anthropometric factors of body weight, height, waist circumference, hip circumference, and blood pressure were obtained by trained examiners. Body mass index (BMI) was calculated as weight (kg) divided by height-squared (m^2).

2.5. Statistical Analysis

We derived dietary patterns that explained the variation in TG/HDL-C ratio using reduced rank regression (RRR) [43]. RRR is a posteriori method used to derive linear combinations of predictor variables (food groups) that explain as much as possible of the variation of response variables (disease-related markers) [43]. When using only one response variable, RRR is identical to multiple linear regression [12,44].

When we derived the dietary patterns of the participants at baseline, we included participants who had never been diagnosed with dyslipidemia and used hyperlipidemia drugs, and participants who had normal HbA1c and plasma glucose levels according to the ADA criteria to avoid the effect of these symptoms on their diet. As a result, 3630 participants (1716 men and 1914 women) were included in the study to derive dietary patterns.

We grouped 103 food items from FFQ and alcohol consumption into 41 groups (g/day) on the basis of similarities in food composition or nutrient content, and these were used as predictor variables to derive dietary patterns. As a response variable, the TG/HDL-C ratio was log-transformed for normality and adjusted for age using a residual method. We then derived dietary patterns that explained as much as possible of the variation of age-adjusted TG/HDL-C using a stepwise linear regression model in men and women separately. A significance level of 0.05 was used for entry and retention in the model. We calculated dietary pattern scores by summing the intakes of selected food groups that were weighted by the regression coefficients for all the study participants.

We used Spearman's correlation coefficients to assess the correlations of dietary pattern and selected foods with the TG/HDL-C ratio. We divided the study participants according to the quintiles of dietary pattern scores and identified the intakes of selected food groups as well as demographic, lifestyle, and clinical characteristics. We used multivariate logistic regression models to calculate the odds ratio (OR) and 95% confidence interval (CI) of type 2 diabetes in each quintile of dietary pattern scores using the lowest quintile as the reference group. In multivariate models, we adjusted for age (continuous, years), living area (Ansan and Ansung), energy intake (continuous, kcal/day), menopausal status (pre and postmenopausal status for women), smoking status (0, >0 and <15, 15–<30, and 30≤ pack-years for men; ever and never smoking for women), alcohol consumption (0, >0 and <5, 5–<15, 15–<30, and 30≤ g/day for men; ever and never drinking for women), family history of diabetes (yes, no), chronic disease status at baseline (yes, no; diagnosis or use of medication for hypertension or hyperlipidemia), and physical activity (continuous, METs-hours/week). We further adjusted for BMI (kg/m^2), which may be an intermediate factor in the causal pathway between dietary patterns related to TG/HDL-C ratio and the risk of type 2 diabetes. We calculated the p value for the trend across quintiles by assigning the median value of each quintile to corresponding participants and treating this value as a continuous variable in the model. We tested for effect modification by age, menopausal status, and BMI at baseline by performing stratified analyses and the likelihood ratio test (LRT) for each variable. We also conducted a sensitivity analysis by excluding incident cases of type 2 diabetes during 2 years of follow up when we examined the association between dietary pattern scores and the risk of type 2 diabetes. All statistical analyses were performed using SAS statistical software version 9.4 (SAS Institute Inc., Cary, NC). All hypothesis tests were evaluated using two-tailed tests of significance at $p < 0.05$.

3. Results

When we derived dietary patterns associated with TG/HDL-C ratio, the list of selected food items differed by sex (Table 1). A high dietary pattern score was characterized in men by higher intakes of noodles, fruits, fermented salted seafood and lower intakes of candy and chocolate, nuts, and pork, whereas that in women was characterized by higher intakes of organ and other meats and lower intakes of dairy products and nuts. The calculated dietary pattern scores were positively associated with TG/HDL-C ratio; the Spearman's correlation coefficients were 0.15 for men and 0.13 for women.

Table 1. Spearman correlation coefficients between dietary pattern scores, selected foods, and the TG/HDL-C ratio, and the mean intake of selected food groups (g/day) according to the quintile of dietary pattern scores.

	Spearman's Correlation with Dietary Pattern Scores		Quintile of TG/HDL-C Ratio-Related Dietary Pattern Scores		
	Dietary Pattern Scores	TG/HDL-C Ratio	Quintile1	Quintile3	Quintile5
Men (n = 2410)					
Diet pattern scores	1.00	0.15 [a]			
Positive associations				Mean ± SD	
Noodles	0.37 [a]	0.07 [a]	63.24 ± 54.12	68.18 ± 47.97	152.57 ± 120.93
Fruits	0.33 [a]	0.03	156.68 ± 150.35	154.63 ± 145.63	426.23 ± 382.61
Fermented salted seafood	0.23 [a]	0.03	1.26 ± 2.66	0.88 ± 1.58	4.91 ± 8.12
Inverse associations					
Candy and chocolate	−0.30 [a]	−0.06 [a]	5.02 ± 8.62	0.68 ± 1.42	0.69 ± 1.90
Nuts	−0.29 [a]	−0.06 [a]	2.46 ± 4.40	0.39 ± 1.02	0.36 ± 1.08
Pork	−0.26 [a]	−0.03	69.70 ± 55.90	32.44 ± 29.14	37.11 ± 34.88
Women (n = 2687)					
Diet pattern scores	1.00	0.13 [a]			
Positive associations				Mean ± SD	
Organ and other meats	0.10 [a]	−0.01	0.94 ± 3.11	0.97 ± 2.44	3.62 ± 16.72
Inverse associations					
Dairy products	−0.88 [a]	−0.12 [a]	292.40 ± 173.30	75.75 ± 40.48	9.51 ± 32.10
Nuts	−0.42 [a]	−0.09 [a]	2.50 ± 5.02	0.33 ± 0.57	0.04 ± 0.17

Abbreviations: TG, triglyceride; HDL-C, high-density lipoprotein cholesterol. [a] Spearman's correlation coefficient was statistically significant ($p < 0.05$).

The baseline characteristics of men and women are presented in Table 2 according to the quintiles of sex-specific dietary pattern associated with TG/HDL-C ratio. Men who had higher dietary pattern scores were more likely to live in a rural area, have a higher energy intake, and be a current smoker. Women who had higher dietary pattern scores were more likely to be older and postmenopausal, live in a rural area, and have a lower energy intake and physical activity. Participants who had higher dietary pattern scores were more likely to have a higher TG/HDL-C ratio, higher TG levels and lower HDL-C levels than those who had lower dietary pattern scores.

Table 2. Baseline characteristics of the study participants according to the quintiles for TG/HDL-C ratio-related dietary pattern scores.

	Quintile of TG/HDL-C Ratio-Related Dietary Pattern Scores		
	Quintile1	Quintile3	Quintile5
Men (n = 2410)	482	482	482
Age (years), mean ± SD	50.38 ± 8.08	50.50 ± 7.99	51.10 ± 8.19
Residential area, n (%)			
Rural (Ansung)	148 (30.71)	209 (43.36)	260 (53.94)
Urban (Ansan)	334 (69.29)	273 (56.64)	222 (46.06)
Energy intake (kcal/day), mean ± SD	2095.97 ± 527.68	1802.31 ± 437.21	2289.32 ± 603.02
BMI (kg/m^2), mean ± SD [a]	24.02 ± 2.88	24.27 ± 2.77	24.37 ± 2.90
Physical activity (METs h/week), mean ± SD	9.65 ± 14.83	8.06 ± 12.29	8.76 ± 12.05
Smoking status, n (%) [a]			
Non-smoker	116 (24.07)	97 (20.12)	99 (20.54)
Past smoker	175 (36.31)	165 (34.23)	130 (26.97)
Current smoker	191 (39.63)	220 (45.64)	253 (52.49)
Alcohol consumption status, n (%)			
Non-drinker	94 (19.50)	101 (20.95)	80 (16.60)
Past drinker	48 (9.96)	32 (6.64)	51 (10.58)
Current drinker	340 (70.54)	349 (72.41)	351 (72.82)
Family history of diabetes, n (%)			
No	434 (90.04)	433 (89.83)	437 (90.66)
Yes	48 (9.96)	49 (10.17)	45 (9.34)
TG/HDL-C ratio, mean ± SD	3.66 ± 2.79	4.14 ± 2.95	4.97 ± 4.06
TG (mg/dL), mean ± SD	150.52 ± 92.96	166.22 ± 92.86	191.56 ± 123.95
HDL-C (mg/dL), mean ± SD	44.88 ± 9.96	43.69 ± 9.27	42.73 ± 10.10

Table 2. *Cont.*

	Quintile of TG/HDL-C Ratio-Related Dietary Pattern Scores		
	Quintile1	Quintile3	Quintile5
Women (n = 2687)	538	531	512
Age (years), mean ± SD	50.02 ± 8.06	50.24 ± 8.26	54.41 ± 8.97
Menopausal status, n (%) [a]			
Pre-menopause	243 (52.83)	263 (55.96)	165 (35.71)
Post-menopause	217 (47.17)	207 (44.04)	297 (64.29)
Residential area, n (%)			
Rural (Ansung)	199 (36.99)	236 (44.44)	358 (69.92)
Urban (Ansan)	339 (63.01)	295 (55.56)	154 (30.08)
Energy intake (kcal/day), mean ± SD	2081.36 ± 513.71	1818.15 ± 480.73	1679.94 ± 517.76
BMI (kg/m^2), mean ± SD [a]	24.21 ± 2.97	24.72 ± 2.97	25.13 ± 3.23
Physical activity (METs h/week), mean ± SD	11.72 ± 16.47	9.46 ± 14.56	6.69 ± 10.16
Smoking status, n (%) [a]			
Non-smoker	510 (96.05)	511 (96.78)	481 (95.06)
Past smoker	4 (0.75)	5 (0.95)	10 (1.98)
Current smoker	17 (3.20)	12 (2.27)	15 (2.96)
Alcohol consumption status, n (%)			
Non-drinker	368 (68.40)	378 (71.19)	371 (72.46)
Past drinker	10 (1.86)	14 (2.64)	18 (3.52)
Current drinker	160 (29.74)	139 (26.18)	123 (24.02)
Family history of diabetes, n (%)			
No	467 (86.80)	469 (88.32)	461 (90.04)
Yes	71 (13.20)	62 (11.68)	51 (9.96)
TG/HDL-C ratio, mean ± SD	3.08 ± 2.24	3.27 ± 2.64	3.74 ± 2.59
TG (mg/dL), mean ± SD	133.63 ± 74.45	136.19 ± 81.17	153.49 ± 82.92
HDL-C (mg/dL), mean ± SD	47.72 ± 10.1	45.59 ± 9.76	45.11 ± 9.95

Abbreviations: BMI, body mass index; METs, metabolic equivalents; TG, triglyceride; HDL-C, high-density lipoprotein cholesterol. [a] Some participants did not provide relevant information (among men, 1 missing for BMI; and among women, 326 missing for menopausal status and 27 missing for smoking status).

A total of 1069 (560 men and 509 women) cases of type 2 diabetes were identified over a mean follow up of 11.54 years. Multivariate adjusted OR (95% CIs) comparing extreme quintiles was 1.53 (1.12–2.09; p for trend = 0.008) among men and 1.33 (0.95–1.86; p for trend = 0.011) among women (Table 3). For women, OR (95% CI) comparing the 3rd versus the 1st quintile was 1.45 (1.06–1.99). After further adjustment for BMI, the association was slightly attenuated in both men and women. We examined whether the associations between dietary pattern scores and incident type 2 diabetes varied by age (≤median, >median), menopausal status, and BMI (<25, ≥25 kg/m^2) at baseline regarding the risk of type 2 diabetes (Table 4). The associations appeared to be stronger among older or postmenopausal women than among younger or premenopausal women; the ORs (95% CI) comparing the extreme quintiles were 1.10 (0.65–1.86) for younger women and 1.61 (1.03–2.54) for older women. For BMI, the association appeared to be stronger among men with lower BMI than among those with higher BMI; the ORs (95% CI) comparing the extreme quintiles were 1.82 (1.19–2.80) for men with lower BMI and 1.17 (0.74–1.85) for men with higher BMI. However, there were no significant interactions by these factors.

In the sensitivity analysis, we excluded incident cases that were identified during 2 years of follow-up (n = 193), and the estimates of the association between the dietary pattern scores and the incidence of type 2 diabetes were similar to those found in the main analysis (Table S1).

Table 3. Odds ratios (ORs) and 95% confidence intervals (CIs) of incident type 2 diabetes according to the quintiles of TG/HDL-C ratio-related dietary pattern scores.

	Quintiles of TG/HDL-C Ratio-Related Dietary Pattern Scores					*p* for Trend
	Quintile1	Quintile2	Quintile3	Quintile4	Quintile5	
Men (*n* = 2410)						
Case/non-case	99/383	110/372	106/376	112/370	133/349	
Unadjusted model	Reference	1.14 (0.84–1.56)	1.09 (0.80–1.49)	1.17 (0.86–1.59)	1.47 (1.10–1.99)	0.010
Age-adjusted model	Reference	1.15 (0.85–1.57)	1.09 (0.80–1.48)	1.17 (0.86–1.60)	1.46 (1.08–1.97)	0.013
Multivariate adjusted model1 [a]	Reference	1.17 (0.85–1.61)	1.12 (0.81–1.54)	1.19 (0.87–1.63)	1.53 (1.12–2.09)	0.008
Multivariate adjusted model2 [b]	Reference	1.16 (0.84–1.59)	1.08 (0.78–1.49)	1.12 (0.82–1.53)	1.48 (1.09–2.03)	0.019
Women (*n* = 2687)						
Case/non-case	89/449	76/461	118/413	114/455	112/400	
Unadjusted model	Reference	0.83 (0.60–1.16)	1.44 (1.06–1.96)	1.26 (0.93–1.72)	1.41 (1.04–1.92)	0.002
Age-adjusted model	Reference	0.83 (0.59–1.15)	1.44 (1.06–1.95)	1.20 (0.88–1.64)	1.27 (0.93–1.74)	0.014
Multivariate adjusted model1 [c]	Reference	0.83 (0.59–1.16)	1.45 (1.06–1.99)	1.23 (0.88–1.71)	1.33 (0.95–1.86)	0.011
Multivariate adjusted model2 [b]	Reference	0.80 (0.57–1.13)	1.37 (1.00–1.89)	1.14 (0.81–1.59)	1.21 (0.86–1.70)	0.053

Abbreviations: TG, triglyceride; HDL-C, high-density lipoprotein cholesterol. [a] Adjusted for age (continuous, years), living area (Ansan and Ansung), energy intake (continuous, kcal/day), pack-years of smoking (0, >0 and <15, 15–<30, and 30≤ pack-years), alcohol consumption (0, >0 and <5, 5–<15, 15–<30, and 30≤ g/day), family history of diabetes (yes, no), hypertension or hyperlipidemia at baseline (yes, no), and physical activity (continuous, metabolic equivalents-hours/week). [b] Further adjusted for body mass index (continuous, kg/m^2) in addition to the variables included in Model 1. [c] Adjusted for age (years), living area (Ansan and Ansung), energy intake (continuous, kcal/day), menopausal status (pre and postmenopausal status), smoking status (ever and never), alcohol consumption (ever and never), family history of diabetes (yes, no), hypertension or hyperlipidemia at baseline (yes, no), and physical activity (continuous, metabolic equivalents-hours/week).

Table 4. Odds ratios (ORs) and 95% confidence intervals (CIs) of incident type 2 diabetes according to the quintiles of dietary pattern scores by age, menopausal status, and BMI at baseline.

	Quintiles of TG/HDL-C Ratio-Related Dietary Pattern Scores						
	Quintile1	Quintile2	Quintile3	Quintile4	Quintile5	*p* for Trend	*p* for Interaction
Men [a]							
≤48 years, median (n = 1229)	Reference	1.26 (0.80–1.98)	1.02 (0.63–1.64)	1.12 (0.71–1.77)	1.65 (1.05–2.61)	0.052	0.788
>48 years (n = 1181)	Reference	1.09 (0.70–1.70)	1.21 (0.79–1.88)	1.26 (0.82–1.94)	1.46 (0.96–2.23)	0.063	
Women [b]							
≤49 years, median (n = 1376)	Reference	0.73 (0.45–1.18)	1.20 (0.76–1.90)	1.02 (0.63–1.66)	1.10 (0.65–1.86)	0.407	0.319
>49 years (n = 1311)	Reference	0.90 (0.55–1.46)	1.75 (1.12–2.73)	1.49 (0.94–2.38)	1.61 (1.03–2.54)	0.004	
Menopausal-status at baseline [c]							
Pre-menopause (n = 1143)	Reference	0.83 (0.49–1.41)	1.47 (0.90–2.41)	1.17 (0.68–2.01)	1.15 (0.64–2.07)	0.236	0.324
Post-menopause (n = 1218)	Reference	0.84 (0.50–1.41)	1.57 (0.97–2.55)	1.43 (0.87–2.33)	1.55 (0.96–2.50)	0.013	
Men [a]							
<25 kg/m^2 (n = 1441)	Reference	1.20 (0.78–1.85)	1.21 (0.78–1.89)	1.20 (0.76–1.89)	1.82 (1.19–2.80)	0.007	0.238
≥25 kg/m^2 (n = 968)	Reference	1.12 (0.69–1.80)	0.92 (0.57–1.50)	0.98 (0.63–1.53)	1.17 (0.74–1.85)	0.593	
Women [b]							
<25 kg/m^2 (n = 1543)	Reference	0.63 (0.38–1.05)	1.53 (0.98–2.39)	1.04 (0.64–1.69)	1.17 (0.71–1.93)	0.138	0.625
≥25 kg/m^2 (n = 1144)	Reference	1.00 (0.62–1.61)	1.31 (0.83–2.07)	1.31 (0.82–2.08)	1.29 (0.81–2.05)	0.133	

Abbreviations: TG, triglyceride; HDL-C, high-density lipoprotein cholesterol; BMI, body mass index. [a] Adjusted for age (continuous, years), living area (Ansan and Ansung), energy intake (continuous, kcal/day), pack-years of smoking (0, >0 and <15, 15–<30, and 30≤ pack-years), alcohol consumption (0, >0 and <5, 5–<15, 15–<30, and 30≤ g/day), family history of diabetes (yes, no), hypertension or hyperlipidemia at baseline (yes, no), and physical activity (continuous, metabolic equivalents-hours/week). [b] Adjusted for age (continuous, years), living area (Ansan and Ansung), energy intake (continuous, kcal/day), menopausal status (pre and postmenopausal status), smoking status (ever and never), alcohol consumption status (ever and never), family history of diabetes (yes, no), hypertension or hyperlipidemia at baseline (yes, no), and physical activity (continuous, metabolic equivalents-hours/week). [c] Adjusted for age (years), living area (Ansan and Ansung), energy intake (kcal/day), smoking status (ever and never), alcohol consumption status (ever and never), family history of diabetes (yes, no), hypertension or hyperlipidemia at baseline (yes, no), and physical activity (continuous, metabolic equivalents-hours/week).

4. Discussion

We derived dietary patterns that explain the variation in the diabetes-related biomarker, the TG/HDL-C ratio, in men and women separately. The dietary pattern was characterized by high intakes of noodles, fruits, fermented salted seafood and low intakes of candy and chocolate, nuts, and pork among men and by high intakes of organ and other meats and low intakes of dairy products and nuts among women. Dietary pattern scores were positively associated with the TG/HDL-C ratio. High dietary pattern score was associated with an increased risk of type 2 diabetes. The associations appeared to be stronger among older or postmenopausal women, albeit without statistical significance.

Insulin resistance is a major risk factor for the development of type 2 diabetes [22,23, 45]. The consequences of insulin resistance and its compensatory hyperinsulinemia include glucose intolerance, dyslipidemia (increased TG and/or decreased HDL-C), high blood pressure, hyperuricemia, and increased plasminogen activator inhibitor (PAI)-1 activity [23]. Several studies have examined the association between risk of type 2 diabetes and dietary patterns that explain the variation of biomarkers that are linked to diabetes [12–21]. Biomarkers linked to diabetes that have been used to derive dietary patterns include inflammatory markers (e.g., PAI-1, tumor necrosis factor-α receptor 2, C-reactive protein (CRP), and Interleukin 6) [12,13,19,21], glucose (e.g., HbA1c, HOMA-IR, and fasting glucose) [12,14,16,20], lipid-related metabolites (e.g., TG, HDL-C, adiponectin, and leptin) [12,16,18,21], and uric acids [17]. Food groups that have been frequently reported to be associated with an increased risk of type 2 diabetes have been characterized by high intakes of sugar-sweetened beverages or soft drinks [12–14,16,17,21], processed meats [12,13,16,21], red meats [12,15,16,21], refined grains [13,16], white rice [21] or bread [14,19] and low intakes of wine [13,15,16], whole grains [16,21], and yellow [13,16,21] and green [16,21] vegetables. In our study, noodles positively contributed to the dietary pattern scores among men. Batis et al. [20] also identified a positive association of wheat noodles with dietary pattern scores that explained variations of HbA1c, HOMA-IR, and fasting glucose levels among Chinese men and women. Additionally, consistent with previous studies that identified a positive contribution of red meats to diabetes-related dietary pattern scores [12,15,16,21], we found a positive contribution of organ and other meats to dietary pattern scores among women.

The estimates of the association between dietary pattern scores and the risk of type 2 diabetes are comparable to those found in previous studies. Jannasch et al. [11] conducted meta-analyses of the association between posteriori-dietary patterns associated with diabetes-related biomarkers and risk of type 2 diabetes [12–14,16,46]; combined relative risks (95% CIs) were 0.51 (0.27–0.98) for dietary pattern related to HbA1c, HDL-C, CRP, and adiponectin [12,16,46], 2.53 (1.56–4.10) for dietary pattern related to inflammatory markers [13,16,46] and 1.39 (1.25–1.54) for dietary patterns associated with HOMA-IR [14,16,46].

Previous studies have identified the TG/HDL-C ratio as a clinically useful surrogate estimate of insulin resistance [25–28]. Methods for estimating TG and HDL-C concentrations are well standardized [26], and the ratio of the two values provides information on the atherogenic lipoprotein profile associated with the risk of CVD [47] as well as insulin resistance. A high TG/HDL-C ratio is associated with an increased risk of type 2 diabetes [29,32,48,49] and with CHD and/or CVD events [50,51] and mortality [29,52]. Tabung et al. [53] developed an empirical dietary index for insulin resistance using the TG/HDL-C ratio as a response variable and food groups as explanatory variables in a stepwise linear regression model in a female cohort, the Nurses' Health Study (NHS). An empirical dietary index for insulin resistance was characterized by high intakes of low-calorie beverages, margarine, red meat, refined grains, processed meats, tomatoes, other vegetables, other fish, fruit juice, and creamy soups and low intakes of coffee, wine, liquor, beer, green leafy vegetables, high-fat dairy products, dark yellow vegetables, and nuts [53]. Consistent with a previous study that developed a dietary index for insulin resistance, our study also found that dietary pattern was positively associated with organ and other meats and negatively associated with dairy products and nuts among women. According to the meta-analysis of prospective cohort studies for individual food groups, a higher consumption of red meats was associated with an increased risk of type 2 diabetes [54], whereas higher consumption of dairy products [55,56] and nuts [57] were associated with a reduced risk of type 2 diabetes.

There were unexpected inverse associations of dietary pattern scores with pork and candy/chocolate among men. Even though we used an age-adjusted TG/HDL-C ratio, a difference in pork by age may exist. Low consumption of pork among older men may explain our finding; mean intake of pork among men aged 40s, 50s, and 60s was 47.19 g/day, 42.25 g/day, and 37.65 g/day, respectively. Further study is needed to examine dietary patterns associated with various biomarkers that have been linked to diabetes and their prediction of type 2 diabetes risk in different study populations.

This study has several limitations. We did not use person-years of follow-up to analyze the association because we did not have information on type 2 diabetes incidence for more than 20% of the original study participants. Therefore, we included participants whose fasting plasma glucose, 2-h plasma glucose after a 75 g OGTT, and HbA1c were available during the follow-up. This may limit the generalizability of our findings; however, we tried to remove the potential bias that could occur from loss to follow-up. We also cannot rule out the possibility of the presence of measurement error in the dietary assessment or residual or unknown confounding factors.

The strengths of our study include the measurement of biomarkers to detect the incidence of type 2 diabetes. Fasting plasma glucose, 2-h plasma glucose after a 75 g OGTT, and HbA1c were measured at baseline and at every biannual follow up. This is the first cohort study in Korea to examine the association between biomarker-related dietary pattern and type 2 diabetes incidence. We were able to examine a temporal relationship between dietary patterns and the risk of type 2 diabetes, given a cohort study design. Information on sociodemographic and lifestyle factors as well as medical status allowed us to adjust for potential confounders. Last, we additionally derived the dietary patterns of men and women separately. Providing sex-specific findings is important because of the sex difference in biological and behavioral characteristics and sex-specific results may provide appropriate evidence on modifiable factors that contributing to disease prevention in men and women [58]. We found that the components of dietary patterns differed by sex, and the results were consistent with previous studies that examined the association in a sex-specific way.

5. Conclusions

The present study derived posteriori-dietary patterns using the TG/HDL-C ratio as a biomarker that is linked to type 2 diabetes, and examined the associations between the dietary pattern scores and the risk of type 2 diabetes among Korean men and women. Among men, dietary pattern was characterized by higher intakes of noodles, fruits, fermented salted seafood and lower intakes of candy and chocolate, nuts, and pork; and the dietary pattern for women was characterized by higher intakes of organ and other meats and lower intakes of dairy products and nuts. Higher dietary pattern scores were associated with an increased risk of type 2 diabetes. Our study provides sex-specific evidence on dietary patterns associated with the risk of type 2 diabetes, which may partly be mediated by the TG/HDL-C ratio. Consideration of TG/HDL-C ratio related dietary patterns to reduce the burden of type 2 diabetes may be needed and our study warrants further replication.

Supplementary Materials:
Figure S1: Flow diagram of inclusion for study participants, Table S1: Odds ratios (ORs) and 95% confidence intervals (CIs) of incident 2 diabetes according to the quintiles of TG/HDLC-related dietary pattern after excluding incident cases during 2 years of follow up.

Author Contributions: Conceptualization, J.E.L. and S.S.; Formal Analysis, S.S.; Writing—Original Draft Preparation, S.S.; Writing—Review & Editing, J.E.L.; Funding Acquisition, J.E.L.

Acknowledgments: Data in this study were from the Korean Genome and Epidemiology Study (KoGES; 4851-302), National Research Institute of Health, Centers for Disease Control and Prevention, Ministry for Health and Welfare, Republic of Korea.

References

1. International Diabetes Foundation. *IDF Diabetes Atlas*, 3rd ed.; International Diabetes Foundation: Brussels, Belgium, 2006.
2. International Diabetes Federation. *IDF Diabetes Atlas*, 8th ed.; International Diabetes Foundation: Brussels, Belgium, 2017.
3. Zimmet, P.; Alberti, K.; Shaw, J. Global and societal implications of the diabetes epidemic. *Nature* **2001**, *414*, 782. [CrossRef]
4. Chen, L.; Magliano, D.J.; Zimmet, P.Z. The worldwide epidemiology of type 2 diabetes mellitus—Present and future perspectives. *Nat. Rev. Endocrinol.* **2012**, *8*, 228. [CrossRef] [PubMed]
5. World Health Organization. *Global Report on Diabetes*; World Health Organization: Geneva, Switzerland, 2016.
6. World Health Organization. *Diet, Nutrition, and the Prevention of Chronic Diseases: Report of a Joint Who/Fao Expert Consultation*; World Health Organization: Geneva, Switzerland, 2003.
7. World Health Organization. *Guideline: Sugars Intake for Adults and Children*; World Health Organization: Geneva, Switzerland, 2015.
8. National Research Council. *Diet and Health: Implications for Reducing Chronic Disease Risk*; National Academies Press: Washington, DC, USA, 1989.
9. Hu, F.B. Dietary pattern analysis: A new direction in nutritional epidemiology. *Curr. Opin. Lipidol.* **2002**, *13*, 3–9. [CrossRef] [PubMed]
10. Ley, S.H.; Hamdy, O.; Mohan, V.; Hu, F.B. Prevention and management of type 2 diabetes: Dietary components and nutritional strategies. *The Lancet* **2014**, *383*, 1999–2007. [CrossRef]
11. Jannasch, F.; Kroger, J.; Schulze, M.B. Dietary Patterns and Type 2 Diabetes: A Systematic Literature Review and Meta-Analysis of Prospective Studies. *J. Nutr.* **2017**, *147*, 1174–1182. [CrossRef]
12. Heidemann, C.; Hoffmann, K.; Spranger, J.; Klipstein-Grobusch, K.; Mohlig, M.; Pfeiffer, A.F.; Boeing, H. A dietary pattern protective against type 2 diabetes in the European Prospective Investigation into Cancer and Nutrition (EPIC)–Potsdam Study cohort. *Diabetologia* **2005**, *48*, 1126–1134. [CrossRef]
13. Schulze, M.B.; Hoffmann, K.; Manson, J.E.; Willett, W.C.; Meigs, J.B.; Weikert, C.; Heidemann, C.; Colditz, G.A.; Hu, F.B. Dietary pattern, inflammation, and incidence of type 2 diabetes in women. *Am. J. Clin. Nutr.* **2005**, *82*, 675–684. [CrossRef]
14. McNaughton, S.A.; Mishra, G.D.; Brunner, E.J. Dietary patterns, insulin resistance, and incidence of type 2 diabetes in the whitehall II study. *Diabetes Care* **2008**, *31*, 1343–1348. [CrossRef]
15. Liese, A.D.; Weis, K.E.; Schulz, M.; Tooze, J.A. Food intake patterns associated with incident type 2 diabetes: The insulin resistance atherosclerosis study. *Diabetes Care* **2009**, *32*, 263–268. [CrossRef]
16. Imamura, F.; Lichtenstein, A.H.; Dallal, G.E.; Meigs, J.B.; Jacques, P.F. Generalizability of dietary patterns associated with incidence of type 2 diabetes mellitus. *Am. J. Clin. Nutr.* **2009**, *90*, 1075–1083. [CrossRef]
17. Sluijs, I.; Beulens, J.W.; van der, A.D.; Spijkerman, A.M.; Schulze, M.B.; van der Schouw, Y.T. Plasma uric acid is associated with increased risk of type 2 diabetes independent of diet and metabolic risk factors. *Am. J. Clin. Nutr.* **2013**, *143*, 80–85. [CrossRef] [PubMed]
18. Frank, L.K.; Jannasch, F.; Kroger, J.; Bedu-Addo, G.; Mockenhaupt, F.P.; Schulze, M.B.; Danquah, I. A Dietary Pattern Derived by Reduced Rank Regression is Associated with Type 2 Diabetes in An Urban Ghanaian Population. *Nutrients* **2015**, *7*, 5497–5514. [CrossRef] [PubMed]
19. McGeoghegan, L.; Muirhead, C.R.; Almoosawi, S. Association between an anti-inflammatory and anti-oxidant dietary pattern and diabetes in British adults: Results from the national diet and nutrition survey rolling programme years 1–4. *Int. J. Food Sci. Nutr.* **2015**, *67*, 553–561. [CrossRef]
20. Batis, C.; Mendez, M.A.; Gordon-Larsen, P.; Sotres-Alvarez, D.; Adair, L.; Popkin, B. Using both principal component analysis and reduced rank regression to study dietary patterns and diabetes in Chinese adults. *Public Health Nutr.* **2016**, *19*, 195–203. [CrossRef]
21. Jacobs, S.; Kroeger, J.; Schulze, M.B.; Frank, L.K.; Franke, A.A.; Cheng, I.; Monroe, K.R.; Haiman, C.A.; Kolonel, L.N.; Wilkens, L.R.; et al. Dietary Patterns Derived by Reduced Rank Regression Are Inversely Associated with Type 2 Diabetes Risk across 5 Ethnic Groups in the Multiethnic Cohort. *Curr. Dev. Nutr.* **2017**, *1*, e000620. [CrossRef] [PubMed]

22. Reaven, G.M. Role of Insulin Resistance in Human Disease. *Diabetes* **1988**, *37*, 1595–1607. [CrossRef] [PubMed]
23. Reaven, G.M. Pathophysiology of insulin resistance in human disease. *Physiol. Rev.* **1995**, *75*, 473–486. [CrossRef]
24. Antuna-Puente, B.; Disse, E.; Rabasa-Lhoret, R.; Laville, M.; Capeau, J.; Bastard, J.-P. How can we measure insulin sensitivity/resistance? *Diabetes Metab.* **2011**, *37*, 179–188. [CrossRef]
25. McLaughlin, T.; Abbasi, F.; Cheal, K.; Chu, J.; Lamendola, C.; Reaven, G. Use of metabolic markers to identify overweight individuals who are insulin resistant. *Ann. Intern. Med.* **2003**, *139*, 802–809. [CrossRef]
26. McLaughlin, T.; Reaven, G.; Abbasi, F.; Lamendola, C.; Saad, M.; Waters, D.; Simon, J.; Krauss, R.M. Is there a simple way to identify insulin-resistant individuals at increased risk of cardiovascular disease? *Am. J. Cardiol.* **2005**, *96*, 399–404. [CrossRef]
27. Li, C.; Ford, E.S.; Meng, Y.-X.; Mokdad, A.H.; Reaven, G.M. Does the association of the triglyceride to high-density lipoprotein cholesterol ratio with fasting serum insulin differ by race/ethnicity? *Cardiovasc. Diabetol.* **2008**, *7*, 4. [CrossRef] [PubMed]
28. Salazar, M.R.; Carbajal, H.A.; Espeche, W.G.; Leiva Sisnieguez, C.E.; Balbín, E.; Dulbecco, C.A.; Aizpurúa, M.; Marillet, A.G.; Reaven, G.M. Relation Among the Plasma Triglyceride/High-Density Lipoprotein Cholesterol Concentration Ratio, Insulin Resistance, and Associated Cardio-Metabolic Risk Factors in Men and Women. *Am. J. Cardiol.* **2012**, *109*, 1749–1753. [CrossRef] [PubMed]
29. Vega, G.L.; Barlow, C.E.; Grundy, S.M.; Leonard, D.; DeFina, L.F. Triglyceride–to–high-density-lipoprotein-cholesterol ratio is an index of heart disease mortality and of incidence of type 2 diabetes mellitus in men. *J. Investig. Med.* **2014**, *62*, 345–349. [CrossRef] [PubMed]
30. Kang, H.-T.; Yoon, J.-H.; Kim, J.-Y.; Ahn, S.-K.; Linton, J.; Koh, S.-B.; Kim, J.-K. The association between the ratio of triglyceride to HDL-C and insulin resistance according to waist circumference in a rural Korean population. *Nutr. Metab. Cardiovasc. Dis.* **2012**, *22*, 1054–1060. [CrossRef] [PubMed]
31. Kim, J.-S.; Kang, H.-T.; Shim, J.-Y.; Lee, H.-R. The association between the triglyceride to high-density lipoprotein cholesterol ratio with insulin resistance (HOMA-IR) in the general Korean population: Based on the National Health and Nutrition Examination Survey in 2007–2009. *Diabetes Res. Clin. Pract.* **2012**, *97*, 132–138. [CrossRef] [PubMed]
32. Sung, K.-C.; Park, H.-Y.; Kim, M.-J.; Reaven, G. Metabolic markers associated with insulin resistance predict type 2 diabetes in Koreans with normal blood pressure or prehypertension. *Cardiovasc. Diabetol.* **2016**, *15*, 47. [CrossRef] [PubMed]
33. Wang, X.; Magkos, F.; Mittendorfer, B. Sex differences in lipid and lipoprotein metabolism: It's not just about sex hormones. *J. Clin. Endocrinol. Metab.* **2011**, *96*, 885–893. [CrossRef]
34. Arganini, C.; Saba, A.; Comitato, R.; Virgili, F.; Turrini, A. Gender differences in food choice and dietary intake in modern western societies. In *Public Health-Social and Behavioral Health*; InTech Open Access Publisher: Rijeka, Croatia, 2012.
35. Kim, Y.; Han, B.-G.; KoGES Group. Cohort Profile: The Korean Genome and Epidemiology Study (KoGES) Consortium. *Int. J. Epidemiol.* **2017**, *46*, e20. [CrossRef]
36. KCDC Center for Genome Sciences. FFQ guideline for Korean Genome and Epidemiology Study (KoGES). 2014. Available online: http://www.cdc.go.kr/NIH_NEW/contents/NihKrContentView.jsp?cid=141857&menuIds=HOME005-MNU2016-MNU1010-MNU1023#menu2_2_2 (accessed on 20 October 2018).
37. Ahn, Y.; Kwon, E.; Shim, J.; Park, M.; Joo, Y.; Kimm, K.; Park, C.; Kim, D. Validation and reproducibility of food frequency questionnaire for Korean genome epidemiologic study. *Eur. J. Clin. Nutr.* **2007**, *61*, 1435. [CrossRef]
38. Korean Nutrition Society. *Recommended Dietary Allowances for Koreans*, 7th ed.; Korean Nutrition Society: Seoul, Korea, 2000.
39. American Diabetes Association. 2. Classification and diagnosis of diabetes. *Diabetes Care* **2015**, *38*, S8–S16. [CrossRef]
40. Korea Centers for Disease Control and Prevention. *The Second Korea National Health and Nutrition Examination Survey (KNHANES II), 2001*; Korea Centers for Disease Control and Prevention: Seoul, Korea, 2002.

41. Ainsworth, B.E.; Haskell, W.L.; Whitt, M.C.; Irwin, M.L.; Swartz, A.M.; Strath, S.J.; O Brien, W.L.; Bassett, D.R.; Schmitz, K.H.; Emplaincourt, P.O. Compendium of physical activities: An update of activity codes and MET intensities. *Med. Sci. Sports Exerc.* **2000**, *32*, S498–S504. [CrossRef] [PubMed]
42. Ainsworth, B.E.; Haskell, W.L.; Herrmann, S.D.; Meckes, N.; Bassett, D.R., Jr.; Tudor-Locke, C.; Greer, J.L.; Vezina, J.; Whitt-Glover, M.C.; Leon, A.S. 2011 Compendium of Physical Activities: A second update of codes and MET values. *Med. Sci. Sports Exerc.* **2011**, *43*, 1575–1581. [CrossRef] [PubMed]
43. Hoffmann, K.; Schulze, M.B.; Schienkiewitz, A.; Nothlings, U.; Boeing, H. Application of a new statistical method to derive dietary patterns in nutritional epidemiology. *Am J. Epidemiol.* **2004**, *159*, 935–944. [CrossRef] [PubMed]
44. Fung, T.T.; Hu, F.B.; Schulze, M.; Pollak, M.; Wu, T.; Fuchs, C.S.; Giovannucci, E. A dietary pattern that is associated with C-peptide and risk of colorectal cancer in women. *Cancer Causes Control* **2012**, *23*, 959–965. [CrossRef]
45. Lillioja, S.; Mott, D.M.; Spraul, M.; Ferraro, R.; Foley, J.E.; Ravussin, E.; Knowler, W.C.; Bennett, P.H.; Bogardus, C. Insulin resistance and insulin secretory dysfunction as precursors of non-insulin-dependent diabetes mellitus: Prospective studies of Pima Indians. *N. Engl. J. Med.* **1993**, *329*, 1988–1992. [CrossRef] [PubMed]
46. InterAct Consortium. Adherence to predefined dietary patterns and incident type 2 diabetes in European populations: EPIC-InterAct Study. *Diabetologia* **2014**, *57*, 321–333. [CrossRef] [PubMed]
47. Dobiásová, M.; Frohlich, J. The plasma parameter log (TG/HDL-C) as an atherogenic index: Correlation with lipoprotein particle size and esterification rate inapob-lipoprotein-depleted plasma (FERHDL). *Clin. Biochem.* **2001**, *34*, 583–588. [CrossRef]
48. Zhang, M.; Zhou, J.; Liu, Y.; Sun, X.; Luo, X.; Han, C.; Zhang, L.; Wang, B.; Ren, Y.; Zhao, Y. Risk of type 2 diabetes mellitus associated with plasma lipid levels: The rural Chinese cohort study. *Diabetes Res. Clin. Pract.* **2018**, *135*, 150–157. [CrossRef]
49. He, S.; Wang, S.; Chen, X.; Jiang, L.; Peng, Y.; Li, L.; Wan, L.; Cui, K. Higher ratio of triglyceride to high-density lipoprotein cholesterol may predispose to diabetes mellitus: 15-year prospective study in a general population. *Metabolism* **2012**, *61*, 30–36. [CrossRef]
50. Hadaegh, F.; Khalili, D.; Ghasemi, A.; Tohidi, M.; Sheikholeslami, F.; Azizi, F. Triglyceride/HDL-cholesterol ratio is an independent predictor for coronary heart disease in a population of Iranian men. *Nutr. Metab. Cardiovasc. Dis.* **2009**, *19*, 401–408. [CrossRef]
51. Bittner, V.; Johnson, B.D.; Zineh, I.; Rogers, W.J.; Vido, D.; Marroquin, O.C.; Bairey-Merz, C.N.; Sopko, G. The triglyceride/high-density lipoprotein cholesterol ratio predicts all-cause mortality in women with suspected myocardial ischemia: A report from the Women's Ischemia Syndrome Evaluation (WISE). *Am. Heart J.* **2009**, *157*, 548–555. [CrossRef] [PubMed]
52. Asia Pacific Cohort Studies Collaboration. A Comparison of Lipid Variables as Predictors of Cardiovascular Disease in the Asia Pacific Region. *Ann. Epidemiol.* **2005**, *15*, 405–413. [CrossRef] [PubMed]
53. Tabung, F.K.; Wang, W.; Fung, T.T.; Hu, F.B.; Smith-Warner, S.A.; Chavarro, J.E.; Fuchs, C.S.; Willett, W.C.; Giovannucci, E.L. Development and validation of empirical indices to assess the insulinaemic potential of diet and lifestyle. *Br. J. Nutr.* **2016**, *116*, 1787–1798. [CrossRef] [PubMed]
54. Pan, A.; Sun, Q.; Bernstein, A.M.; Schulze, M.B.; Manson, J.E.; Willett, W.C.; Hu, F.B. Red meat consumption and risk of type 2 diabetes: 3 cohorts of US adults and an updated meta-analysis. *Am. J. Clin. Nutr.* **2011**, *94*, 1088–1096. [CrossRef] [PubMed]
55. Tong, X.; Dong, J.; Wu, Z.; Li, W.; Qin, L. Dairy consumption and risk of type 2 diabetes mellitus: A meta-analysis of cohort studies. *Eur. J. Clin. Nutr.* **2011**, *65*, 1027. [CrossRef] [PubMed]
56. Gijsbers, L.; Ding, E.L.; Malik, V.S.; de Goede, J.; Geleijnse, J.M.; Soedamah-Muthu, S.S. Consumption of dairy foods and diabetes incidence: A dose-response meta-analysis of observational studies. *Am. J. Clin. Nutr.* **2016**, *103*, 1111–1124. [CrossRef] [PubMed]
57. Afshin, A.; Micha, R.; Khatibzadeh, S.; Mozaffarian, D. Consumption of nuts and legumes and risk of incident ischemic heart disease, stroke, and diabetes: A systematic review and meta-analysis. *Am. J. Clin. Nutr.* **2014**, *100*, 278–288. [CrossRef] [PubMed]
58. Song, S.; Kim, S.; Lee, J.E. Sex consideration in diet–biomarker-related indices: A systematic review. *Public Health Nutr.* **2018**, 1–13. [CrossRef]

14

Daily Intake of Grape Powder Prevents the Progression of Kidney Disease in Obese Type 2 Diabetic ZSF1 Rats

Salwa M. K. Almomen [1], Qiunong Guan [1,2], Peihe Liang [1,3], Kaidi Yang [1], Ahmad M. Sidiqi [1,4], Adeera Levin [4] and Caigan Du [1,2,*]

1 Department of Urologic Sciences, University of British Columbia, Vancouver, BC V6H3Z6, Canada; sa.momen@windowslive.com (S.M.K.A.); qiunong@hotmail.com (Q.G.); lph1972@163.com (P.L.); kaidiyang1994@gmail.com (K.Y.); ahmad.sidiqi@alumni.ubc.ca (A.M.S.)

2 Immunity and Infection Research Centre, Vancouver Coastal Health Research Institute, Vancouver, BC V6H3Z6, Canada

3 Department of Urology, The Second Affiliated Hospital, Chongqing Medical University, Chongqing 400010, China

4 Division of Nephrology, Department of Medicine, University of British Columbia, Vancouver, BC V6Z1Y6, Canada; alevin@providencehealth.bc.ca

* Correspondence: caigan@mail.ubc.ca

Abstract: Individuals living with metabolic syndrome (MetS) such as diabetes and obesity are at high risk for developing chronic kidney disease (CKD). This study investigated the beneficial effect of whole grape powder (WGP) diet on MetS-associated CKD. Obese diabetic ZSF1 rats, a kidney disease model with MetS, were fed WGP (5%, *w/w*) diet for six months. Kidney disease was determined using blood and urine chemical analyses, and histology. When compared to Vehicle controls, WGP intake did not change the rat bodyweight, but lowered their kidney, liver and spleen weight, which were in parallel with the lower serum glucose and the higher albumin or albumin/globin ratio. More importantly, WGP intake improved the renal function as urination and proteinuria decreased, or it prevented kidney tissue damage in these diabetic rats. The renal protection of WGP diet was associated with up-regulation of antioxidants (*Dhcr24, Gstk1, Prdx2, Sod2, Gpx1 and Gpx4*) and downregulation of *Txnip* (for ROS production) in the kidneys. Furthermore, addition of grape extract reduced H_2O_2-induced cell death of cultured podocytes. In conclusion, daily intake of WGP reduces the progression of kidney disease in obese diabetic rats, suggesting a protective function of antioxidant-rich grape diet against CKD in the setting of MetS.

Keywords: metabolic syndrome; chronic kidney disease; grape powder; antioxidants; natural products; dietary supplements

1. Introduction

Chronic kidney disease (CKD) is multifactorial, and is defined as abnormalities of kidney structure or function that is present for more than three months. While not progressive in all, it can lead to end-stage renal disease (ESRD)—total and permanent kidney failure [1,2]. CKD places a major public health burden on our community as it affects more than 10% of adults aged 20 years or older, or more than 40% in those aged 65 years or older in the United States (source: Centers for Disease Control and Prevention), and 12.5% of adults, representing approximately three million, in Canada [3,4]. Like other chronic diseases, many cases of CKD are not curable, but there are substantial numbers of people who can benefit from prevention or delay of progression [5], suggesting that an effective and feasible preventive strategy is expected to reduce the burden of CKD in our community. However, there are a limited number of these that are proven or used in our daily practice. Recently, there is an increasing interest in diet, the interaction of gut microbiome and CKD progression. Dietary supplements or natural health products is definitely an attractive and feasible strategy for CKD prevention.

Metabolic syndrome (MetS) is a collective term for several clinical measures, which include insulin resistance, high serum glucose, overweight or obesity, high triglyceride or low high-density lipoprotein cholesterol and hypertension [6]. Literature suggests that MetS may increase the risk of the development of CKD [7–9], mainly seen as hypertensive and diabetic nephropathy (DN). While the etiology for MetS-induced CKD remains unknown [9], oxidative stress is theorized to a play a role [8,10,11]. The oxidative stress is induced by the imbalance between the level of reactive oxygen species (ROS, free radicals) and the capacity of antioxidant defenses, which leads to the generation of excessive ROS and consequently tissue damage [11,12]. One of major antioxidant defense mechanisms in our body is exogenous antioxidants, such as flavonoids, vitamins, resveratrol, anthocyanine, curcumin and phenolic acid that come from our food and other dietary sources [11,13–15]. There are some data that antioxidant rich berry diet has benefit in preventing or mitigating MetS [15,16], suggesting that a dietary strategy of using antioxidant-rich food may be a novel strategy to employ to reduce the incidence of CKD among individuals who are living with MetS.

Grapes are one of the most widely cultivated and popularly consumed fruits in the world, and contain over 1600 phytonutrients including some major antioxidant flavonoids, such as catechins (catechin and epicatechin), anthocyanins (peonidin, cyaniding, and malvidin), flavonols (quercetin, kaempferol, and isorhamnetin) and resveratrol (source: the California Table Grape Commission report, Fresno, CA, USA). The renoprotective activities of these compounds have been demonstrated in various experimental models. For example, epicatechin, quercetin or resveratrol has been shown to lower the oxidative stress in the kidneys and reduce renal damage in animals with cisplatin nephropathy [17–19], and feeding with anthocyanin-rich food reduces diabetes-associated kidney failure in db/db mice [20]. A recent study shows that daily drinking of whole grape powder (WGP) prevents age-related decline of kidney function in rats [21], but its beneficial effect on MetS-associated CKD, a common public health problem in our community [22], has not been investigated. Obese ZSF1 male rats are generated by a cross between a Zucker diabetic fatty (ZDF) female and a spontaneously hypertensive heart failure (SHHF) male rat, which have MetS similar to humans, including hypertension, type 2 diabetes, hyperlipidemia and nephropathy [23–27]. Hence, these rats have been widely used as a disease model for renal failure in the condition of MetS [27–30]. The objective of this study was to examine the effect of daily feeding with the WGP on the progression of kidney disease in obese ZSF1 rats, as compared to control animals.

2. Materials and Methods

2.1. Animals and Cells

Obese ZSF1 male rats (~300 g bodyweight, 8 weeks old) were purchased from Charles River Laboratories International, Inc. (Wilmington, MA, USA). These rats were F1 hybrids from a cross between a female ZDF rat and a male SHHF rat [27], and were maintained in the animal facility of the Jack Bell Research Centre (Vancouver, BC, Canada). All animal experiments were performed in accordance with the Canadian Council on Animal Care guidelines under protocols approved by the Animal Use Subcommittee at the University of British Columbia (Vancouver, BC, Canada).

Heat-sensitive mouse podocyte (HSMP) cell line was a gift from Dr. Stuart Shankland (University of Washington School of Medicine, Seattle, WA, USA). HSMP cells were maintained and grown in RPMI 1640 culture medium supplemented with 10% fetal bovine serum and 0.2 $ng \cdot mL^{-1}$ of IFN-γ in a CO_2 incubator at 33 °C as described previously [31]. To induce quiescence and the differentiated phenotype for experiments, HSMP cells were grown at 37 °C in the same medium but in the absence of IFN-γ (growth restrictive conditions) [31].

2.2. *Whole Grape Powder (WGP)*

WGP was provided by the California Table Grape Commission (CTGC), and was a freeze-dried grape product developed for the usage of research purposes only. WGP was composed of seeded and seedless varieties of fresh green, red and black California grapes that were initially frozen, and then ground with food-quality dry ice. The processing and storage of the WGP were done properly for preserving the bioactivities of the compounds found in the grapes. Approximately 90% of the WGP by weight was sugars (glucose and fructose found in a 1:1 ratio), and the remainder consisted of organic acids, phenolic compounds, nitrogenous compounds, aroma compounds, and minerals and pectic substances. Antioxidants, such as resveratrol, flavans (including catechin), flavonols (including quercetin), anthocyanins and many simple phenolics (as per the CTGC report) were also found. This product was stored at −80 °C in moisture-proof containers until it was mixed with regular rat chow for the animal experiments.

2.3. *Food Supplements*

According to the CTGC guideline of the usage of WGP as food supplements for animal studies, WGP supplement food (denoted as WGP here) was prepared for this study by mixing regular chow (95%, *w*/*w*) with WGP (5%, *w*/*w*), and its Vehicle control the regular chow (95.5%, *w*/*w*) with 2.25% (*w*/*w*) glucose and 2.25% (*w*/*w*) fructose. Rats were randomly assigned to two groups (WGP and Vehicle), in which they were fed with either WGP or sugar control. The animal experiment was repeated twice with total 15 rats in each group. One rat in WGP group suffered a urinary tract infection diagnosed early during the second month of the feeding experiment, and was consequently excluded from the experiment and data analysis.

2.4. *Preparation of WGP Extract*

The WGP extract was prepared for both cell culture experiments to determine its antioxidative activity. In brief, WGP (4 g) was dissolved in 200 mL of methanol (anhydrous, 99.8%) and was stirred for 72 h at room temperature, followed by centrifugation at 3000 rpm for 15 min. The resultant supernatant fraction was subsequently dried by lyophilization using a centrifugal evaporator. Around 3.3 g of WGP-methanol extract was produced from 4 g of WGP by this procedure. The stock solution of WGP extract was prepared by dissolving the dried extract pellet in culture medium at the concentration of 5 mg·mL^{-1}.

2.5. *Primary Outcomes from This Study*

Our primary outcomes were to measure renal function through assessment of urine volume, proteinuria, urine protein to creatinine ratio (uPCR), and estimated glomerular filtration rate (GFR). Renal injury was also measured via the kidney organ index and histological analysis.

2.6. *Urine Collection and Determination of Kidney Function*

A 24-h urine sample was collected using metabolic caging, in which the rat had unrestricted access to food and drinking water. The collected urine was immediately centrifuged at 3000 rpm for 15 min to remove any food scraps and fecal matters. After its volume was measured, the sample was stored in aliquots at −20 °C until all the samples were collected for the determination of both protein and creatinine levels at the same time.

The levels of urine creatinine (UCr) were measured in the Chemistry Laboratory at the Vancouver Coastal Health Regional Laboratory Medicine (Vancouver, BC, Canada) by using the Dimension Vista® System with CRE2 reagent cartridges (Siemens Healthcare Diagnostics Inc., Newark, DE, USA). The levels of urine protein were determined using Bio-Rad protein assay following manufacturer's instruction (Bio-Rad Laboratories-Canada, Mississauga, ON, Canada). In brief, the protein in the urine was precipitated using 10% trichloroacetic acid, followed by centrifugation at 10,000 rpm for 10 min.

The protein pellet was suspended in 3% sodium hydroxide (NaOH) solution, and 1 μL of this protein solution was added to 200 μL of Bio-Rad dye (10 × dilution). The optical density (OD) of urine protein samples, background control and bovine serum albumin (BSA) standards at 595 nm was measured using an ELx808 Ultra Microplate Reader (BioTek, Winooski, VT, USA), and protein concentration ($mg{\cdot}mL^{-1}$) in the urine sample was calculated based on the BSA standard curve.

2.7. Blood Collection and Chemical Analysis

Blood samples were collected from the tail vein using a lithium heparin tube after 1, 3 and 6 months of WGP feeding. A comprehensive metabolic panel of 14 blood substances, including alanine aminotransferase (ALT), albumin (ALB), alkaline phosphatase (ALP), amylase (AMY), total calcium (Ca^{2+}), creatinine (CRE), globulin (GLOB), glucose (GLU), phosphorus (PHOS), potassium (K^+), sodium (Na^+), total bilirubin (TBIL), total protein (TP), and urea nitrogen (BUN), were determined using the VetScan® Comprehensive Diagnostic Profile reagent rotor with the VetScan Chemistry Analyzer VS2 (Abaxis, Inc., Union City, CA, USA) in the Animal Unit Hematology Diagnostic Laboratory at Jack Bell Research Centre (Vancouver, BC, Canada).

2.8. Glomerular Filtration Rate (GFR)

The renal function was estimated using GFR that was calculated based on the creatinine clearance using the following: GFR = (UCr × V)/SCr, where UCr was creatinine level in urine sample, V the volume of the 24-h urine sample, and SCr the creatinine in serum.

2.9. Renal Histopathology

The kidney tissues (6 rats/group) were randomly selected. The tissues were fixed in 10% neutral buffered formalin, followed by embedding in paraffin wax. Sections were cut at 4-μm thickness, and were stained with hematoxylin and eosin (HE) or periodic acid-Schiff (PAS). The stained tissue sections were scanned with Leica SCN400 Slide scanner (Leica Microsystens Inc., Concord, ON, Canada), and the pathological parameters of renal disease were determined in two separate sections of each kidney using the Digital Image Hub—A slidepath Software Solution (Leica Microsystems Inc.) in a blinded fashion.

The number of intratubular protein cast formation or glomerular atrophy in each microscopic view was counted in HE-stained section, and the average number of at least 20 randomly selected views under 40× magnification represented these two parameters in each kidney.

A semi-quantitative scoring system using a 0 to 4 scale was established to determine the severity of the tubular atrophy (including tubular dilution and/or cellular flatting) in the renal cortex of HE-stained kidney sections. The scale/score was measured based on the percentage of damaged tubules occupying a microscopic view: 1 (0%–24% of the area affected with damaged tubules), 2 (25%–49%), 3 (50%–74%), and 4 (>75%). The average of at least 30 randomly selected views under 200× magnification represented the tubular atrophy in each kidney.

The mesangial expansion was also determined using a 0 to 4 scale based on the percentage of the area stained strongly with PAS, indicating the mesangial expansion in an affected glomerulus: 1 (0%–24% of the area affected with densely stain, minimal), 2 (25%–49%, mild), 3 (50%–74%, moderate), and 4 (>75%, severe). A range of 180 to 250 glomeruli were counted and averaged for each kidney.

2.10. PCR Array Analysis of Oxidative Stress

The expression of 84 oxidative stress-associated genes in kidney tissues was quantitatively examined using PCR Arrays kits (Cat. No.: PARN-065Z, SABiosciences—QIAGEN Inc., Valencia, CA, USA) following manufacturer's instruction. Four samples/rats (one from each rat) were randomly selected from each group. In brief, one piece of kidney cortex was snap-frozen in liquid nitrogen and stored at −80 °C until all the samples were ready for the experiment. The total RNA from the tissues was extracted and purified using the RNeasy Microarray Tissue Mini kit

(QIAGEN), and converted to cDNA using RT^2 First Strand Kit (QIAGEN). The expression of selected genes was amplified by real-time PCR using RT^2 Profile PCR arrays (QIAGEN). Data were analyzed using Web-based PCR Array Data Analysis Software at the website of the manufacturer (http://www.SABiosciences.com/pcrarraydataanalysis.php).

2.11. Flow Cytometric Analysis

Cell death or viability was quantitatively determined by using fluorescence-activated cell sorter (FACS) analysis following the manufacturer's protocol (BD Biosciences, Mississauga, ON, Canada). Annexin-V conjugated with phycoerythrin (Annexin-V-PE) stained apoptotic cells, and 7-amino-actinomycin D (7-AAD) positivity indicated late apoptotic and necrotic cells. Briefly, cells were stained with both Annexin-V-PE and 7-AAD for 15 min in the dark, and cell apoptosis and necrosis were detected by using a flow cytometry and further quantified using FlowJo software (Tree Star Inc., Ashland, OR, USA). In a FACS graph, the lower right quadrant—only Annexin V positive indicated early apoptosis; the upper right quadrant—Annexin V/7-AAD double positive showed late apoptosis; and the upper left quadrant—7-AAD positive cells were necrosis. Finally, negative staining (the lower left quadrant—Annexin V/7-AAD double negative) showed the population of viable cells.

2.12. Statistical Analysis

Data were presented as mean ± standard derivation (SD) of each group. Statistical analysis of difference between groups was performed using GraphPad Prism software (GraphPad, San Diego, CA, USA) by *t*-test or analysis of variance (ANOVA) as indicated in the text. A p value of $\leq$0.05 was considered statistically significant.

3. Results

3.1. Daily Intake of WGP Is Associated with Lower Organ Index of the Kidney, Liver and Spleen but Does Not Affect Bodyweight in Obese Diabetic Rats

Both bodyweight and diet consumption were monitored once a week. As shown in Figure 1, the weight gain of rats during six months of WGP feeding was the same as sugar-fed Vehicle control group, indicated by a complete overlap of growth curves between these two groups (WGP vs. Vehicle: p = 0.7701, two-way ANOVA). This observation was correlated with their diet consumption, which remained the same at 25 ± 2 g·day^{-1}·animal^{-1} between these two groups throughout the experiment. Interestingly, at the end of feeding experiment, significantly lower organ weight index was seen in the kidney (WGP vs. Vehicle: p = 0.0127, two-tailed *t*-test), liver (WGP vs. Vehicle: p < 0.0001, two-tailed *t*-test) and spleen (WGP vs. Vehicle: p = 0.0341, two-tailed *t*-test) of WGP-fed rats compared to Vehicle controls, whereas both the heart and the lung remained the same (Table 1). The data suggested that daily intake of WGP reduced the weight/size of these three organs—the liver, kidney and spleen—as compared to those in control group in these obese diabetic rats.

The bodyweight of rats in both Vehicle (n = 15) and WGP (n = 14) groups was recorded during a period of six months of dietary supplements. Data were presented as mean ± SD of each group. Vehicle vs. WGP: p = 0.7701 (two-way ANOVA).

Table 1. Organ index (organ weight/bodyweight) after six months of feeding sugar (Vehicle) or whole grape powder (WGP).

	Kidneys	Liver	Spleen	Heart	Lung
Vehicle (n = 15)	0.0070 ± 0.00072	0.0627 ± 0.00418	0.00135± 0.00010	0.00289 ± 0.00115	0.00356 ± 0.00096
WGP (n = 14)	0.0063 ± 0.00069	0.0544 ± 0.00546	0.00129 ± 0.00001	0.00251 ± 0.00022	0.00371 ± 0.00103
p value *	0.0127	<0.0001	0.0341	0.2351	0.6880

* The difference between Vehicle and WGP was compared using two-tailed *t*-test.

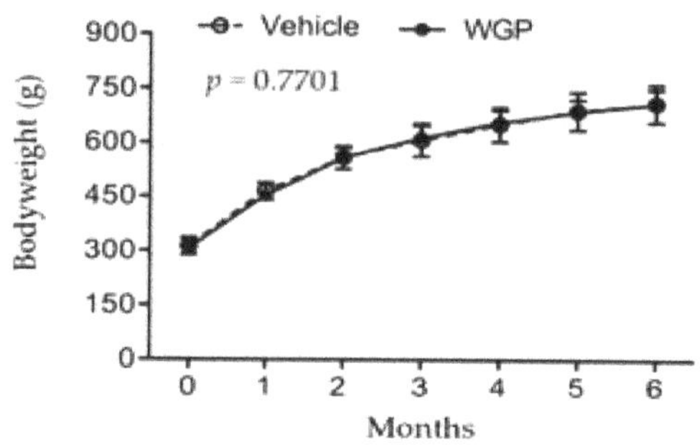

Figure 1. No effect of daily intake of whole grape powder (WGP) on bodyweight gain or obesity in obese diabetic ZSF1 rats.

3.2. Daily Intake of WGP Is Associated with Higher Serum Albumin and Lower Blood Glucose in Obese Diabetic Rats

The overall metabolism status of these rats was determined by using the changes in a comprehensive metabolic panel of 14 blood substances that represent the basic metabolism (GLU), electrolytes (Na^+, K^+, Ca^{2+}, and PHOS) and both kidney and liver functions (BUN, CRE, ALB, GLOB. ALB/GLOB ratio, ALP, ALT, AMY, TP and TBIL). Over six months of feeding experiment, the rats in both groups experienced a significant decline in ALB (including ALB/GLOB ratio), ALP, BUN, K^+ and PHOS, and at the same time an increase in GLU, AMY, TBIL, GLOB, TP, Ca^{2+} and Na^+ (Table S1). Only CRE and ALT remained unchanged (Table S1). The importance for this examination was that as compared to the Vehicle group, WGP-fed rats had significantly higher levels of serum ALB ($p = 0.0013$, two-way ANOVA) or ALB/GLOB ratio ($p = 0.0092$, two-way ANOVA), and lower levels of blood GLU ($p = 0.0276$, two-way ANOVA) (Table S1 and Figure 2), at the end of the six-month period.

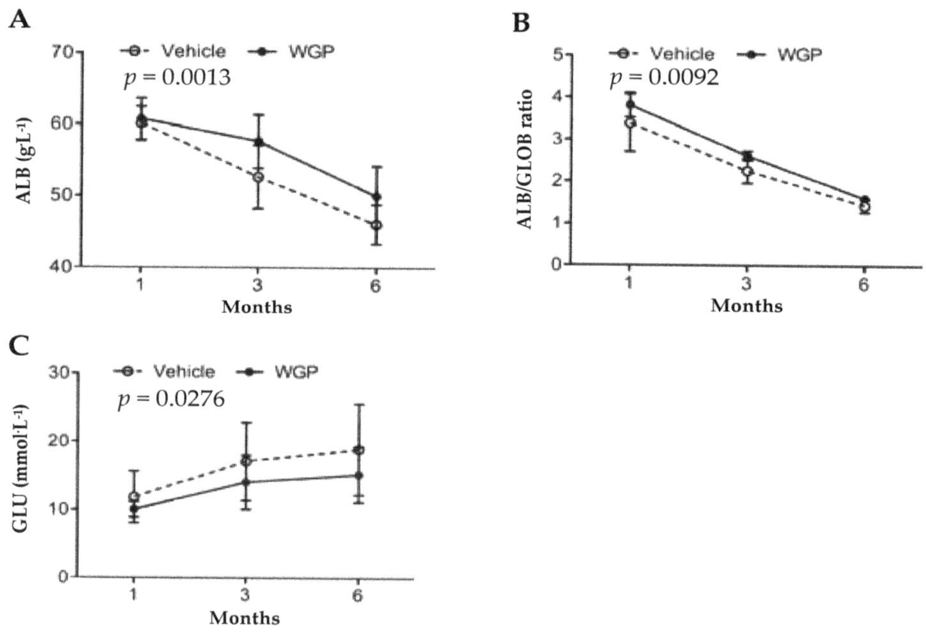

Figure 2. Daily intake of WGP has beneficial effect on the maintenance of blood albumin and the reduction of blood glucose in obese diabetic ZSF1 rats. The blood levels of albumin (ALB), globulin (GLOB) and glucose (GLU) were measured in randomly selected rats in Vehicle ($n = 8$–12) or WGP ($n = 8$–11) group after one, three or six months of dietary supplements. Data were presented as mean ± SD of each group. (**A**) Blood ALB levels. Vehicle vs. WGP: $p = 0.0013$ (two-way ANOVA); (**B**) ALB/GLOB ratio. Vehicle vs. WGP: $p = 0.0092$ (two-way ANOVA); (**C**) Blood GLU levels. Vehicle vs. WGP: $p = 0.0276$ (two-way ANOVA).

3.3. Daily Intake of WGP Significantly Is Associated with Lower Urine Volume and Urine Protein Excretion but Does Not Impact GFR after Six Months in Obese Diabetic Rats

The baseline ranges for renal function in obese ZSF1 rats at the age of eight weeks were 164.8 ± 14.5 mL·kg^{-1}·day^{-1} of urine volume, 307 ± 23 mg·kg^{-1}·day^{-1} of proteinuria or 5.98 ± 0.41 of urine protein to creatinine ratio (uPCR) [28], and the average of bodyweight of the rats at this age was approximately 300 g (Figure 1). After six months of feeding, a 24-h urine sample was collected from each rat. As shown in Figure 3A, WGP-fed rats had lower urine output than Vehicle controls ($p = 0.0092$, one-tailed t-test). Similarly, the WGP group had significantly lower proteinuria ($p = 0.0412$, one-tailed t-test) (Figure 3B), and uPCR ($p = 0.0084$, one-tailed t-test) (Figure 3C), when compared to the Vehicle controls. When GFR (mL·24 h^{-1}) between these two groups was compared, no significant difference was found between the WGP-fed and control groups ($p = 0.3474$, one-tailed t-test) (Figure 3D).

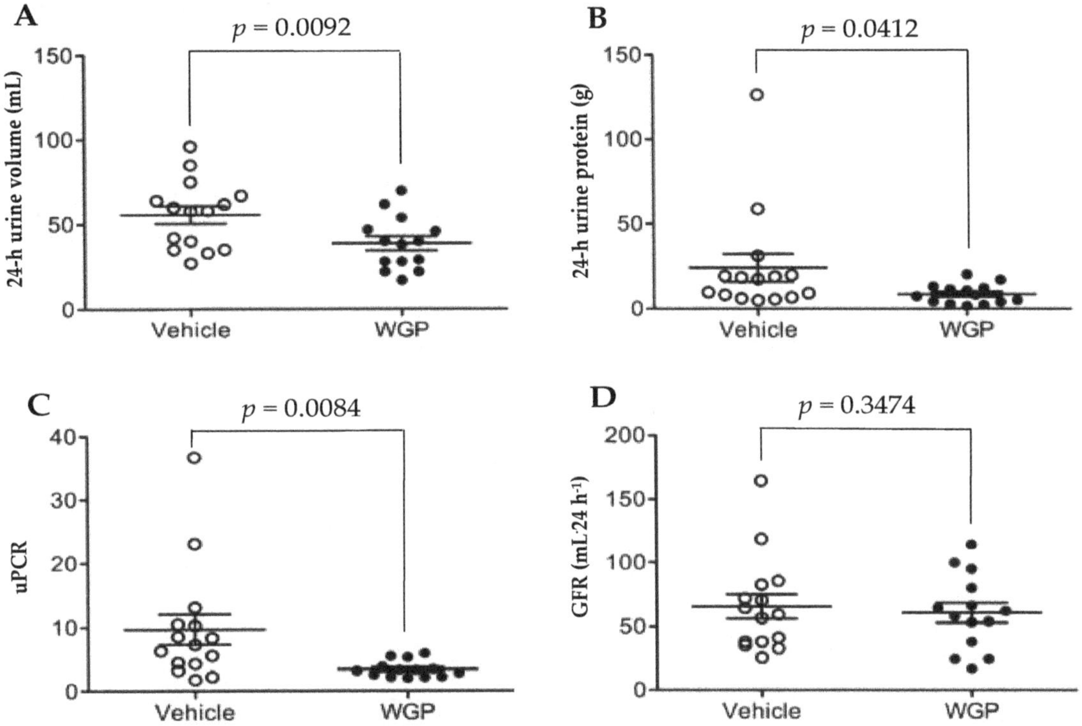

Figure 3. Daily intake of WGP reduces urine production and proteinuria but no effect on GFR in obese diabetic ZSF1 rats. A 24-h urine sample was collected from each rat in both Vehicle ($n = 15$) and WGP ($n = 14$) at the end of six months of dietary supplements. (**A**) Total volume of urine production from each rat during 24 h. Vehicle vs. WGP: $p = 0.0092$ (one-tailed t-test); (**B**) Total amount of protein in 24-h urine sample of each rat. Vehicle vs. WGP: $p = 0.0412$ (one-tailed t-test); (**C**) Protein to creatinine ratio (uPCR) in the urine sample of each rat. Vehicle vs. WGP: $p = 0.0084$ (one-tailed t-test); (**D**) GFR of each rat calculated based on creatinine clearance. Vehicle vs. WGP: $p = 0.3474$ (one-tailed t-test). Line: mean with the standard error of the mean (SEM).

3.4. Daily Intake of WGP Partially Prevents Renal Pathological Changes in Obese Diabetic Rats

To further explore the beneficial effect of daily intake of WGP on the prevention of kidney damage in obese diabetic rats, histological analysis of kidney sections was performed and compared between these two groups. The histological score of all four renal pathological parameters in WGP group were significantly lower than that in Vehicle group (Figure 4A–E). The WGP group had lower scores of glomerular atrophy per view ($p = 0.0225$, two-tailed t-test, $n = 9$) (Figure 4B), reduced mesangial expansion ($p < 0.0001$, two-tailed t-test, $n = 9$) (Figure 4C), fewer tubular protein cast formation per view ($p = 0.0006$, two-tailed t-test, $n = 12$) (Figure 4D), and less severe tubular dilation and atrophy ($p = 0.0036$, two-tailed t-test, $n = 12$) (Figure 4E), when compared to the Vehicle controls. Together, the histological data indicated less kidney injury in all compartments of the kidneys in WGP-fed rats.

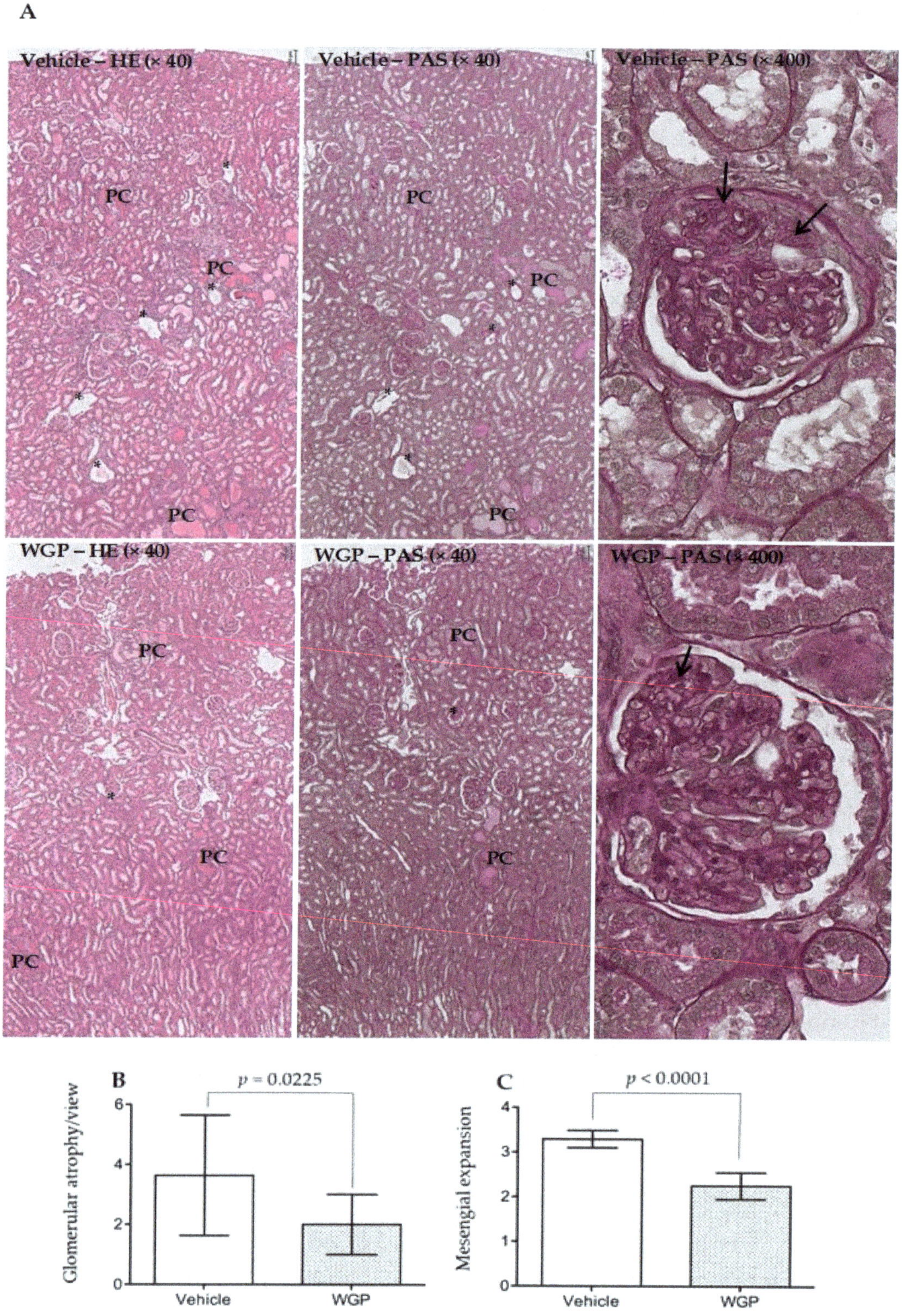

Figure 4. *Cont.*

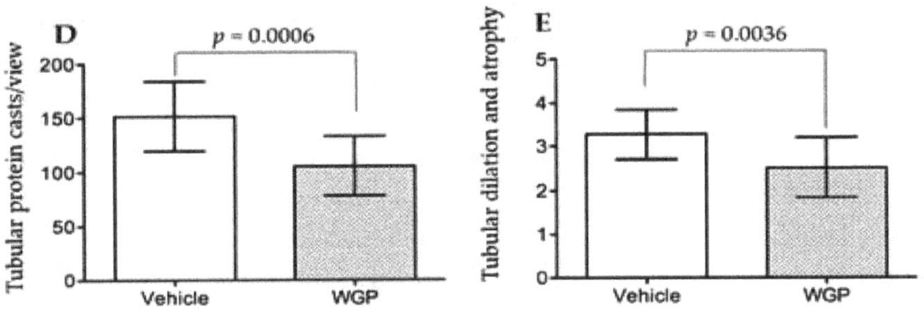

Figure 4. Daily intake of WGP reduces kidney injury in obese diabetic ZSF1 rats. At the end of six months of dietary supplements, six kidneys/rats were randomly selected from each group (Vehicle vs. WGP), and kidney sections were stained with either hematoxylin and eosin (HE) or Periodic acid-Schiff (PAS). (**A**) Typical microscopic images of renal cortex, outer medulla and a glomerulus in each group (Vehicle: top panel; WGP: bottom panel); data showed the same area of renal cortex and outer medulla stained with either HE or PAS. PC: protein cast formation; black stars (*): damaged glomerulus (glomerular atrophy); arrows: PAS-stained mesangial expansion; (**B**) The glomerular atrophy was scored in at least 20 randomly selected views in two separate sections of each kidney, and was presented in average per view; data are presented as mean ± SD of each group ($n = 9$); vehicle vs. WGP: $p = 0.0225$ (two-tailed t-test); (**C**) The mesangial expansion was determined using a 0 to 4 scale based on the percentage of the area stained strongly with PAS; a range of 180 to 250 glomeruli were counted and averaged for each kidney. Data are presented as mean ± SD of each group ($n = 9$); vehicle vs. WGP: $p < 0.0001$ (two-tailed t-test); (**D**) The number of intratubular protein cast formation in each microscopic view was counted in HE-stained section, and the average number of at least 20 randomly selected views under 40× magnification represented in each kidney; data are presented as mean ± SD of each group ($n = 12$); vehicle vs. WGP: $p = 0.0006$ (two-tailed t-test); (**E**) Tubular dilation and atrophy were determined using a 0–4 scale based on the percentage of damaged tubules occupying an area in each microscopic view; the average of at least 30 randomly selected views under 200× magnification represented the tubular atrophy in each kidney; data are presented as mean ± SD of each group ($n = 12$). Vehicle vs. WGP: $p = 0.0036$ (two-tailed t-test).

3.5. Daily Intake of WGP Is Associated with Increasing Local Antioxidant Defense in the Kidney of Obese Diabetic Rats

To understand the mechanisms by which the daily intake of WGP reduced the progression of kidney disease in these rats, the transcriptional profile of 84 genes that are involved in oxidative stress and antioxidant defense in the kidney was examined using PCR array. In the kidneys of WGP-fed rats compared to Vehicle controls, the expression levels of antioxidants (*Gpx1, Gpx4, Gstk1 and Prdx2*) and reactive oxygen species (ROS) metabolism (*Sod2, Cyba, Dhcr24 and Park7*) were significantly up-regulated while oxidative stress response genes (*Hmox1, Ercc6, Gstp1 and Txnip*) downregulated (Table S2 and Table 2). These results suggest an increase in antioxidant defense in the kidneys by WGP diet.

Table 2. Significant changes of oxidative stress-related gene expression in renal cortex of WGP-fed rats as compared to Vehicle controls, analyzed using PCR array.

Gene Symbol	Gene Names	Functions	Fold Change *	p Value ($n = 4$)
Dhcr24	24-dehydrocholesterol reductase	H_2O_2 scavenger, preventing H_2O_2-induced cell death	4.265	0.00222
Cyba	Cytochrome *b*-245, alpha polypeptide	NADPH oxidase subunit, optimizing immunity	4.215	0.00875
Gstk1	Glutathione S-transferase kappa 1	Cellular detoxification (lipid peroxide detoxification)	1.1475	0.01279
Prdx2	Peroxiredoxin 2	H_2O_2 and Alkyl hydroperoxide antioxidant	1.7625	0.02746
Sod2	Superoxide dismutase, mitochondrial	Limiting ROS detrimental effect, and moderating ROS release	2.3375	0.02983

Table 2. *Cont.*

Gene Symbol	Gene Names	Functions	Fold Change *	*p* Value ($n = 4$)
Park7	Parkinson disease (autosomal recessive, early onset) 7	Redox-sensitive chaperone	1.24	0.03723
Gpx4	Glutathione peroxidase 4	H_2O_2, lipid peroxide and hydroperoxide reduction	1.96	0.03756
Gpx1	Glutathione peroxidase 1	H_2O_2 antioxidant	3.235	0.04614
Hmox1	Heme oxygenase (decycling) 1	Heme degradation to CO	−101.533	0.01283
Ercc6	Excision repair cross-complementing rodent repair deficiency, complementation group 6	Damaged DNA repair	−3.9575	0.02908
Gstp1	Glutathione S-transferase pi 1	Cellular detoxification	−22.4875	0.0405
Txnip	Thioredoxin interacting protein	Increasing ROS production	−37.8825	0.04436

* Minus: decreased.

3.6. Addition of WGP Extract Reduced H_2O_2-Induced Cell Death in Cultured Podocytes

Podocyte injury plays a key role in the initiation and early progression of DN [32]. To investigate if the antioxidant compounds from WGP prevented podocyte injury under oxidative stress, the protective activity of WGP extract was tested in cultured podocytes in the presence of H_2O_2. Methanol extraction of WGP exhibited a high antioxidative activity, indicated by the equivalence of approximately 1.7 mg of the extract to 5 μg of ascorbic acid in all three different assays (Figure S1). H_2O_2 induced significant podocyte cell death through apoptosis (positive stain with Annexin-V) (Figure 5A). However, cells that were co-treated with WGP extract (200 mg·mL^{-1}) and H_2O_2 had significantly more cell viability than cells that were treated with H_2O_2 only ($p = 0.037$, two-tailed *t*-test, $n = 8$). The viability of cells treated with both H_2O_2 and WGP extract was not different from that in cultures treated with the extract only ($p = 0.2732$, two-tailed *t*-test. $n = 8$), suggesting that the extract significantly inhibited H_2O_2-induced cell death under this condition.

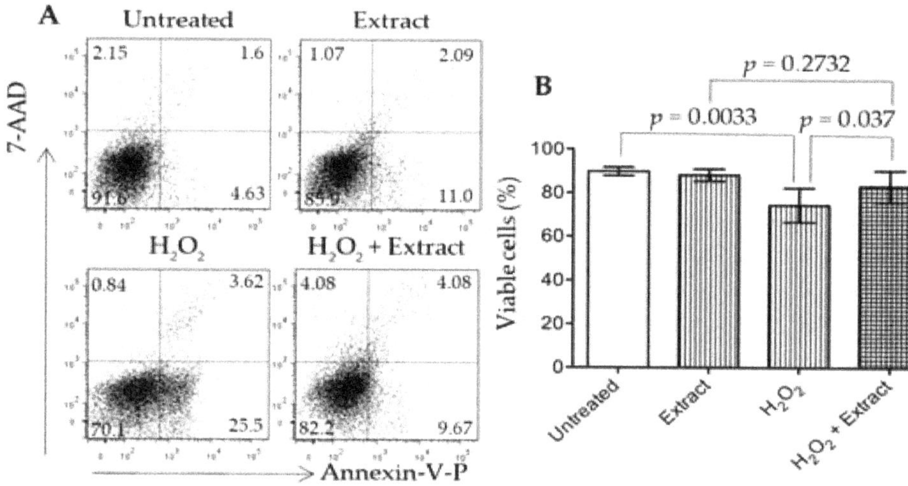

Figure 5. Grape extract protects cultured podocytes from H_2O_2-induced cell death. Grape extract was prepared by using methanol extraction. HSMP cells (0.25×10^6 cells/well) were grown in RPMI 1640 culture medium in 24-well plates at 37 °C overnight, followed by grape extract treatment (200 mg·mL^{-1}) in the presence or absence of H_2O_2 (1 μM). (**A**) Cell viability or apoptosis was determined by FACS analysis with Annexin-V-PE and 7-AAD staining after 24-h treatment with the grape extract. Data were represented as a typical FACS graph in each group; (**B**) Cell viability represented the percentage of viable cells (double-Annexin-V-PE/7-AAD negative cells in lower left quadrant). Data were presented as mean ± SD of eight separate experiments in each group. Untreated vs. H_2O_2, $p = 0.0033$ (two-tailed *t*-test); H_2O_2 vs. H_2O_2 + Extract, $p = 0.037$ (two-tailed *t*-test); or Extract vs. H_2O_2 + Extract, $p = 0.2732$ (two-tailed *t*-test).

4. Discussion

CKD is a major health problem in our society. In addition to pharmacological therapy, such as through angiotensin converting enzyme (ACE) inhibitors or angiotensin receptor blockers (ARB) for proteinuria and/or hypertension control, nutritional interventions have been widely recommended in the management of CKD [33]. A low-protein diet is a popular and practical nutritional management of CKD [34–36]. Interestingly, a recent pilot clinical study shows that dietary supplementation with two gram of grape seed extract a day for six months can improve some kidney function parameters of 2–4 stage CKD in patients, in which the grape seed extract likely acts through the strong antioxidative activity and anti-inflammation of phytochemicals [37]. This study may suggest that a diet containing the antioxidative grape extract can potentially become a nutritional management strategy for the prevention of CKD.

In the present study, when the rats started diet supplement at 8 weeks old, compared to the reference range [38] (Table S3), they had significant higher levels of blood GLU, BUN, TBIL, ALT, ALP and AMY, which may represent a sign of mild diabetes (higher GLU), pancreatic (higher AMY) and nonalcoholic fatty liver disease (higher ALT, ALP, TBIL and BUN). During six months of feeding experiments, the serum levels of AMY, Ca^{2+}, GLOB, GLU, Na^+, TBIL and TB were increased and of ALB (including ALB/GLOB ratio), ALP, BUN, K^+ and PHOS decreased in both groups (Table S1). These data may suggest progressively worsening diabetic (high GLU) and pancreatic (high AMY), fatty liver (high GLOB, TB and TBIL, low ALB and BUN), and kidney disease (low ALB or ALB/GLOB ratio for albumin loss, and the imbalance of Na^+, Ca^{2+}, K^+ and PHOS). When compared to the vehicle control group, with no difference in their bodyweight (Figure 1) the lower organ index of WGP-fed rats may indicate the reduced fatty liver, kidney hypertrophy and perhaps low-degree systemic immune response activity (indicated by the smaller size of the spleens) (Table 1). Further chemical tests showed that daily intake of WGP improved blood ALB and ALB/GLOB ratio and decreased GLU levels (Figure 2), and lower proteinuria, uPCR and urination (probably due to higher renal water reabsorption) (Figure 3). Histologically, we found that glomerular atrophy, mesangial expansion, tubular injury and protein cast formation, all of which are elevated in early stages of diabetic related CKD [39,40], were reduced in the WGP-fed rats (Figure 4). In vitro, the grape extract inhibited H_2O_2-induced cell death in cultured podocytes and exhibited a high antioxidative activity (Figure 5). In consistent with our study, a recently study demonstrates similar benefits of the grape powder to age-related kidney functions in Fischer 344 rats [21].

We described higher urine volumes in the vehicle fed rats versus WGP fed rats (Figure 3A), which may be due to either a manifestation of higher glycemic levels (Figure 2C) or worsened MetS, resulting in increasing hyperfiltration and renal injury. Hyperglycemia-induced hyperfiltration is an early manifestation of diabetes that causes polyuria and is an early predictor of glomerular damage in late stages of kidney disease [41–43]. While there was no evidence of better renal function (eGFR levels) in the WGP group (Figure 3D), this may have been due to the short duration of the study, since decline in GFR is a late marker of nephropathy when around 50% of nephrons are already lost [39,44]. The obese ZSF1 rats in this study indeed show the signs of early stages of CKD where an evidence of kidney damage such as proteinuria is present with normal or slightly decreased eGFR.

The renal protective pathway of WGP diet in obese diabetic ZSF1 rats is not fully understood. A previous study has demonstrated that the kidney disease of these rats is mostly independent on hypertension and/or hypertensive nephropathy [45], suggesting the attribution of renal pathophysiology strictly to other components of MetS, such as obesity and/or hyperglycemia. Indeed, many studies in literature use these rats as an appropriate model for the purposes of investigating MetS-related kidney disease or DN [28,46]. Our data show that the daily intake of WGP had no impact on the bodyweight or obesity of these rats (Figure 1). Therefore, the beneficial effect of WGP diet on the diseased kidney may act through direct and/or indirect pathways, which include the improvement of glucose metabolism and/or fatty liver disease (Figure 2), and the probability of suppressing low-degree immune response activity as indicated by the smaller size of the spleens

(Table 1), but not relate to hypertension and obesity. The mechanism by which a WGP diet protects the kidney under the influence of both diabetic mellitus and fatty liver disease remains unknown and requires further investigation.

Oxidative stress is induced by the excess levels of ROS that are generated in many different situations, including the mitochondrial injury [47], the increased activity of oxidases (e.g., cytochrome p450s, xanthine oxidase, 5-lipoxygenase, and NADPH oxidase) in the response to inflammatory stimuli (e.g., hypoxia and immunologic stimuli) [48–50] and the loss of antioxidant defense system that includes enzymes (e.g., SOD, CAT and GSH-Px) and small molecular antioxidant scavengers (e.g., vitamin E, *N*-acetylcysteine and α-lipoic acid) [51,52]. The oxidative stress or ROS causes cellular damage by reacting with and/or denaturing cellular macromolecules including lipid, protein and nucleic acids, and/or even mediating or activating intracellular death signaling pathways [53], which plays an important role in the pathogenesis and progression of diabetes, fatty liver disease and their associated CKD including DN [52,54–56]. Grape products are rich in antioxidant chemicals, such as phenolic, flavonoid, and anthocyanidin [57–59], and exhibit anti-oxidative activities in both humans and animals [37,60,61]. Our study showed that each gram of WGP extract from methanol extraction contained approximately 21.5 mg of phenolics (reference: tannic acid), 0.25 mg of total flavonoids (reference: quercetin) and 5.2 mg of proanthocyandins (reference: catechine). The antioxidative activity of approximately 1.7 mg of this extract was equivalent to that of 5 μg of ascorbic acid in all three different assays (ABTS, DPPH, and FRAP) (Figure S1), and addition of this extract prevented H_2O_2-induced podocyte injury in cultures (Figure 5). Consist with these data, the anti-oxidative stress system in the kidneys of the rats receiving WGP diet was improved (Table 2). Taken together, these findings from both the literature and our study imply that WGP diet may improve antioxidant capability not only systemically (e.g., in the liver and the immune system/spleen and glucose metabolism) but also locally specific in the kidneys, resulting in less cellular damage in the setting of MetS and CKD.

The US Department of Agriculture considers 1.5 to 2 cups (250 g to 340 g, or 3.125 $g{\cdot}kg^{-1}$ to 4.25 $g{\cdot}kg^{-1}$ based on 80 kg, an average bodyweight of an adult) of fresh grapes per day as a standard serving size. In this experimental study, each ZSF1 rat (300 g to 600 g) consumed an average of approximately 25 g of food or 1.25 g of WGP a day that was equal to 2.8 $g{\cdot}kg^{-1}{\cdot}day^{-1}$. There are two simple ways to converse this dose between rats and humans [62]; one is based on the equivalent surface area (1 for rats = 1/7 for humans), so that the equivalent dose for humans will be $2.8 \times 1/7 = 0.4$ $g{\cdot}kg^{-1}$; the other is based on the representative surface area to weight ratio (Km), whereas rat Km = 5.9 and human (adult) Km = 37, then the dose for adult humans will be $2.8 \times (5.9/37) = 0.45$ $g{\cdot}kg^{-1}$. The result from both calculations is similar. Given that grapes are approximately 80% water by weight, 0.45 $g{\cdot}kg^{-1}$ of WGP dose equals to 2.25 $g{\cdot}kg^{-1}$ of fresh grapes, indicating that the dose we used in this experimental study was less than the standard serving size recommended by the US Department of Agriculture.

There are several limitations of this study. First, this is an experimental study using a relatively small number of animals from one strain, so the results may just limit to this strain and disease type. It is not certain if the same results would be seen in different species, or in different models of kidney disease. Second, a relatively short duration of this study may not represent the most of metabolic conditions and strategies that require life-long exposure and long duration of intervention. Finally, if the findings of the renoprotective effects of WGP diet are possibly attributable to better glycemic control, so there is a need to test the WGP diet in non-diabetic animal models.

5. Conclusions

CKD has been known as an initially silent condition where clinical manifestations are usually underreported at its early stages. By the time SCr reaches abnormally high levels, there already is 50% nephron loss in the kidneys [44]. This highlights the importance of early stage management, such as lifestyle and dietary modifications, which may be able to improve disease prognosis [63]. In this experimental study, we demonstrate that a daily intake of WGP for six months shows renoprotection in a MetS animal model (obese diabetic ZSF1 rats), as evidenced by decreased proteinuria, lower uPCR, improved diabetic uremia and reduced renal injury in DN (early stages of CKD). Our findings suggest that a daily intake of grape product rich in antioxidants may delay the progression of early CKD to late or ESRD in humans, and warrants further investigation.

Supplementary Materials:
Figure S1: Antioxidant activity of WGP extract, Table S1: The blood chemistry of obese male ZSF1 rats over six months of daily intake of whole grape powder (WGP) compared to sugar (Vehicle) group, Table S2: Oxidative stress-related gene expression in kidney cortex of WGP-fed rats compared to Vehicle controls at the end of six months of feeding experiment, Table S3: Blood chemistry of metabolism of obese male ZSF1 rats (approximately eight weeks old) compared with a reference in the literature [36].

Acknowledgments: This study was supported by a grant from the California Table Grape Commission (CA, USA); S.M.K.A. received the scholarship from King Abdullah Scholarship Program of the Kingdom of Saudi Arabia; P.L. the funding support from the Second Affiliated Hospital of Chongqing Medical University; and K.Y. the Canadian Mitacs Globalink Internship.

Author Contributions: A.L. and C.D. were responsible for the concept and design of the study; S.M.K.A., Q.G., P.L. and K.Y. for the lab work; S.M.K.A., Q.G., A.M.S., A.L. and C.D. for the data analysis and interpretation; S.M.K.A., A.M.S., A.L. and C.D. for drafting the article; and A.M.S., A.L. and C.D. for revising the article critically for intellectual content. All authors gave the approval of the final version to the manuscript.

References

1. Coresh, J.; Astor, B.C.; Greene, T.; Eknoyan, G.; Levey, A.S. Prevalence of chronic kidney disease and decreased kidney function in the adult us population: Third national health and nutrition examination survey. *Am. J. Kidney Dis.* **2003**, *41*, 1–12. [CrossRef] [PubMed]
2. Levin, A.; Hemmelgarn, B.; Culleton, B.; Tobe, S.; McFarlane, P.; Ruzicka, M.; Burns, K.; Manns, B.; White, C.; Madore, F.; et al. Guidelines for the management of chronic kidney disease. *CMAJ* **2008**, *179*, 1154–1162. [CrossRef] [PubMed]
3. Stigant, C.; Stevens, L.; Levin, A. Nephrology: 4. Strategies for the care of adults with chronic kidney disease. *CMAJ* **2003**, *168*, 1553–1560. [PubMed]
4. Arora, P.; Vasa, P.; Brenner, D.; Iglar, K.; McFarlane, P.; Morrison, H.; Badawi, A. Prevalence estimates of chronic kidney disease in canada: Results of a nationally representative survey. *CMAJ* **2013**, *185*, E417–E423. [CrossRef] [PubMed]
5. Levey, A.S.; Coresh, J. Chronic kidney disease. *Lancet* **2012**, *379*, 165–180. [CrossRef]
6. Kaur, J. A comprehensive review on metabolic syndrome. *Cardiol. Res. Pract.* **2014**, *2014*, 943162. [CrossRef] [PubMed]
7. Singh, A.K.; Kari, J.A. Metabolic syndrome and chronic kidney disease. *Curr. Opin. Nephrol. Hypertens.* **2013**, *22*, 198–203. [CrossRef] [PubMed]
8. Prasad, G.V. Metabolic syndrome and chronic kidney disease: Current status and future directions. *World J. Nephrol.* **2014**, *3*, 210–219. [CrossRef] [PubMed]
9. Thomas, G.; Sehgal, A.R.; Kashyap, S.R.; Srinivas, T.R.; Kirwan, J.P.; Navaneethan, S.D. Metabolic syndrome and kidney disease: A systematic review and meta-analysis. *Clin. J. Am. Soc. Nephrol.* **2011**, *6*, 2364–2373. [CrossRef] [PubMed]
10. Nashar, K.; Egan, B.M. Relationship between chronic kidney disease and metabolic syndrome: Current perspectives. *Diabetes Metab. Syndr. Obes.* **2014**, *7*, 421–435. [CrossRef] [PubMed]
11. Asmat, U.; Abad, K.; Ismail, K. Diabetes mellitus and oxidative stress-a concise review. *Saudi Pharm. J.* **2016**, *24*, 547–553. [CrossRef] [PubMed]
12. Betteridge, D.J. What is oxidative stress? *Metabolism* **2000**, *49*, 3–8. [CrossRef]
13. Sadowska-Bartosz, I.; Bartosz, G. Effect of antioxidants supplementation on aging and longevity. *Biomed. Res. Int.* **2014**, *2014*, 404680. [CrossRef] [PubMed]
14. Williamson, G.; Faulkner, K.; Plumb, G.W. Glucosinolates and phenolics as antioxidants from plant foods. *Eur. J. Cancer Prev.* **1998**, *7*, 17–21. [PubMed]
15. Vendrame, S.; Del Bo, C.; Ciappellano, S.; Riso, P.; Klimis-Zacas, D. Berry fruit consumption and metabolic syndrome. *Antioxidants (Basel)* **2016**, *5*, 34. [CrossRef] [PubMed]

16. Kowalska, K.; Olejnik, A. Current evidence on the health-beneficial effects of berry fruits in the prevention and treatment of metabolic syndrome. *Curr. Opin. Clin. Nutr. Metab. Care* **2016**, *19*, 446–452. [CrossRef] [PubMed]
17. El-Mowafy, A.M.; Salem, H.A.; Al-Gayyar, M.M.; El-Mesery, M.E.; El-Azab, M.F. Evaluation of renal protective effects of the green-tea (EGCG) and red grape resveratrol: Role of oxidative stress and inflammatory cytokines. *Nat. Prod. Res.* **2011**, *25*, 850–856. [CrossRef] [PubMed]
18. Sanchez-Gonzalez, P.D.; Lopez-Hernandez, F.J.; Perez-Barriocanal, F.; Morales, A.I.; Lopez-Novoa, J.M. Quercetin reduces cisplatin nephrotoxicity in rats without compromising its anti-tumour activity. *Nephrol. Dial. Transplant.* **2011**, *26*, 3484–3495. [CrossRef] [PubMed]
19. Tanabe, K.; Tamura, Y.; Lanaspa, M.A.; Miyazaki, M.; Suzuki, N.; Sato, W.; Maeshima, Y.; Schreiner, G.F.; Villarreal, F.J.; Johnson, R.J.; et al. Epicatechin limits renal injury by mitochondrial protection in cisplatin nephropathy. *Am. J. Physiol. Ren. Physiol.* **2012**, *303*, F1264–F1274. [CrossRef] [PubMed]
20. Li, J.; Kang, M.K.; Kim, J.K.; Kim, J.L.; Kang, S.W.; Lim, S.S.; Kang, Y.H. Purple corn anthocyanins retard diabetes-associated glomerulosclerosis in mesangial cells and db/db mice. *Eur. J. Nutr.* **2012**, *51*, 961–973. [CrossRef] [PubMed]
21. Pokkunuri, I.; Ali, Q.; Asghar, M. Grape powder improves age-related decline in mitochondrial and kidney functions in fischer 344 rats. *Oxid. Med. Cell. Longev.* **2016**, *2016*, 6135319. [CrossRef] [PubMed]
22. Laguardia, H.A.; Hamm, L.L.; Chen, J. The metabolic syndrome and risk of chronic kidney disease: Pathophysiology and intervention strategies. *J. Nutr. Metab.* **2012**, *2012*, 652608. [CrossRef] [PubMed]
23. Tofovic, S.P.; Kusaka, H.; Kost, C.K., Jr.; Bastacky, S. Renal function and structure in diabetic, hypertensive, obese ZDFxSHHF-hybrid rats. *Ren. Fail.* **2000**, *22*, 387–406. [CrossRef] [PubMed]
24. Baynes, J.; Murray, D.B. Cardiac and renal function are progressively impaired with aging in zucker diabetic fatty type II diabetic rats. *Oxid. Med. Cell. Longev.* **2009**, *2*, 328–334. [CrossRef] [PubMed]
25. Rafikova, O.; Salah, E.M.; Tofovic, S.P. Renal and metabolic effects of tempol in obese ZSF1 rats—Distinct role for superoxide and hydrogen peroxide in diabetic renal injury. *Metab. Clin. Exp.* **2008**, *57*, 1434–1444. [CrossRef] [PubMed]
26. Vora, J.P.; Zimsen, S.M.; Houghton, D.C.; Anderson, S. Evolution of metabolic and renal changes in the ZDF/DRT-fa rat model of type II diabetes. *J. Am. Soc. Nephrol.* **1996**, *7*, 113–117. [PubMed]
27. Tofovic, S.P.; Jackson, E.K. Rat models of the metabolic syndrome. *Methods Mol. Med.* **2003**, *86*, 29–46. [PubMed]
28. Bilan, V.P.; Salah, E.M.; Bastacky, S.; Jones, H.B.; Mayers, R.M.; Zinker, B.; Poucher, S.M.; Tofovic, S.P. Diabetic nephropathy and long-term treatment effects of rosiglitazone and enalapril in obese ZSF1 rats. *J. Endocrinol.* **2011**, *210*, 293–308. [CrossRef] [PubMed]
29. Tofovic, S.P.; Kusaka, H.; Jackson, E.K.; Bastacky, S.I. Renal and metabolic effects of caffeine in obese (fa/fa(cp)), diabetic, hypertensive ZSF1 rats. *Ren. Fail.* **2001**, *23*, 159–173. [CrossRef] [PubMed]
30. Zhang, X.; Jia, Y.; Jackson, E.K.; Tofovic, S.P. 2-methoxyestradiol and 2-ethoxyestradiol retard the progression of renal disease in aged, obese, diabetic ZSF1 rats. *J. Cardiovasc. Pharmacol.* **2007**, *49*, 56–63. [CrossRef] [PubMed]
31. Griffin, S.V.; Hiromura, K.; Pippin, J.; Petermann, A.T.; Blonski, M.J.; Krofft, R.; Takahashi, S.; Kulkarni, A.B.; Shankland, S.J. Cyclin-dependent kinase 5 is a regulator of podocyte differentiation, proliferation, and morphology. *Am. J. Pathol.* **2004**, *165*, 1175–1185. [CrossRef]
32. Brosius, F.C.; Coward, R.J. Podocytes, signaling pathways, and vascular factors in diabetic kidney disease. *Adv. Chronic Kidney Dis.* **2014**, *21*, 304–310. [CrossRef] [PubMed]
33. Anderson, C.A.; Nguyen, H.A.; Rifkin, D.E. Nutrition interventions in chronic kidney disease. *Med. Clin. N. Am.* **2016**, *100*, 1265–1283. [CrossRef] [PubMed]
34. Chan, M. Protein-controlled versus restricted protein versus low protein diets in managing patients with non-dialysis chronic kidney disease: A single centre experience in Australia. *BMC Nephrol.* **2016**, *17*, 129. [CrossRef] [PubMed]
35. Shah, B.V.; Patel, Z.M. Role of low protein diet in management of different stages of chronic kidney disease—Practical aspects. *BMC Nephrol.* **2016**, *17*, 156. [CrossRef] [PubMed]

36. Wang, M.; Chou, J.; Chang, Y.; Lau, W.L.; Reddy, U.; Rhee, C.M.; Chen, J.; Hao, C.; Kalantar-Zadeh, K. The role of low protein diet in ameliorating proteinuria and deferring dialysis initiation: What is old and what is new. *Panminerva Med.* **2017**, *59*, 157–165. [PubMed]
37. Turki, K.; Charradi, K.; Boukhalfa, H.; Belhaj, M.; Limam, F.; Aouani, E. Grape seed powder improves renal failure of chronic kidney disease patients. *EXCLI J.* **2016**, *15*, 424–433. [PubMed]
38. Bernardi, C.; Moneta, D.; Brughera, M.; DiSalvo, M.; Lamparelli, D.; Mazue, G.; Iatropoulos, M.J. Haematology and clinical chemistry in rats: Comparison of different blood collection sites. *Comp. Haematol. Int.* **1996**, *6*, 160–166. [CrossRef]
39. Vassalotti, J.A.; Stevens, L.A.; Levey, A.S. Testing for chronic kidney disease: A position statement from the national kidney foundation. *Am. J. Kidney Dis.* **2007**, *50*, 169–180. [CrossRef] [PubMed]
40. Arici, M. *Management of Chronic Kidney Disease: A Clinician's Guide*; Springer: Berlin/Heidelberg, Germany, 2014.
41. Spira, A.; Gowrishankar, M.; Halperin, M.L. Factors contributing to the degree of polyuria in a patient with poorly controlled diabetes mellitus. *Am. J. Kidney Dis.* **1997**, *30*, 829–835. [CrossRef]
42. Ahloulay, M.; Schmitt, F.; Dechaux, M.; Bankir, L. Vasopressin and urinary concentrating activity in diabetes mellitus. *Diabetes Metab.* **1999**, *25*, 213–222. [PubMed]
43. Mogensen, C.E. Early glomerular hyperfiltration in insulin-dependent diabetics and late nephropathy. *Scand. J. Clin. Lab. Investig.* **1986**, *46*, 201–206. [CrossRef]
44. Ahmed, S.; Lowder, G. Severity and stages of chronic kidney disease. *Age* **2012**, *140*, 13–25.
45. Griffin, K.A.; Abu-Naser, M.; Abu-Amarah, I.; Picken, M.; Williamson, G.A.; Bidani, A.K. Dynamic blood pressure load and nephropathy in the ZSF1 (fa/fa cp) model of type 2 diabetes. *Am. J. Physiol. Renal. Physiol.* **2007**, *293*, F1605–F1613. [CrossRef] [PubMed]
46. Tofovic, S.P.; Salah, E.M.; Jackson, E.K.; Melhem, M. Early renal injury induced by caffeine consumption in obese, diabetic zsf1 rats. *Ren. Fail.* **2007**, *29*, 891–902. [CrossRef] [PubMed]
47. Rocha, M.; Hernandez-Mijares, A.; Garcia-Malpartida, K.; Banuls, C.; Bellod, L.; Victor, V.M. Mitochondria-targeted antioxidant peptides. *Curr. Pharm. Des.* **2010**, *16*, 3124–3131. [CrossRef] [PubMed]
48. Novo, E.; Parola, M. Redox mechanisms in hepatic chronic wound healing and fibrogenesis. *Fibrogenesis Tissue Repair* **2008**, *1*, 5. [CrossRef] [PubMed]
49. Babior, B.M. NADPH oxidase: An update. *Blood* **1999**, *93*, 1464–1476. [PubMed]
50. Forman, H.J.; Torres, M. Redox signaling in macrophages. *Mol. Aspects Med.* **2001**, *22*, 189–216. [CrossRef]
51. Birben, E.; Sahiner, U.M.; Sackesen, C.; Erzurum, S.; Kalayci, O. Oxidative stress and antioxidant defense. *World Allergy Organ. J.* **2012**, *5*, 9–19. [CrossRef] [PubMed]
52. Du, C.; Wang, X.; Chen, H. Oxidative stress to renal tubular epithelial cells—A common pathway in renal pathologies. In *Systems Biology of Free Radicals and Anti-Oxidants*; Laher, I., Ed.; Springer: Berlin/Heidelberg, Germany, 2014; pp. 2606–2624.
53. Rhee, S.G. Redox signaling: Hydrogen peroxide as intracellular messenger. *Exp. Mol. Med.* **1999**, *31*, 53–59. [CrossRef] [PubMed]
54. Turkmen, K. Inflammation, oxidative stress, apoptosis, and autophagy in diabetes mellitus and diabetic kidney disease: The four horsemen of the apocalypse. *Int. Urol. Nephrol.* **2016**. [CrossRef] [PubMed]
55. Sunny, N.E.; Bril, F.; Cusi, K. Mitochondrial adaptation in nonalcoholic fatty liver disease: Novel mechanisms and treatment strategies. *Trends Endocrinol. Metab.* **2017**, *28*, 250–260. [CrossRef] [PubMed]
56. Newsholme, P.; Cruzat, V.F.; Keane, K.N.; Carlessi, R.; de Bittencourt, P.I., Jr. Molecular mechanisms of ROS production and oxidative stress in diabetes. *Biochem. J.* **2016**, *473*, 4527–4550. [CrossRef] [PubMed]
57. Yilmaz, Y.; Toledo, R.T. Major flavonoids in grape seeds and skins: Antioxidant capacity of catechin, epicatechin, and gallic acid. *J. Agric. Food Chem.* **2004**, *52*, 255–260. [CrossRef] [PubMed]
58. Ross, C.F.; Hoye, C., Jr.; Fernandez-Plotka, V.C. Influence of heating on the polyphenolic content and antioxidant activity of grape seed flour. *J. Food Sci.* **2011**, *76*, C884–C890. [CrossRef] [PubMed]
59. Yang, J.; Xiao, Y.Y. Grape phytochemicals and associated health benefits. *Crit. Rev. Food Sci. Nutr.* **2013**, *53*, 1202–1225. [CrossRef] [PubMed]
60. Aloui, F.; Charradi, K.; Hichami, A.; Subramaniam, S.; Khan, N.A.; Limam, F.; Aouani, E. Grape seed and skin extract reduces pancreas lipotoxicity, oxidative stress and inflammation in high fat diet fed rats. *Biomed. Pharmacother.* **2016**, *84*, 2020–2028. [CrossRef] [PubMed]

61. Oueslati, N.; Charradi, K.; Bedhiafi, T.; Limam, F.; Aouani, E. Protective effect of grape seed and skin extract against diabetes-induced oxidative stress and renal dysfunction in virgin and pregnant rat. *Biomed. Pharmacother.* **2016**, *83*, 584–592. [CrossRef] [PubMed]
62. Freireich, E.J.; Gehan, E.A.; Rall, D.P.; Schmidt, L.H.; Skipper, H.E. Quantitative comparison of toxicity of anticancer agents in mouse, rat, hamster, dog, monkey, and man. *Cancer Chemother. Rep.* **1966**, *50*, 219–244. [PubMed]
63. Johnson, D.W. Evidence-based guide to slowing the progression of early renal insufficiency. *Intern. Med. J.* **2004**, *34*, 50–57. [CrossRef] [PubMed]

15

Insulin in Type 1 and Type 2 Diabetes—Should the Dose of Insulin Before a Meal be Based on Glycemia or Meal Content?

Janusz Krzymien and Piotr Ladyzynski *

Nalecz Institute of Biocybernetics and Biomedical Engineering of the Polish Academy of Sciences, 4 Trojdena Street, 02-109 Warsaw, Poland; janusz.krzymien@hotmail.com

* Correspondence: pladyzynski@ibib.waw.pl

Abstract: The aim of this review was to investigate existing guidelines and scientific evidence on determining insulin dosage in people with type 1 and type 2 diabetes, and in particular to check whether the prandial insulin dose should be calculated based on glycemia or the meal composition, including the carbohydrates, protein and fat content in a meal. By exploring the effect of the meal composition on postprandial glycemia we demonstrated that several factors may influence the increase in glycemia after the meal, which creates significant practical difficulties in determining the appropriate prandial insulin dose. Then we reviewed effects of the existing insulin therapy regimens on glycemic control. We demonstrated that in most existing algorithms aimed at calculating prandial insulin doses in type 1 diabetes only carbohydrates are counted, whereas in type 2 diabetes the meal content is often not taken into consideration. We conclude that prandial insulin doses in treatment of people with diabetes should take into account the pre-meal glycemia as well as the size and composition of meals. However, there are still open questions regarding the optimal way to adjust a prandial insulin dose to a meal and the possible benefits for people with type 1 and type 2 diabetes if particular parameters of the meal are taken into account while calculating the prandial insulin dose. The answers to these questions may vary depending on the type of diabetes.

Keywords: carbohydrate counting; protein and fat counting; insulin dosage; glucose monitoring; diabetes mellitus; type 1 diabetes; type 2 diabetes

---

1. Introduction

In healthy people, fasting plasma glucose rarely reaches 5.5 mmol/L (100 mg/dL) and the highest values after meals do not exceed 7.8 mmol/L (140 mg/dL), and quickly return to the starting level [1]. Hyperglycemia defines diabetes, and glycemic control plays an important role in the treatment of diabetes. Type 1 and type 2 diabetes are the two main types of the disease, which affects more than 425 million people worldwide [2]. Consistent hyperglycemia can lead to serious micro- and macrovascular complications, which cause diseases affecting the heart and blood vessels, kidneys, eyes, nerves and teeth. In addition, people with diabetes also have a higher risk of developing infections. In almost all high-income countries, diabetes is a leading cause of cardiovascular disease, blindness, kidney failure, and lower limb amputation. The premature morbidity, mortality, reduced life expectancy, and financial and social costs of diabetes make it one of the most important public health conditions [3]. The goals of treatment for diabetes are to prevent or delay complications, decrease mortality and maintain quality of life. An adequate glycemic control is a way of achieving these goals. In the American Diabetes Association (ADA) recommendations [4] for the majority of adults with diabetes (excluding pregnant women), the glycated hemoglobin A1c (HbA1c) below 7.0% (53 mmol/mol), preprandial blood glucose concentration in the range from 4.4 to 7.2 mmol/L (from

80 to 130 mg/dL) and after meals—below 10.0 mmol/L (180 mg/dL) were accepted as target values. At the same time, the recommendations underline that more or less stringent targets may be taken into account. They should be individualized depending on the duration of diabetes, age, life expectancy, co-morbid medical conditions, cardiovascular complications or advanced microvascular complications, occurrence of the hypoglycemic unawareness, as well as the individual expectations of the person with diabetes. It should be noted that in recent years, organizations such as The National Institute for Health and Care Excellence (NICE) [5], Institute for Clinical Systems Improvement (ICSI) [6], American Association of Clinical Endocrinologists and American College of Endocrinology (AACE/ACE) [7,8], Scottish Intercollegiate Guidelines Network (SIGN) [9], and the U.S Veterans Affairs/Department of Defense (SIGN) [10] have indicated that the target values of HbA1c are differentiated depending on the individual characteristics of people with diabetes. In its recently published recommendations, the American College of Physicians proposed target values of HbA1c for most people with type 2 diabetes in the range of 7.0% to 8.0% (53 to 64 mmol/mol) [11]. In a commentary from Diabetes Care, Matthew C. Riddle and colleagues [12] indicate the necessity to evaluate established and newer therapeutic options based on many years of observation, which will optimize the individualization of both goals and methods of therapy. The therapeutic goals set by ADA seem balanced and reasonable, they are broadly in line with the guidelines of other scientific societies. The HbA1c concentration below 7.0% (53 mmol/mol) is the accepted target value for the majority of patients with diabetes, excluding pregnant women. The possibility of achieving a more stringent goal of treatment, i.e., HbA1c below 6.5% (48 mmol/mol) for a group of patients who can achieve this goal without an increased risk of hypoglycemia or other adverse effects of the treatment as well as taking into account less stringent values of HbA1c, e.g., below 8.0% (64 mmol/mol) for older people are good examples of individualized therapeutic goals. Recommendations of the Polish Diabetes Association include similar individualized therapeutic goals [13]. Therapy adjustments should be made to maximize the proportion of time that glycemia is within the optimal range, i.e., between 3.9 and 10.0 mmol/L (70 and 180 mg/dL) for most patients [14]. A study of Bode et al. in people with type 1 and type 2 diabetes with HbA1c of 7.5% (58 mmol/mol) showed that 29% of blood glucose values exceeded 10.0 mmol/L (180 mg/dL) [15]. The postprandial blood glucose testing and evaluation is particularly important if the HbA1c target is not achieved despite satisfactory pre-meal glycemia. The postprandial glucose measurements should be made 1–2 h after the beginning of the meal and using treatments aimed at reducing postprandial plasma glucose values to <10.0 mmol/L (180 mg/dL) may help to lower HbA1c [4].

What is the real effect of the diet on the postprandial glycemia? Can we assess the effect of carbohydrates, fat and protein, and meals with a high or low glycemic index (GI) on postprandial glycemia? Are there differences that are related to the type of diabetes? In this review, we have attempted to answer these questions, based on the existing guidelines and available scientific evidence, to see if the prandial insulin dose should be calculated based on glycemia or the size and composition of a meal including carbohydrates, protein and fat content in the meal. We investigated the effect of macronutrient content in a meal on postprandial glycemia and we identified factors that may make it difficult to determine the appropriate dose of insulin to compensate for food intake in people with diabetes. Then we reviewed effects of the existing insulin therapy regimens on glycemic control and we assessed existing algorithms aimed at calculating prandial insulin doses in people with type 1 and type 2 diabetes. Finally, we concluded the work and asked questions which are still waiting for answers.

2. Effect of Fat, Protein and Carbohydrates in a Meal on Postprandial Glycemia

In type 1 diabetes, fat reduces the early glucose response (the first 2–3 h after the meal) and delays the peak blood glucose due to the delayed gastric emptying. In type 1 diabetes, fat leads to late post meal (>3 h) hyperglycemia [16]. In children with type 1 diabetes, adding 35 g of fat to the meal can increase the blood glucose level by 2.3 mmol/L (41 mg/dL) [17]. Fat consumption increases the need for insulin and requires an individual increase of the insulin dose with caution, and the calculation of the necessary insulin dose should take into account the duration of insulin action [18]. While paying attention to prevent late after-meal hyperglycemia, one should remember the risk of early hypoglycemia immediately after the meal. Campbell et al. demonstrated in type 1 diabetic patients that increasing the mealtime insulin is not an efficient strategy alone because it may increase the risk of early postprandial hypoglycemia [19].

Total and saturated fat intake were associated with a higher risk of type 2 diabetes, but these associations were not independent of obesity [20]. Dietary fat and free fatty acids (FFA) are known to impair insulin sensitivity and enhance hepatic glucose production [21]. Limited results are available on the fat effects on gastric emptying and postprandial glycemia in people with type 2 diabetes. Gentilcore et al. demonstrated that ingestion of fat before a carbohydrate meal resulted in slower gastric emptying and attenuated postprandial rises in glucose, insulin, and glucose-dependent insulinotropic polypeptide but it stimulated glucagon-like peptide-1 (GLP-1) in type 2 diabetes [22].

Protein consumption affects the blood glucose concentration in the late postprandial period. In people with type 1 diabetes using intensive insulin therapy 75 g or more of protein alone significantly increases postprandial glycemia from 3 to 5 h in people with type 1 diabetes [23]. Moreover, protein has different effects when consumed with and without carbohydrates, e.g., 30 g of protein with carbohydrates will affect blood glucose [16,17].

In type 2 diabetes, protein when consumed without carbohydrates has a very small effect on the level of glucose in the blood. In people with type 2 diabetes, after ingesting 50 g of protein the glucose response to protein remains stable for 2 h and then begins to decline [24]. Protein does not result in an increase of the blood glucose concentration, and it results in only a modest increase in the rate of glucose disappearance [25].

Meals with a high GI cause a rapid increase in glycemia. An inadequate insulin dose that does not take into account the rapid absorption of carbohydrates after consuming foods with a high GI may lead to a rapid increase in the blood glucose concentration.

Foods with a low GI cause a smaller increase in the glucose level, reducing the peak of glycemia, but at the same time it was demonstrated that such foods increase the risk of hypoglycemia after the meal in people with type 1 diabetes if taken with inadequate doses of insulin [16]. Three studies in people with type 1 diabetes suggested that the risk of mild hypoglycemia is greater with low GI than with high GI foods when the usual carbohydrate-to-insulin ratio is used [26–28]. However, low GI diets can significantly improve metabolic control in less than optimally controlled people with type 1 and type 2 diabetes, as indicated by the results of a meta-analysis reported by Thomas and Elliott [29]. The twelve included studies in this meta-analysis involved a total of 612 participants. Three studies had participants with type 1 diabetes, 8 studies had participants with type 2 diabetes, and one study had participants with either type 1 or type 2 diabetes. Low GI diets lower HbA1c levels by 0.4% compared with comparison diets, i.e., high GI diet in 10 studies, measured carbohydrate exchange diet in one study, and a high-cereal fiber diet in another study. Nevertheless, it should be remembered that eating a large amount of high carbohydrate foods with a low GI can lead to a significant increase in glycemia. A similar effect is observed after eating foods with a low GI but with a high content of fructose or sucrose, e.g., fruit juices.

The following questions should be asked: what do we know about the effects of individual components of the diet on postprandial glycemia in people with diabetes and is this knowledge necessary for us to effectively control it?

In a study reported in 2004, the effect of two diets on a 24-h glycemia and insulinemia profiles was compared in people with untreated type 2 diabetes [30]. The control diet was developed in accordance with the recommendations of the American Heart Association and the US Department of Agriculture, and it consisted of 55% carbohydrates with emphasis on products containing starch, 15% protein and 30% fat, including 10% monounsaturated, 10% polyunsaturated and 10% saturated fatty acids. The test diet was designed to consist of 20% carbohydrates, 30% protein and 50% fat. The content of saturated fatty acids in this diet was ~10% of the total food energy. Mean blood glucose values determined after 5 weeks of the dietary treatment were significantly lower in patients using the test diet compared to those using the control diet, 7.0 mmol/L (126 mg/dL) vs. 10.5 mmol/L (190 mg/dL). The control diet caused a higher increase of the insulin concentration in the blood. Thus, the diet with the carbohydrate restriction consumed for 5 weeks dramatically reduced blood glucose levels in people with type 2 diabetes. However, it should be emphasized that the study was conducted in people with untreated diabetes. Studies on the effect of various diets on glycemic control in people with type 2 diabetes treated with insulin have not been conducted so far, and thus—are required. Low-carbohydrate diets (LCD) are recognized as "no side effects" diets in the newest consensus report of ADA and the European Association for the Study of Diabetes (EASD) [31]. However, in the same consensus report the systematic literature review and meta-analysis of Sainsbury et al. is cited, which indicates that LCDs (26% of total energy) in people with type 1 and type 2 diabetes produce substantial reductions in HbA1c at 3 months and 6 months, with diminishing effects at 12 and 24 months and that no benefit of moderate carbohydrate restriction (26%–45%) was observed in 25 randomized controlled trials involving 2415 participants that were included in the meta-analysis [32]. Moreover, Mizidi et al. demonstrated the unfavorable effect of LCDs on total and cause-specific mortality, based on both individual data and pooling previous cohort studies. These authors concluded that given the fact that LCDs may be unsafe, it would be currently preferable not to recommend such diets [33]. On the other hand, several cohort studies showed that high carbohydrate diets (HCD) might be associated with higher risk of total mortality and cardiovascular disease [34,35].

The composition of the diet isn't the only factor that affects the blood glucose after a meal. In people with poorly controlled type 2 diabetes, reducing consumption of carbohydrates during breakfast and increasing it during lunch helps to improve glycemic control. By choosing one of meals with the highest carbohydrate content, while keeping the same daily intake of carbohydrates, a different therapeutic effect can be obtained [36].

The order in which foods containing various amounts of carbohydrates, protein and fat are consumed also affects the postprandial glucose level. Shukla et al. studied people with type 2 diabetes, who have been receiving the same meal consisting of carbohydrates, protein and vegetables for three days and consumed it in a random order: first carbohydrates, then after 10 min protein and vegetables or first protein and vegetables, then after 10 min carbohydrates or all components of the meal at the same time. It was shown that peaks of the glucose rise after the meal were more than 50% lower, with a simultaneously lower increase of insulinemia and higher secretion of GLP-1 when carbohydrates had been consumed as the last part of the meal in comparison with consumption of carbohydrates at the beginning of the meal [37]. The order of consuming food products affects also concentration of ghrelin—the "hunger hormone" which has orexigenic and adipogenic properties and is thought to play an important role in regulating food intake and body weight. Shukla et al. showed that the intake of carbohydrates at the beginning of the meal led to the restoration of postprandial ghrelin concentration in the postprandial period [38]. This effect was not found when the meal was started by serving protein and vegetables. Ghrelin secretion is suppressed immediately after a meal, the depth and duration of the suppression being proportional to the energy intake. Insulin may suppress circulating ghrelin independently of glucose [39]. Taking carbohydrates at the beginning of a meal shortens the period of suppression of ghrelin, which may result in shortening the period of feeling satiety, speeding up the next meal, and consequently leading to weight gain.

All these data indicate that a few factors may influence the increase in glycemia after the meal, which creates significant practical difficulties in determining the appropriate dose of insulin to compensate for food intake in people with diabetes.

3. Automatic Bolus Calculators in People with Type 1 Diabetes

People with type 1 diabetes treated with insulin pumps may use an automatic bolus calculator that allows them to determine the insulin dose based on the amount of carbohydrates consumed in the meal and an individual insulin sensitivity. The use of the bolus calculator in patients treated with multiple insulin injections resulted in a significant improvement of the metabolic control while the number of hypoglycemic episodes was slightly reduced [40]. There are some promising new applications of the emerging technologies in this field like the expert system using the automatic speech-to-text conversion, which is able to determine the caloricity, the content of carbohydrates, fat and protein in the meal in a fairly accurate way based on its voice description provided by the user. Such a system is an easy-to-use support tool in the type 1 diabetes treatment that makes it possible to improve the postprandial glycemic control [41,42]. This system can also be useful in people with type 2 diabetes to control the amount of food consumed or adjust insulin dosage. Other systems that attempt to calculate the meal content based on its digital image [43,44] or the monitoring of activities related to consumption of the meal, e.g., swallowing or chewing [45] are also under development and testing. Regardless of how the meal content is determined and entered, each automatic bolus calculator must implement an algorithm determining the insulin dose, which should be able to control postprandial glucose concentration. The review of such algorithms for people with type 1 diabetes can be found for example in a report of Krzymien et al. [46].

In people with type 1 diabetes, prandial insulin doses are individualized using parameters such as the insulin-to-carbohydrates ratio, and much less frequently, the circadian fluctuations of this parameter. However, in most algorithms the meal is characterized just by carbohydrate content despite the fact that new insights concerning the effect of dietary macronutrients on postprandial glycemia confirm that fat and protein content should be taken into consideration while calculating prandial insulin doses [16,47,48]. Pankowska and Blazik showed that the insulin bolus calculator with an algorithm accounting for carbohydrates and protein and/or fat in the meal could effectively suggest a normal or a square-wave bolus and indicate the timing of the square-wave bolus in the insulin pump users [49]. The same authors demonstrated in a 3-month open label randomized control study that the use of this system by educated children and adolescents with type 1 diabetes was safe and reduced 2-h postprandial blood glucose level and glucose variability [50].

Summing up, the improvement in the postprandial plasma glucose control in people with type 1 diabetes depends primarily on properly adjusting the insulin dose to the meal being consumed.

4. Inter-Subject Variability of a Response to Meals

The algorithms that have been implemented in automatic bolus calculators so far have not accounted for variability in the response to meals with identical carbohydrate content. In 2015, Zeevi et al. demonstrated on an 800-person cohort of individuals aged 18–70 not previously diagnosed with diabetes that people eating identical meals presented high variability in post-meal blood glucose responses. These authors showed that personalized diets created with the help of an accurate predictor of the blood glucose response integrating parameters such as dietary habits, physical activity, and gut microbiota might successfully lower postprandial blood glucose concentration and its long-term metabolic consequences [51]. In the same report authors developed a machine-learning algorithm accurately predicting personalized postprandial glycemic responses to real-life meals based on blood parameters, dietary habits, anthropometrics, physical activity, and the gut microbiota. These results indicate that it may be beneficial to incorporate such a personalized meal-dependent predictor of the postprandial glycemia into automatic insulin bolus calculators. However, we must emphasize that in the work of Zeevi et al., the study group consisted of a healthy population and it should be confirmed that the findings are equally valid in people with diabetes before they can be used to optimize the diabetes treatment. Recently, Rozendaal et al. demonstrated that the large variability in postprandial glycemic response dynamics to different types of food is inadequately predicted by existing glycemic measures such as the Glycemic Index, the Glycemic Load and the Glycemic Glucose Equivalents [52]. They quantitatively described the postprandial glycemic response dynamics using a physiology-based dynamic model. Although both these reports were based on data of people without diabetes, their conclusions admittedly should be applicable also to people with type 1 diabetes. The conclusions from the recent studies on variability of postprandial glucose response, if confirmed in people with diabetes, should result in more personalized algorithms for prandial insulin dose calculation in the future.

5. Insulin Therapy in People with Type 2 Diabetes

Insulin therapy in people with type 2 diabetes is significantly different from that used to treat people with type 1 diabetes. Typically, the treatment starts with the basal insulin and is directed to the fasting blood glucose control [53]. The fasting glucose is closely controlled by regulating hepatic glucose production with variable release of insulin into the portal vein, and with modulation of insulin action in the liver by glucagon and FFA [54,55]. In type 2 diabetes, the basal insulin secretion is impaired, and FFA and the fasting glucagon levels are high. An injection of long-acting insulin inhibits glucose production in the liver by acting directly on the liver and indirectly by reducing the release of FFA from adipose tissue [56,57]. In untreated type 2 diabetes, the HbA1c level depends primarily on fasting glycemia. The postprandial glucose concentration is less influential, especially in cases where the HbA1c level is greater than 8.0% (64 mmol/mol) [58]. In type 2 diabetes, most of the hypoglycemic agents used allow effective control of the fasting blood glucose. Metformin, sulfonylureas, thiazolidinediones and basal insulins (human NPH and insulin glargine, detemir, degludec) have little effect on postprandial hyperglycemia. Starting the basal insulin therapy is very simple. Normally, oral medications that have been used before initiation of the insulin therapy are given with insulin at a dose of 10 U or 0.1–0.2 U/kg of the body weight. The daily dose is then adjusted based on the fasting glycemia to obtain an individually determined fasting glucose target by increasing it in steps of 10% to 15% or 2 to 4 U once or twice a week. In the case of hypoglycemia, the dose is usually reduced by 4 U or 10% to 15% [59]. Yki-Järvinen et al. performed a study in patients with type 2 diabetes treated with one or two oral preparations with an average baseline HbA1c value of 9.5% (80 mmol/mol). After 36 weeks of active administration of insulin glargine and metformin, a significant improvement in metabolic control and a reduction in the fasting glucose was achieved. During the last 12 weeks the fasting plasma glucose averaged 5.8 mmol/L (104 mg/dL), and the mean HbA1c value was 7.14% (54 mmol/mol) at the end of the study period implying that half of the study group remained inadequately controlled (HbA1c > 7%), mainly due to hyperglycemia during the day [60]. The insulin treatment of people with type 2 diabetes requires normalization of both fasting and postprandial glycemia [61]. Failure to achieve HbA1c targets requires intensification of the therapy by choosing one of two therapeutic options, administering insulin mixtures twice a day, or administering fast-acting insulin before the largest meal.

For the treatment with insulin mixtures, the following principles established by ADA should be followed in the majority of people with type 2 diabetes [59]:

- Initially, the usual dose of the basal insulin should be divided, and 2/3 of the dose should be administered before the morning and 1/3 of the dose before the evening meal.
- The insulin dose should be adjusted by adding 1 to 2 U or 10% to 15% once or twice a week until the target values in the glucose self-monitoring are obtained. In case of 4 blood glucose measurements per day, the insulin dose before the breakfast should be adjusted to control the blood glucose concentration after lunch and before supper, and the dose administered before the dinner should be changed to control the blood glucose measured before bedtime and before breakfast.
- If hypoglycemia occurs, the appropriate insulin dose should be reduced by 2 to 4 U or 10% to 20%.

Recommendations for choosing dosage of insulin mixtures are similar to those of basal insulin, and dose adjustments depend on the results of blood glucose measurements. It is assumed that patients treated with insulin mixtures should eat meals at a similar rate of calories. It should also be noted what part of the mixture is short-acting or fast-acting insulin. A randomized study performed by Chen et al. showed that insulin mixtures containing 50% of the fast-acting analogue are much more effective in treating patients using higher carbohydrate diets [62]. This is reflected in the summary of clinical recommendations on the use of insulin mixtures in the treatment of type 2 diabetes, indicating that in some patients Mix50 mixtures may be more appropriate than Mix25/30 mixtures, and clinicians should consider not only efficacy and safety, but also traits and patient preferences during insulin treatment of people with type 2 diabetes [63].

In healthy people after eating a meal, insulin releases quickly and significantly increases, which is accompanied by an increase in the secretion of amylin (another hormone besides insulin, which is produced by β cells), which inhibits the secretion of glucagon, slows gastric emptying and causes a feeling of satiety. An important role is also played by various gastro-intestinal peptides, including GLP-1, which also inhibit the release of glucagon, such as amylin, and slow the emptying of the stomach and lead to a feeling of fullness. In people with type 2 diabetes, the release of insulin after a meal is slower, no increase is observed as in healthy people, the peak of insulin secretion occurs 90 to 120 min after starting the meal whereas in healthy people it is observed within the first 30 min. The increase in amylin secretion is also delayed and reduced, which, as a consequence, does not lead to suppression of glucagon, slowing gastric emptying and limiting food intake (no feeling of fullness). The secretion or action of GLP-1 may also be impaired [64]. Many individuals with type 2 diabetes may require mealtime bolus insulin dosing in addition to basal insulin. The dose and duration of action of prandial insulin should correspond to the need for adequate glycemic control. In many cases, meals vary greatly in terms of composition, size and time of consumption. Inappropriate therapeutic decisions regarding insulin dosing may lead to significant hyperglycemia or hypoglycemia. It should also be remembered that the exogenous insulin injection leads to inhibition of endogenous insulin and amylin secretion, reducing the feeling of satiety, leading to increased food intake and the body weight gain. In the case of a significant reduction in endogenous insulin and amylin secretion, treatment with insulin administered before meals is very difficult.

A lack of ability to achieve adequate glycemic control (HbA1c) during the treatment with basal insulin is a signal, besides the possibility of treatment with insulin mixtures, for administration of a fast-acting analogue before the largest meal, i.e., the use of the basal-plus insulin regimen. Usually an analogue is administered at a dose of 4 U, 0.1 U/kg or 10% of the basal insulin dose. If HbA1c is lower than 8.0% (64 mmol/mol) during this period, a reduction in the basal insulin dose should be considered. Then the dose should be adjusted by 1 to 2 U or 10% to 15% once or twice a week until the target values in self- control are achieved. In the presence of hypoglycemia and the diagnosis of the cause, the dose is reduced by 2 to 4 U or by 10% to 20%. It is a simple treatment that is easily accepted by patients [59]. On average, after adding a single dose before one meal, a reduction of HbA1c by 0.3 to 0.5% (3.3 to 5.5 mmol/mol) is observed. At the beginning of the treatment, the addition of a single injection of insulin is usually just as effective as using two injections, but with a lower risk of hypoglycemia and similar glycemic control is achievable as in the case of insulin delivery in multiple injections [65,66]. A good therapeutic effect can be obtained regardless of the rate of change in adjusting insulin doses [67]. Hence, just like in the case of insulin mixtures, the dose setting depends on the results of glycemic measurements and it is not based on adjusting the doses to the meal. Along with the time from the diagnosis of type 2 diabetes, the postprandial hyperglycemia control becomes more and more difficult. Many patients require early significant intensification of therapy to ensure further decades of active life. In particular, earlier intensification of the treatment due to a rapid deterioration of metabolic control is required in relatively young people with type 2 diabetes [68]. However, intensification of insulin therapy increases the risk of weight gain and hypoglycemia. Many patients reach a state where further insulin dose increase does not improve glycemic control. In addition, as demonstrated in studies evaluating the results of intensification of insulin therapy in people with type 2 diabetes, the basal-bolus regimen provides a small further improvement in HbA1c levels compared to simpler insulin delivery regimens [69,70].

The ADA states in its recommendations that the postprandial glucose increase may be better controlled by adjusting the time of insulin administration before a meal, indicating that the type of insulin used (short acting insulin or a fast-acting analog) should be taken into account while adjusting the time of insulin administration. Insulin doses set before meals should depend on the measured blood glucose levels and meal times. In this case, ADA also draws attention to the adjustment of the dose according to the carbohydrates consumed. However, this is only a note, because in the published recommendations the results of glycemia have a major impact on the setting of insulin doses [59].

For over a dozen years, research has been undertaken to assess the effectiveness of insulin therapy in people with type 2 diabetes based on adjusting insulin doses to meals. In 2008, Bergenstal et al. published the results of a multicenter, controlled, open label, randomized study that compared the use of two algorithms, i.e., Simple Algorithm vs. Carbohydrates Count, for adjusting mealtime insulin along with a simple algorithm for adjusting glargine insulin in a group of people with type 2 diabetes. The study involved 273 participants aged 18–70 years, with type 2 diabetes for at least 6 months, with HbA1c in the range of 7.0 to 10.0% (53 to 86 mmol/mol), taking at least 2 insulin injections per day for at least 3 months before the study. All patients recorded results of the self-monitored blood glucose before meals and at bedtime, insulin doses, menus, information on hypoglycemia, physical activity levels as well as the results of a 7-point blood glucose profile performed on week 0, 12, 18, and 24. The study established fairly stringent blood glucose targets that were as follows: fasting < 5.3 mmol/L (95 mg/dL), preprandial (before lunch and dinner) < 5.6 mmol/L (100 mg/dL) and before sleep < 7.2 mmol/L (130 mg/dL). In the Carbohydrates Count group, depending on the sensitivity to insulin, from 1 U per 20 g of carbohydrates to 3 U per 15 g of carbohydrates were given. In this group, a slightly greater but not statistically significant reduction in HbA1c, i.e., −1.59 vs. −1.46% (−17.5 vs. −16.1 mmol/mol) was obtained, lower daily doses of insulin were used, and a tendency towards less weight gain was observed [71]. In AACE/ACE Consensus Statement it has been declared that "carbohydrate counting was not more effective than a simplified bolus insulin dosage algorithm based on pre-meal and bedtime glucose patterns" based on results of this trial [8]. However, Hirose et al. conducted tests in a hospital setting in a small group of patients comparing the results of dose setting based on glycemia and based on carbohydrate content counting. After 14 days of treatment, better glycemic control was obtained in the carbohydrate counting group ($p < 0.001$) [72]. These results were not confirmed by the authors of another randomized study, which compared the fixed meal insulin dosing with flexible meal dosing based on carbohydrate counting in hospitalized people with type 2 diabetes requiring at least 20 U of insulin per day. In the flexible meal dosing group, the algorithm used to treat type 1 diabetes with insulin pumps was adopted. The constant dose group required much larger amounts of basal insulin, but both groups achieved similar glycemic control [73]. During the last EASD meeting in Berlin (2018), a group of Danish researchers announced the results of the evaluation of efficacy of advanced carbohydrate counting and the use of an automated bolus calculator compared with mental insulin bolus calculation in people with type 2 diabetes on the basal-bolus insulin therapy. In conclusion they stated that the advanced carbohydrate counting and insulin bolus calculation is an efficient, low cost tool to reduce HbA1c in people with type 2 diabetes on the basal-bolus insulin regimen. Similar effects were observed regardless of whether the automated bolus calculator or the mental bolus calculations were used. The blinded continuous glucose monitoring revealed decreased glycemic variability with both options, whereas only the group using the automated bolus calculator increased the time in the euglycemic range [74].

Practically, the system based on the results of both glycemic and glycemic-after-prone tests is a combined treatment with GLP-1 agonist and the basal insulin. However, this treatment is effective only in those people with type 2 diabetes who have preserved endogenous insulin secretion.

6. Conclusions

It seems reasonable to conclude that in the insulin treatment of people with diabetes prandial doses of insulin should take into account the result of pre-meal glycemia as well as the composition and size of meals. There are still open questions regarding the optimal way to adjust a prandial insulin dose to a meal and the possible benefits for people with type 1 and type 2 diabetes if particular parameters of the meal are taken into account while calculating the prandial insulin dose (e.g., content of all macronutrients in a meal, the proportion and order of consumption of various foods during a meal, inter-subject variability of response to the meal in respect to the postprandial blood glucose etc.). It should be emphasized that the answers to these questions may vary depending on the type of diabetes. In type 1 diabetes, it is generally accepted and considered to be beneficial to take into account the carbohydrate content of the meals when adjusting the prandial insulin doses. There is also evidence that protein and fat counting is advantageous in children and adolescents with type 1 diabetes treated with insulin pumps. However, there is no data available on this topic for adults with type 1 diabetes or people with type 2 diabetes. Hence, we should emphasize that the following questions are still waiting for answers:

- Is the calculation of carbohydrate exchangers sufficient to achieve improved postprandial glycemic control in adults with type 1 diabetes and people with type 2 diabetes or should the intake of protein and fat be also taken into account?
- What other factors should be taken into consideration when determining doses of insulin administered before meals in people with diabetes?
- Is it possible to develop a simple algorithm for prandial insulin dose adjustment based on the blood glucose measurements and counting all macronutrients in the meal?

Author Contributions: Conceptualization, writing—original draft preparation, J.K.; data curation, investigation, methodology, validation, J.K. and P.L.; project administration, supervision, writing—review and editing, P.L. Both authors approved the final version of the paper.

References

1. Mazze, R.S.; Strock, E.; Wesley, D.; Borgman, S.; Morgan, B.; Bergenstal, R.; Cuddihy, R. Characterizing glucose exposure for individuals with normal glucose tolerance using continuous glucose monitoring and ambulatory glucose profile analysis. *Diabetes Technol.* **2008**, *10*, 149–159. [CrossRef] [PubMed]
2. International Diabetes Federation. Diabetes Atlas Eighth Edition 2018. Available online: http://diabetesatlas.org/resources/2017-atlas.html (accessed on 15 February 2019).
3. Forouhi, N.G.; Wareham, N.J. Epidemiology of diabetes. *Medicine (Abingdon)* **2014**, *42*, 698–702. [CrossRef]
4. American Diabetes Association. Glycemic targets: Standards of medical care in diabetes—2019. *Diabetes Care* **2019**, *42*, S61–S70. [CrossRef] [PubMed]
5. National Institute for Health and Care Excellence. Type 2 Diabetes in Adults: Management. Available online: http://www.nice.org.uk/guidance/ng28/resources/type-2-diabetes-in-adults-management-pdf-1837338615493 (accessed on 28 January 2019).
6. Redmon, B.; Caccamo, D.; Flavin, P.; Michels, R.; Myers, C.; O'Connor, P.; Roberts, J.; Setterlund, L.; Smith, S.; Sperl-Hillen, J.; Institute for Clinical Systems Improvement. Diagnosis and Management of Type 2 Diabetes Mellitus in Adults. Updated July 2014. Available online: https://www.icsi.org/_asset/3rrm36/Diabetes.pdf (accessed on 28 January 2019).
7. Handelsman, Y.; Bloomgarden, Z.T.; Grunberger, G.; Umpierrez, G.; Zimmerman, R.S.; Bailey, T.S.; Blonde, L.; Bray, G.A.; Cohen, A.J.; Dagogo-Jack, S.; et al. American Association of Clinical Endocrinologists and American College of Endocrinology—Clinical practice guidelines for developing a diabetes mellitus comprehensive care plan—2015. *Endocr. Pract.* **2015**, *21*, 1–87. [CrossRef] [PubMed]
8. Consensus Statement by the American Association of Clinical Endocrinologists and American College of Endocrinology on the comprehensive type 2 diabetes management algorithm—2018 Executive summary. *Endocr. Pract.* **2018**, *24*, 91–120. [CrossRef] [PubMed]
9. Scottish Intercollegiate Guidelines Network Management of Diabetes. *A National Clinical Guidelinei*; SIGN Publication No. 116; Scottish Intercollegiate Guidelines Network: Edinburgh, UK, 2013; pp. 1–161.
10. The Management of Type 2 Diabetes Mellitus in Primary Care Work Group. VA/DoD Clinical Practice Guideline for the Management of Type 2 Diabetes Mellitus in Primary Care. April 2017. Available online: http://www.healthquality.va.gov/guidelines/CD/diabetes/VADoDDMCPGFinal508.pdf (accessed on 28 January 2019).
11. Qaseem, A.; Wilt, T.J.; Kansagara, D.; Horwitch, C.; Barry, M.J.; Forciea, M.A.; Clinical Guidelines Committee of the American College of Physicians. Hemoglobin A1c Targets for glycemic control with pharmacologic therapy for nonpregnant adults with type 2 diabetes mellitus: A Guidance Statement Update from the American College of Physicians. *Ann. Intern. Med.* **2018**, *168*, 569–576. [CrossRef] [PubMed]

12. Riddle, M.C.; Gerstein, H.C.; Holman, R.R.; Inzucchi, S.E.; Zinman, B.; Zoungas, S.; Cefalu, W.T. A1c targets should be personalized to maximize benefits while limiting risks. *Diabetes Care* **2018**, *41*, 1121–1124. [CrossRef] [PubMed]
13. Polish Diabetes Association. Guidelines on the management of diabetic patients. Diabetes and pregnancy. *Clin. Diabetes* **2017**, *3*, A53–A56.
14. Fonseca, V.A.; Grunberger, G.; Anhalt, H.; Bailey, T.S.; Blevins, T.; Garg, S.K.; Handelsman, Y.; Hirsch, I.B.; Orzeck, E.A.; Consensus Conference Writing Committee; et al. Continuous glucose monitoring: A consensus conference of the American Association of Clinical Endocrinologists and American College of Endocrinology. *Endocr. Pract.* **2016**, *22*, 1008–1021. [CrossRef]
15. Bode, B.W.; Schwartz, S.; Stubbs, H.A.; Block, J.E. Glycemic characteristics in continuously monitored patients with type 1 and type 2 diabetes. *Diabetes Care* **2005**, *28*, 2361–2366. [CrossRef]
16. Bell, K.J.; Carmel, E.; Smart, C.E.; Steil, G.M.; Brand-Miller, J.C.; King, B.; Wolper, H.A. Impact of fat, protein, and glycemic index on postprandial glucose control in type 1 diabetes: Implications for intensive diabetes management in the continuous glucose monitoring era. *Diabetes Care* **2015**, *38*, 1008–1015. [CrossRef]
17. Smart, C.E.; Evans, M.; O'Connell, S.M.; McElduff, P.; Lopez, P.E.; Jones, T.W.; Davis, E.A.; King, B.R. Both dietary protein and fat increase postprandial glucose excursions in children with type 1 diabetes, and the effect is additive. *Diabetes Care* **2013**, *36*, 3897–3902. [CrossRef]
18. Wolpert, H.A.; Atakov-Castillo, A.; Smith, S.A.; Steil, G.M. Dietary fat acutely increases glucose concentrations and insulin requirements in patients with type 1 diabetes: Implications for carbohydrate-based bolus dose calculation and intensive diabetes management. *Diabetes Care* **2013**, *36*, 810–816. [CrossRef]
19. Campbell, M.D.; Walker, M.; King, D.; Gonzalez, J.T.; Allerton, D.; Stevenson, E.J.; Shaw, J.A.; West, D.J. Carbohydrate counting at meal time followed by a small secondary postprandial bolus injection at 3 hours prevents late hyperglycemia, without hypoglycemia, after a high-carbohydrate, high-fat meal in type 1 diabetes. *Diabetes Care* **2016**, *39*, e141–e142. [CrossRef]
20. Van Dam, R.M.; Willett, W.C.; Rimm, E.B.; Stampfer, M.J.; Hu, F.B. Dietary fat and meat intake in relation to risk of type 2 diabetes in men. *Diabetes Care* **2002**, *25*, 417–424. [CrossRef]
21. Savage, D.B.; Petersen, K.F.; Shulman, G.I. Disordered lipid metabolism and the pathogenesis of insulin resistance. *Physiol. Rev.* **2007**, *87*, 507–520. [CrossRef]
22. Gentilcore, D.; Chaikomin, R.; Jones, K.L.; Russo, A.; Feinle-Bisset, C.; Wishart, J.M.; Rayner, C.K.; Horowitz, M. Effects of fat on gastric emptying of and the glycemic, insulin, and incretin responses to a carbohydrate meal in type 2 diabetes. *J. Clin. Endocrinol. Metab.* **2006**, *91*, 2062–2067. [CrossRef]
23. Paterson, M.A.; Smart, C.E.; Lopez, P.E.; McElduff, P.; Attia, J.; Morbey, C.; King, B.R. Influence of pure protein on postprandial blood glucose levels in individuals with type 1 diabetes mellitus. *Diabet Med.* **2016**, *33*, 592–598. [CrossRef]
24. Nuttall, F.Q.; Mooradian, A.D.; Gannon, M.C.; Billington, C.J.; Krezowski, P.A. Effect of protein ingestion on the glucose and insulin response to a standardized oral glucose load. *Diabetes Care* **1984**, *7*, 465–470. [CrossRef]
25. Gannon, M.C.; Nuttall, J.A.; Damberg, G.; Gupta, V.; Nuttall, F.Q. Effect of protein ingestion on the glucose appearance rate in people with type 2 diabetes. *J. Clin. Endocrinol. Metab.* **2001**, *86*, 1040–1047. [CrossRef]
26. Lafrance, L.; Rabasa-Lhoret, R.; Poisson, D.; Ducros, F.; Chiasson, J.L. Effects of different glycaemic index foods and dietary fibre intake on glycaemic control in type 1 diabetic patients on intensive insulin therapy. *Diabet Med.* **1998**, *15*, 972–978. [CrossRef]
27. Mohammed, N.H.; Wolever, T.M.S. Effect of carbohydrate source on post-prandial blood glucose in subjects with type 1 diabetes treated with insulin lispro. *Diabetes Res. Clin. Pract.* **2004**, *65*, 29–35. [CrossRef]
28. Nansel, T.R.; Gellar, L.; McGill, A. Effect of varying glycemic index meals on blood glucose control assessed with continuous glucose monitoring in youth with type 1 diabetes on basal-bolus insulin regimens. *Diabetes Care* **2008**, *31*, 695–697. [CrossRef]
29. Thomas, D.E.; Elliott, E.J. The use of low-glycaemic index diets in diabetes control. *Br. J. Nutr.* **2010**, *104*, 797–802. [CrossRef]
30. Gannon, M.C.; Nuttall, F.Q. Effect of a high-protein, low-carbohydrate diet on blood glucose control in people with type 2 diabetes. *Diabetes* **2004**, *53*, 2375–2382. [CrossRef]

31. Davs, M.J.; D'Alessio, D.A.; Fradkin, J.; Kernan, W.N.; Mathieu, C.; Mingrone, G.; Rossing, P.; Tsapas, A.; Wexler, D.J.; Buse, J.B. Management of hyperglycemia in type 2 diabetes, 2018. A Consensus Report by the American Diabetes Association (ADA) and the European Association for the Study of Diabetes (EASD). *Diabetes Care* **2018**, *41*, 2669–2701. [CrossRef]
32. Sainsbury, E.; Kizirian, N.V.; Partridge, S.R.; Gill, T.; Colagiuri, S.; Gibson, A.A. Effect of dietary carbohydrate restriction on glycemic control in adults with diabetes: A systematic review and metaanalysis. *Diabetes Res. Clin. Pract.* **2018**, *139*, 239–252. [CrossRef]
33. Mazidi, M.; Katsiki, N.; Mikhailidis, D.P.; Banach, M.; International Lipid Expert Panel (ILEP). Low-carbohydrate diets and all-cause and cause-specific mortality: A population-based cohort study and pooling prospective studies. *Eur. Heart J.* **2018**, *39*, 289–298. [CrossRef]
34. Yu, D.; Shu, X.-O.; Li, H.; Xiang, Y.B.; Yang, G.; Gao, Y.T.; Zheng, W.; Zhang, X. Dietary carbohydrates, refined grains, glycemic load, and risk of coronary heart disease in Chinese adults. *Am. J. Epidemiol.* **2013**, *178*, 1542–1549. [CrossRef]
35. Dehghan, M.; Mente, A.; Zhang, X.; Swaminathan, S.; Li, W.; Mohan, V.; Iqbal, R.; Kumar, R.; Wentzel-Viljoen, E.; Rosengren, A.; et al. Associations of fats and carbohydrate intake with cardiovascular disease and mortality in 18 countries from five continents (PURE): A prospective cohort study. *Lancet* **2017**, *390*, 2050–2062. [CrossRef]
36. Pearce, K.L.; Noakes, M.; Keogh, J.; Clifton, P.M. Effect of carbohydrate distribution on postprandial glucose peaks with the use of continuous glucose monitoring in type 2 diabetes. *Am. J. Clin. Nutr.* **2008**, *87*, 638–644. [CrossRef] [PubMed]
37. Shukla, A.P.; Andono, J.; Touhamy, S.H.; Casper, A.; Iliescu, R.G.; Mauer, E.; Zhu, Y.S.; Ludwig, D.S.; Aronne, L.J. Carbohydrate-last meal pattern lowers postprandial glucose and insulin excursions in type 2 diabetes. *BMJ Open Diab. Res. Care* **2017**, *5*, e000440. [CrossRef] [PubMed]
38. Shukla, A.P.; Mauer, E.; Igel, L.I.; Truong, W.; Casper, A.; Kumar, R.B.; Saunders, K.H.; Aronne, L.J. Effect of food order on ghrelin suppression. *Diabetes Care* **2018**, *41*, e76–e77. [CrossRef] [PubMed]
39. Flanagan, D.E.; Evans, M.L.; Monsod, T.P.; Rife, F.; Heptulla, R.A.; Tamborlane, W.V.; Sherwin, R.S. The influence of insulin on circulating ghrelin. *Am. J. Physiol. Endocrinol. Metab.* **2003**, *284*, E313–E316. [CrossRef] [PubMed]
40. Vallejo-Mora, M.D.; Carreira-Soler, M.; Linares-Parrado, F.; Olveira, G.; Rojo-Martínez, G.; Domínguez-López, M.; Ruiz-de-Adana-Navas, M.S.; González-Romero, M.S. The Calculating Boluses on Multiple Daily Injections (CBMDI) study: A randomized controlled trial on the effect on metabolic control of adding a bolus calculator to multiple daily injections in people with type 1 diabetes. *J. Diabetes* **2017**, *9*, 24–33. [CrossRef] [PubMed]
41. Ladyzynski, P.; Krzymien, J.; Foltynski, P.; Rachuta, M.; Bonalska, B. Accuracy of automatic carbohydrate, protein, fat and calorie counting based on voice descriptions of meals in people with type 1 diabetes. *Nutrients* **2018**, *10*, 518. [CrossRef] [PubMed]
42. Foltynski, P.; Ladyzynski, P.; Pankowska, E.; Mazurczak, K. Efficacy of automatic bolus calculator with automatic speech recognition in patients with type 1 diabetes: A randomized cross-over trial. *J. Diabetes* **2018**, *10*, 600–608. [CrossRef] [PubMed]
43. Bally, L.; Dehais, J.; Nakas, C.T.; Anthimopoulos, M.; Laimer, M.; Rhyner, D.; Rosenberg, G.; Zueger, T.; Diem, P.; Mougiakakou, S.; et al. Carbohydrate estimation supported by the GoCARB system in individuals with type 1 diabetes: A randomized prospective pilot study. *Diabetes Care* **2017**, *40*, e6–e7. [CrossRef] [PubMed]
44. Wang, Y.; He, Y.; Boushey, C.J.; Zhu, F.; Delp, E.J. Context based image analysis with application in dietary assessment and evaluation. *Multimed. Tools Appl.* **2018**, *77*, 19769–19794. [CrossRef] [PubMed]
45. Schiboni, G.; Amft, O. Automatic dietary monitoring using wearable accessories. In *Seamless Healthcare Monitoring. Advances in Wearable, Attachable and Invisible Devices*; Tamura, T., Chen, W., Eds.; Springer Int. Publ.: Cham, Switzerland, 2018; pp. 369–412. [CrossRef]
46. Krzymien, J.; Rachuta, M.; Kozlowska, I.; Ladyzynski, P.; Foltynski, P. Treatment of patients with type 1 diabetes—Insulin pumps or multiple injections? *Biocybern. Biomed. Eng.* **2016**, *29*, 1–8. [CrossRef]
47. Tascini, G.; Berioli, M.G.; Cerquiglini, L.; Santi, E.; Mancini, G.; Rogari, F.; Toni, G.; Esposito, S. Carbohydrate counting in children and adolescents with type 1 diabetes. *Nutrients* **2018**, *10*, 109. [CrossRef] [PubMed]

48. Kordonouri, O.; Hartmann, R.; Remus, K.; Bläsig, S.; Sadeghian, E.; Danne, T. Benefit of supplementary fat plus protein counting as compared with conventional carbohydrate counting for insulin bolus calculation in children with pump therapy. *Pediatr. Diabetes* **2012**, *13*, 540–544. [CrossRef] [PubMed]
49. Pankowska, E.; Blazik, M. Bolus calculator with nutrition database software, a new concept of prandial insulin programming for pump users. *J. Diabetes Sci. Technol.* **2010**, *4*, 571–576. [CrossRef] [PubMed]
50. Blazik, M.; Pankowska, E. The effect of bolus and food calculator Diabetics on glucose variability in children with type 1 diabetes treated with insulin pump: The results of RCT. *Pediatr. Diabetes* **2012**, *13*, 534–539. [CrossRef] [PubMed]
51. Zeevi, D.; Korem, T.; Zmora, N.; Israeli, D.; Rothschild, D.; Weinberger, A.; Ben-Yacov, O.; Lador, D.; Avnit-Sagi, T.; Lotan-Pompan, M.; et al. Personalized nutrition by prediction of glycemic responses. *Cell* **2015**, *163*, 1079–1094. [CrossRef] [PubMed]
52. Rozendaal, Y.J.; Maas, A.H.; van Pul, C.; Cottaar, E.J.; Haak, H.R.; Hilbers, P.A.; van Riel, N.A. Model-based analysis of postprandial glycemic response dynamics for different types of food. *Clin. Nutr. Exp.* **2018**, *19*, 32–45. [CrossRef]
53. Blonde, L.; Merilainen, M.; Karwe, V.; Raskin, P.; TITRATE Study Group. Patient-directed titration for achieving glycaemic goals using a once-daily basal insulin analogue: An assessment of two different fasting plasma glucose targets—the TITRATE study. *Diabetes Obes. Metab.* **2009**, *11*, 623–631. [CrossRef] [PubMed]
54. Faerch, K.; Borch-Johnsen, K.; Holst, J.J.; Vaag, A. Pathophysiology and aetiology of impaired fasting glycaemia and impaired glucose tolerance: Does it matter for prevention and treatment of type 2 diabetes? *Diabetologia* **2009**, *52*, 1714–1723. [CrossRef] [PubMed]
55. Varghese, R.T.; Dalla Man, C.; Sharma, A.; Viegas, I.; Barosa, C.; Marques, C.; Shah, M.; Miles, J.M.; Rizza, R.A.; Jones, J.G.; et al. Mechanisms underlying the pathogenesis of isolated impaired glucose tolerance in humans. *J. Clin. Endocrinol. Metab.* **2016**, *101*, 4816–4824. [CrossRef] [PubMed]
56. Porcellati, F.; Lucidi, P.; Cioli, P.; Candeloro, P.; Andreoli, A.M.; Marzotti, S.; Ambrogi, M.; Bolli, G.B.; Carmine, G.; Fanelli, C.G. Pharmacokinetics and pharmacodynamics of insulin glargine given in the evening as compared with in the morning in type 2 diabetes. *Diabetes Care* **2015**, *38*, 503–512. [CrossRef] [PubMed]
57. Wang, Z.; Hedrington, M.S.; Gogitidze Joy, N.; Briscoe, V.J.; Richardson, M.A.; Younk, L.; Nicholson, W.; Tate, D.B.; Davis, S.N. Dose-response effects of insulin glargine in type 2 diabetes. *Diabetes Care* **2010**, *33*, 1555–1560. [CrossRef] [PubMed]
58. Monnier, L.; Lapinski, H.; Colette, C. Contributions of fasting and postprandial plasma glucose increments to the overall diurnal hyperglycemia of type 2 diabetic patients. *Diabetes Care* **2003**, *26*, 881–885. [CrossRef] [PubMed]
59. The American Diabetes Association (ADA). Pharmacologic approaches to glycemic treatment: Standards of medical care in diabetes—2018. *Diabetes Care* **2018**, *41*, S73–S85. [CrossRef] [PubMed]
60. Yki-Järvinen, H.; Kauppinen-Mäkelin, R.; Tiikkainen, M.; Vähätalo, M.; Virtamo, H.; Nikkilä, K.; Tulokas, T.; Hulme, S.; Hardy, K.; McNulty, S.; et al. Insulin glargine or NPH combined with metformin in type 2 diabetes: The LANMET study. *Diabetologia* **2006**, *49*, 442–451. [CrossRef] [PubMed]
61. Matthew Riddle, M.; Umpierrez, G.; DiGenio, A.; Zhou, R.; Rosenstock, J. Contributions of basal and postprandial hyperglycemia over a wide range of A1c levels before and after treatment intensification in type 2 diabetes. *Diabetes Care* **2011**, *34*, 2508–2514. [CrossRef] [PubMed]
62. Chen, W.; Qian, L.; Watada, H.; Li, P.F.; Iwamoto, N.; Imori, M.; Yang, W.Y. Impact of diet on the efficacy of insulin lispro mix 25 and insulin lispro mix 50 as starter insulin in East Asian patients with type 2 diabetes: Subgroup analysis of the comparison between low mixed insulin and mid mixed insulin as starter insulin for patients with type 2 diabetes mellitus (CLASSIFY Study) randomized trial. *J. Diabetes Investig.* **2017**, *8*, 75–83. [PubMed]
63. Deed, G.; Kilov, G.; Dunning, T.; Cutfield, R.; Overland, J.; Wu, T. Use of 50/50 Premixed insulin analogs in type 2 diabetes: Systematic review and clinical recommendations. *Diabetes* **2017**, *8*, 1265–1296. [CrossRef] [PubMed]
64. Aronoff, S.L.; Berkowitz, K.; Shreiner, B.; Want, L. Glucose metabolism and regulation: Beyond insulin and glucagon. *Diabetes Spectr.* **2004**, *17*, 183–190. [CrossRef]
65. Meece, J. Basal insulin intensification in patients with type 2 diabetes: A review. *Diabetes Ther.* **2018**, *9*, 877–890. [CrossRef] [PubMed]

66. Rodbard, H.W.; Visco, V.E.; Andersen, H.; Hiort, L.C.; Shu, D.H.W. Treatment intensification with stepwise addition of prandial insulin aspart boluses compared with full basal-bolus therapy (FullSTEP Study): A randomised.; treat-to-target clinical trial. *Lancet Diabetes Endrocinol.* **2014**, *2*, 30–37. [CrossRef]
67. Edelman, S.V.; Liu, R.; Johnson, J.; Glass, L.C. AUTONOMY: The first randomized trial comparing two patient-driven approaches to initiate and titrate prandial insulin lispro in type 2 diabetes. *Diabetes Care* **2014**, *37*, 2132–2140. [CrossRef] [PubMed]
68. Donnelly, L.A.; Zhou, K.; Doney, A.S.F.; Jennison, C.; Franks, P.W.; Pearson, E.R. Rates of glycaemic deterioration in a real-world population with type 2 diabetes. *Diabetologia* **2018**, *61*, 607–615. [CrossRef] [PubMed]
69. Holman, R.R.; Farmer, A.J.; Davies, M.J.; Levy, J.C.; Darbyshire, J.L.; Keenan, J.F.; Paul, S.K.; 4-T Study Group. Three-year efficacy of complex insulin regimens in type 2 diabetes. *N. Engl. J. Med.* **2009**, *361*, 1736–1747. [CrossRef] [PubMed]
70. Riddle, M.C.; Rosenstock, J.; Vlajnic, A.; Gao, L. Randomized, 1-year comparison of three ways to initiate and advance insulin for type 2 diabetes: Twice-daily premixed insulin versus basal insulin with either basal-plus one prandial insulin or basal-bolus up to three prandial injections. *Diabetes Obes. Metab.* **2014**, *16*, 396–402. [CrossRef] [PubMed]
71. Bergenstal, R.M.; Johnson, M.; Powers, M.A.; Wynne, A.; Vlajnic, A.; Hollander, P.; Rendell, M. Adjust to target in type 2 diabetes: Comparison of a simple algorithm with carbohydrate counting for adjustment of mealtime insulin glulisine. *Diabetes Care* **2008**, *31*, 1305–1310. [CrossRef]
72. Hirose, M.; Yamanaka, H.; Ishikawa, E.; Sai, A.; Kawamura, T. Easy and flexible carbohydrate counting sliding scale reduces blood glucose of hospitalized diabetic patient in safety. *Diabetes Res. Clin. Pract.* **2011**, *93*, 404–409. [CrossRef] [PubMed]
73. Dungan, K.M.; Sagrilla, C.; Abdel-Rasoul, M.; Osei, K. Prandial insulin dosing using the carbohydrate counting technique in hospitalized patients with type 2 diabetes. *Diabetes Care* **2013**, *36*, 3476–3482. [CrossRef]
74. Christensen, M.B.; Serifovski, N.; Herz, A.M.; Schmidt, S.; Gaede, P.; Hommel, E.; Raimond, L.; Gotfredsen, A.; Nørgaard, K. Efficacy of advanced carbohydrate counting and automated insulin bolus calculators in type 2 diabetes: The BolusCal2 study. An open-label randomised controlled trial. *Diabetologia* **2018**, *61*, 819.

Permissions

All chapters in this book were first published by MDPI; hereby published with permission under the Creative Commons Attribution License or equivalent. Every chapter published in this book has been scrutinized by our experts. Their significance has been extensively debated. The topics covered herein carry significant findings which will fuel the growth of the discipline. They may even be implemented as practical applications or may be referred to as a beginning point for another development.

The contributors of this book come from diverse backgrounds, making this book a truly international effort. This book will bring forth new frontiers with its revolutionizing research information and detailed analysis of the nascent developments around the world.

We would like to thank all the contributing authors for lending their expertise to make the book truly unique. They have played a crucial role in the development of this book. Without their invaluable contributions this book wouldn't have been possible. They have made vital efforts to compile up to date information on the varied aspects of this subject to make this book a valuable addition to the collection of many professionals and students.

This book was conceptualized with the vision of imparting up-to-date information and advanced data in this field. To ensure the same, a matchless editorial board was set up. Every individual on the board went through rigorous rounds of assessment to prove their worth. After which they invested a large part of their time researching and compiling the most relevant data for our readers.

The editorial board has been involved in producing this book since its inception. They have spent rigorous hours researching and exploring the diverse topics which have resulted in the successful publishing of this book. They have passed on their knowledge of decades through this book. To expedite this challenging task, the publisher supported the team at every step. A small team of assistant editors was also appointed to further simplify the editing procedure and attain best results for the readers.

Apart from the editorial board, the designing team has also invested a significant amount of their time in understanding the subject and creating the most relevant covers. They scrutinized every image to scout for the most suitable representation of the subject and create an appropriate cover for the book.

The publishing team has been an ardent support to the editorial, designing and production team. Their endless efforts to recruit the best for this project, has resulted in the accomplishment of this book. They are a veteran in the field of academics and their pool of knowledge is as vast as their experience in printing. Their expertise and guidance has proved useful at every step. Their uncompromising quality standards have made this book an exceptional effort. Their encouragement from time to time has been an inspiration for everyone.

The publisher and the editorial board hope that this book will prove to be a valuable piece of knowledge for researchers, students, practitioners and scholars across the globe.

List of Contributors

Aron M. Troen
The Nutrition and Brain Health Laboratory, The Institute of Biochemistry, Food and Nutrition Science, The Robert H. Smith Faculty of Agriculture Food and the Environment, The Hebrew University of Jerusalem, 7610001 Rehovot, Israel

Roni Lotan
The Nutrition and Brain Health Laboratory, The Institute of Biochemistry, Food and Nutrition Science, The Robert H. Smith Faculty of Agriculture Food and the Environment, The Hebrew University of Jerusalem, 7610001 Rehovot, Israel
The Joseph Sagol Neuroscience Center, Sheba Medical Center, 5265601 Tel Hashomer, Israel

Moran Zacharia
The Joseph Sagol Neuroscience Center, Sheba Medical Center, 5265601 Tel Hashomer, Israel

Ithamar Ganmore
The Joseph Sagol Neuroscience Center, Sheba Medical Center, 5265601 Tel Hashomer, Israel
Memory Clinic, Sheba Medical Center, 5265601 Tel Hashomer, Israel
Sheba Medical Center, Neurology Department, 5265601 Tel Hashomer, Israel
Sackler Faculty of Medicine, Tel Aviv University, 6997801 Tel Aviv, Israel

Shahar Shelly
The Joseph Sagol Neuroscience Center, Sheba Medical Center, 5265601 Tel Hashomer, Israel
Department of Neurology, Mayo Clinic, Rochester, MN 55905, USA

Michal Schnaider Beeri
The Joseph Sagol Neuroscience Center, Sheba Medical Center, 5265601 Tel Hashomer, Israel
Icahn School of Medicine at Mount Sinai, New York, NY 10029, USA

Jaime Uribarri and Weijing Cai
Icahn School of Medicine at Mount Sinai, New York, NY 10029, USA

Paul Beisswenger
PreventAGE Healthcare, Lebanon, NH 03766, USA

Stina Ramne, Isabel Drake, Ulrika Ericson, Jan Nilsson, Marju Orho-Melander, Gunnar Engström and Emily Sonestedt
Department of Clinical Sciences Malmö, Lund University, 214 28 Malmö, Sweden

Hye Jeong Yang, Min Jung Kim and Dae Young Kwon
Research Division of Food Functionality, Korean Food Research Institutes, Wanjoo 55365, Korea

Da Sol Kim, Ting Zhang and Sunmin Park
Department of Food and Nutrition, Obesity/Diabetes Center, Hoseo University, Asan 31499, Korea

Chulgyu Ha
Department of Bioprocess Technology, Bio Campus Korea Polytechnic, Nonsan 32943, Korea

Christophe Kosinski
Service of Endocrinology, Diabetes and Metabolism, Lausanne University Hospital (CHUV), Avenue de la Sallaz 8, 1011 Lausanne, Switzerland

François R. Jornayvaz
Service of Endocrinology, Diabetes, Hypertension and Nutrition, Geneva University Hospitals, Rue Gabrielle-Perret-Gentil 4, 1205 Geneva, Switzerland

Khaleal Almusaylim, Maggie Minett, Teresa L. Binkley, Tianna M. Beare and Bonny Specker
EA Martin Program in Human Nutrition, South Dakota State University, SWC, Brookings, SD 57007, USA

Tinashe Chikowore, Tertia van Zyl and Karin R. Conradie
Centre for Excellence in Nutrition, North-West University, Potchefstroom 2520, North West Province, South Africa

Pedro T. Pisa
Wits Reproductive Health and HIV Institute, University of the Witwatersrand, Johannesburg 2000, South Africa

Edith J. M. Feskens
Division of Human Nutrition,Wageningen University, AA Wageningen, The Netherlands

Edelweiss Wentzel-Viljoen
Centre for Excellence in Nutrition, North-West University, Potchefstroom 2520, North West Province, South Africa
Medical Research Council Research Unit for Hypertension and Cardiovascular Disease, Faculty of Health Sciences, North-West University, Potchefstroom 2520, South Africa

Yun-Ying Hou, Li-Li Wang, Qi Wang and Xiao-Hua Wang
School of Nursing, Medical College, Soochow University, Suzhou 215006, China

Omorogieva Ojo
Faculty of Education and Health, University of Greenwich, London SE9 2UG, UK

Qing Jiang and Xin-Yu Shao
Medical College, Soochow University, Suzhou 215006, China

Alejandra Contreras-Manzano, Salvador Villalpando, Claudia García-Díaz and Mario Flores-Aldana
Center for Nutrition and Health Research, National Institute of Public Health, Cuernavaca 62100, Mexico

Vibeke H. Telle-Hansen, Line Gaundal and Mari C.W. Myhrstad
Faculty of Health Sciences, Oslo Metropolitan University, St. Olavsplass, 0130 Oslo, Norway

Jesse Bertinato
Nutrition Research Division, Food Directorate, Health Products and Food Branch, Health Canada, Sir Frederick G. Banting Research Centre, 251 Sir Frederick Banting Driveway, Ottawa, ON K1A 0K9, Canada
Department of Biochemistry, Microbiology and Immunology, University of Ottawa, Ottawa, ON K1H 8M5, Canada

Kuan Chiao Wang and Stephen Hayward
Bureau of Food Surveillance and Science Integration, Food Directorate, Health Products and Food Branch, Health Canada, Ottawa, ON K1A 0K9, Canada

Lisse Angarita Dávila and Ma. Cristina Escobar
Escuela de Nutrición y Dietética, Facultad de Medicina, Universidad Andres Bello, Sede Concepción 4260000, Chile

Valmore Bermúdez
Facultad de Ciencias de la Salud, Universidad Simón Bolívar, Barranquilla 080003, Colombia

Nadia Reyna and Daniel Aparicio
Centro de Investigaciones Endocrino-Metabólicas "Dr. Félix Gómez", Escuela de Medicina. Facultad de Medicina, Universidad del Zulia, Maracaibo 4001, Venezuela

Virginia Céspedes
Departamento de Medicina Física y Rehabilitación, Hospital "12 de Octubre", Madrid 28041, Spain

Samuel Durán-Agüero
Escuela de Nutrición y Dietética, Facultad de Ciencias para el Cuidado de la Salud, Universidad San Sebastián, Santiago 7500000, Chile

Silvana Cisternas
Escuela de Salud, Universidad Tecnológica de Chile, INACAP, Sede Concepción, Talcahuano 4260000, Chile

Jorge de Assis Costa
Faculty of Medicine/UniFAGOC, Ubá 36506-022, Minas Gerais, Brazil
Universidade do Estado de Minas Gerais (UEMG), Barbacena 36202-284, Minas Gerais, Brazil

Diana Rojas-Gómez
Escuela de Nutrición y Dietética, Facultad de Medicina, Universidad Andres Bello, Santiago 8370321, Chile

Jose López-Miranda
Lipids and Atherosclerosis Unit, Maimonides Institute for Biomedical Research in Cordoba, Reina Sofia University Hospital, University of Córdoba, 14004 Córdoba, Spain
CIBER Physiopathology of Obesity and Nutrition (CIBEROBN), Institute of Health Carlos III, 28029 Madrid, Spain

Ewa Jablonska, Edyta Reszka and Edyta Wieczorek
Nofer Institute of Occupational Medicine, Department of Toxicology and Carcinogenesis, Sw. Teresy 8 Street, 91-348 Lodz, Poland

Jolanta Gromadzinska, Magdalena B. Krol and Wojciech Wasowicz
Nofer Institute of Occupational Medicine, Department of Biological and Environmental Monitoring, Sw. Teresy 8 Street, 91-348 Lodz, Poland

Sara Raimondi
European Institute of Oncology, Division of Epidemiology and Biostatistics, via Ripamonti 435, Milan 20139, Italy

Katarzyna Socha and Maria H. Borawska
The Medical University of Bialystok, Department of Bromatoloy, A. Mickiewicza 2D Street, 15-222 Bialystok, Poland

Sihan Song
Department of Food and Nutrition, College of Human Ecology, Seoul National University, 1 Gwanak-ro, Gwanak-gu, Seoul 08826, Korea

Jung Eun Lee
Department of Food and Nutrition, College of Human Ecology, Seoul National University, 1 Gwanak-ro, Gwanak-gu, Seoul 08826, Korea
Research Institute of Human Ecology, Seoul National University, 1 Gwanak-ro, Gwanak-gu, Seoul 08826, Korea

Peihe Liang
Department of Urologic Sciences, University of British Columbia, Vancouver, BC V6H3Z6, Canada
Department of Urology, The Second Affiliated Hospital, Chongqing Medical University, Chongqing 400010, China

Qiunong Guan and Caigan Du
Department of Urologic Sciences, University of British Columbia, Vancouver, BC V6H3Z6, Canada
Immunity and Infection Research Centre, Vancouver Coastal Health Research Institute, Vancouver, BC V6H3Z6, Canada

Salwa M. K. Almomen and Kaidi Yang
Department of Urologic Sciences, University of British Columbia, Vancouver, BC V6H3Z6, Canada

Ahmad M. Sidiqi
Department of Urologic Sciences, University of British Columbia, Vancouver, BC V6H3Z6, Canada
Division of Nephrology, Department of Medicine, University of British Columbia, Vancouver, BC V6Z1Y6, Canada

Adeera Levin
Division of Nephrology, Department of Medicine, University of British Columbia, Vancouver, BC V6Z1Y6, Canada

Janusz Krzymien and Piotr Ladyzynski
Nalecz Institute of Biocybernetics and Biomedical Engineering of the Polish Academy of Sciences, 4 Trojdena Street, 02-109 Warsaw, Poland

Index